Anticoagulation

Christian Doutremepuich
Editor

Anticoagulation

With 29 Figures

Springer-Verlag
New York Berlin Heidelberg London Paris
Tokyo Hong Kong Barcelona Budapest

Dr. Christian Doutremepuich
Laboratoire d'Hematologie
3, Place de la Victoire
33076 Bordeaux cedex
France

Library of Congress Cataloging-in-Publication Data
Anticoagulation / Christian Doutremepuich [editor].
Includes bibliographical references.
ISBN 0-387-94318-8. -- ISBN 3-540-94318-8
1. Anticoagulants (Medicine) 2. Thrombolytic therapy.
I. Doutremepuich, Christian
[DNLM: 1. Anticoagulants--therapeutic use. 2. Thrombosis--prevention & control. QV 193 A6287 1994]
RC684.A6A58 1994
615'.718--dc20
DNLM/DLC
for Library of Congress 94-16729

Printed on acid-free paper.

Production managed by Jim Harbison; manufacturing supervised by Vincent Scelta.
Camera-ready copy provided by the editor.
Printed and bound by Braun-Brumfield, Inc., Ann Arbor, MI.
Printed in the United States of America.

9 8 7 6 5 4 3 2 1

ISBN 0-387-94318-8 Springer-Verlag New York Berlin Heidelberg
ISBN 3-540-94318-8 Springer-Verlag Berlin Heidelberg New York

PREFACE

Thrombosis is common to all medical specialities which become aware of the dramatic consequences of this disease.

Thrombosis often leads to considerable morbidity and in some circumstances mortality. So it is important to prevent, to diagnose and to treat as far as possible.

In this book, the procedure of anticoagulation has been evaluated in each particular or disease group. Using this approach we hoped clinicians and biologists will be able to readly utilize this book as a working resource to management principles.

We have tried to cover prevention and curative treatment of thrombosis in a logical and very practical manner.

AKNOWLEDGMENTS

The author wishes to thank his staff Dr F. AZOUGAGH OUALANE, Dr D. PINTIGNY, Dr A. JOURDAN and Dr F. DOUTREMEPUICH for their editing, compiling of the references, preparation of tables and final preparation of the book.

Lastly, a personal and very friendly thank to all contributors.

CONTENTS

Anticoagulation and Heart

Anticoagulation and Vessel

Anticoagulation and Surgery

Anticoagulation and Medecine

Contributors

1. **M. Aparicio**, Professor, Laboratoire d'Hématologie, Faculté de Médecine, Université Bordeaux II, 146, rue Léo Saignat, Bordeaux, France

2. **F. Azougagh Oualane**, Doctorant, Laboratoire d'Hématologie, Université Bordeaux II, 3 Place de la Victoire, 33076 Bordeaux, France

3. **J.C. Baste**, Professor, Service de Chirurgie Générale et Vasculaire, Hôpital Saint André, 1 rue Jean Burguet 33075 Bordeaux, France

4. **I.P. Baskova**, Doctor, Laboratory of Blood Coagulation, Department of Biology, State University, Moscow 119899

5. **E. Baudet** Professor, Service de Chirurgie Cardio-Vasculaire, Hôpital Cardiologique Haut-Lévêque, 33600 Pessac, France

6. **F. Beaufils**, Doctor, Laboratoire d'Hématologie, Service de Réanimation Polyvalente Pédiatrique, Hôpital Robert Debré, Paris, France

7. **J. Bianchini**, Professor, Opocrin S.P.A. - Biofarmaci-Via Pacinotti 3-41040 Corlo di Formigine-Modena-Italy

8. **M. Boisseau**, Professor, Laboratoire d'Hématologie, Faculté de Médecine, Université Bordeaux II, 146, rue Léo Saignat, Bordeaux, France

9. **H.K. Breddin**, Professor, Department of Internal Medicine, Division of Angeology, J.W. Goethe-University, Frankfurt am Main, Germany

10. **J. Choay**, Doctor, Sanofi Recherche, Centre Choay, 9, rue du président Salvador Allende, 94256 Gentilly, France

11. **C. Combe**, Professor, Laboratoire d'Hématologie, Faculté de Médecine, Université Bordeaux II, 146, rue Léo Saignat, Bordeaux, France

12. **P. Couzigou**, Professor, Service d'Hépatogastroentérologie, Hôpital Haut-Lévêque, Avenue Magellan, 33604 Pessac, France

13. **C. Deville**, Professor, Hôpital Cardiologique, Avenue de Magellan, 33604 Pessac, France

14. **J. Di Maio**, Doctor, Protein Chemistry Group, Protein Engineering Section, NRC Biotechnology Research Institute, 6100 Royalmount Avenue, Montreal, Quebec, H4P 2R2 Canada

15. **C. Doutremepuich**, Professor, Laboratoire d'Hématologie, Université Bordeaux II, 3 Place de la Victoire, 33076 Bordeaux, France

16. **F. Doutremepuich**, M.D., Laboratoire d'Hématologie, Université Bordeaux II, 3 Place de la Victoire, 33076 Bordeaux, France

17. **J.P. Emeriau**, Professor, Laboratoire d'Hématologie, Faculté de Médecine, Université Bordeaux II, 146, rue Léo Saignat, Bordeaux, France

18. **J. Fareed**, Professor, Hemostasis Research Laboraories, Departments of Pathology and Thoracic and Cardiovascular Surgery, Loyola University Medical Center, Maywood, Illinois, U.S.A.

19. **O. Gauthier**, M.D., Service de Dermatologie, Hôpital Robert Boulin, BP 199, 33505 Libourne, France

20. **P.M. Garcia**, M.D., Service de Chirurgie Vasculaire Hôpital Pellegrin, Place Amélie Raba Léon, 33076 Bordeaux, France

21. **M. Haissaguerre**, M.D., Hôpital Saint-André, 1 rue Jean Burguet, 33075 Bordeaux, France

22. **F. Hayek**, M.D., Service de Chirurgie Vasculaire Hôpital Pellegrin, Place Amélie Raba Léon, 33076 Bordeaux, France

23. **M.F. Hurtaud-Roux**, Doctor, Laboratoire d'Hématologie, Service de Réanimation Polyvalente Pédiatrique, Hôpital Robert Debré, Paris, France

24. **I.Iturbe Alessio**, Doctor, San Diego Oncology Medical Clinic,7930 Frost Street, Suite 405, San Diego, CA, USA

25. **G. Janvier**, M.D. Département Anesthésie-Réanimation Hôpital Pellegrin, Centre Hospitalier Régional, Université de Bordeaux II, Bordeaux, France

26. **M.C. Lalanne**, Doctor, Laboratoire d'Hématologie, Université Bordeaux II, 3 Place de la Victoire, 33076 Bordeaux, France

27. **J.J Leng**, Professor, Service de Gynécologie Obstétrique - Maternité A - Hôpital Pellegrin, Place Amélie Raba Léon, 33076 Bordeaux, France

28. **P.J. Louvet**, M.D., Clinique Universitaire de Chirurgie Cardio-Vasculaire, Hôpital Cardiologique Haut-Lévêque, 33600 Pessac, France

29. **F. Madonna**, M.D., Hôpital Cardiologique, Avenue de Magellan 33604 Pessac, France

30. **PH. Le Métayer**, M.D., Hôpital Saint-André, 1 rue Jean Burguet, 33075 Bordeaux, France

31. **D. Midy**, Professor, Service de Chirurgie Générale et Vasculaire, Hôpital Saint André, 1 rue Jean Burguet 33075 Bordeaux, France

32. **J. Morser**, Doctor, Berlex Biosciences, 213 East Grand Avenue, South San Francisco, California, CA 94080, USA

33. **G. Pinganaud**, M.D., Laboratoire d'Hématologie, Faculté de Médecine, Université Bordeaux II, 146, rue Léo Saignat, Bordeaux, France

34. **A. Planes**, M.D., Clinique Radio - Chirurgicale du Mail, 96 Allées du Mail, 17028 La Rochelle, France

35. **V. Puel**, M.D, Hôpital Saint-André, 1 rue Jean Burguet, 33075 Bordeaux, France

36. **F. Roques**, M.D., Service de Chirurgie Cardio-Vasculaire, Hôpital Cardiologique Haut-Lévêque, 33600 Pessac, France

37. **X. Roques**, Professor, Service de Chirurgie Cardio-Vasculaire, Hôpital Cardiologique Haut-Lévêque, 33600 Pessac, France

38. **M. Sarret**, Doctor, Sanofi Pharma, Paris, France

39. **G. Sassoust**, M.D., Service de Chirurgie Vasculaire, Hôpital Pellegrin, Place Amélie Raba Léon, 33076 Bordeaux, France

40. **N. Schlegel**, M.D., Laboratoire d'Hématologie, Service de Réanimation Polyvalente Pédiatrique, Hôpital Robert Debré, Paris, France

41. **S. Shouler**, M.D., Service d'Hépatogastroentérologie, Hôpital Haut-Lévêque, Avenue Magellan, 33604 Pessac, France

42. **F. Toulemonde**, M.D. Departement de Pharmacologie Clinique, Sanofi Recherche, Gentilly, France

43. **N. Vochelle**, M.D., Clinique Radio-Chirurgicale du Mail, 96 Allées du Mail, 17028 La Rochelle, France

44. **J.F. Warin**, Professor, Hôpital Saint-André, 1 rue Jean Burguet, 33075 Bordeaux, France

45. **S. Winnock**, M.D. Département Anesthésie-Réanimation Hôpital Pellegrin, Centre Hospitalier Régional, Université de Bordeaux II, Bordeaux, France

1

Current trends in antithrombotic drug device development

J. Fareed

Many significant developments in the diagnosis and clinical management of thrombotic disorders have occurred recently [1- 24, 26]. Basic medical sciences have contributed remarkably in both the areas of therapeutics and diagnosis of arterial and venous thrombosis. Many newer approaches for the diagnosis and treatment of thrombotic disorders have been introduced [10, 14, 16]. This has only been possible due to the understanding of the molecular mechanisms involved in the development of thrombotic processes.

The pathophysiology of thrombosis is multicomponent and involves several components of the blood, vascular and humoral origin. Initially, artherosclerotic masking or endothelial injury results in the activation of platelets. Activated platelets mediate several direct or signal transduction induced processes on other cellular responses. Cellular activation results in the release of various mediators which amplify vascular spasm and the coagulation process. Thus, anaphylotoxins (C_3a and C_5a), superoxide, leukotrienes (LTC4), thromboxane B_2 (TxB_2), serotonin, platelet factor 3 (PF-3), platelet factor 4 (PF-4), platelet activating factor (PAF), endothelin-1 and numerous cytokines play a major role in the overall pathophysiology of myocardial infarction. Drugs that target various sites of the activation process can be developed to control the thrombotic events in the arterial system. The events leading to the formation of an arterial thrombus are shown in the following figure. As can be readily realized, a single drug may not be able to target these sites to produce therapeutic actions. Furthermore, many of these mediators produce localized actions at cellular and subcellular levels. The feedback amplification process plays an important role. This understanding has lead to the concept of polytherapy.

Venous insufficiency, blood plasma related disorders, fibrinolytic deficit and an imbalance of the regulatory proteins result.

Pathophysiology of arterial thrombosis

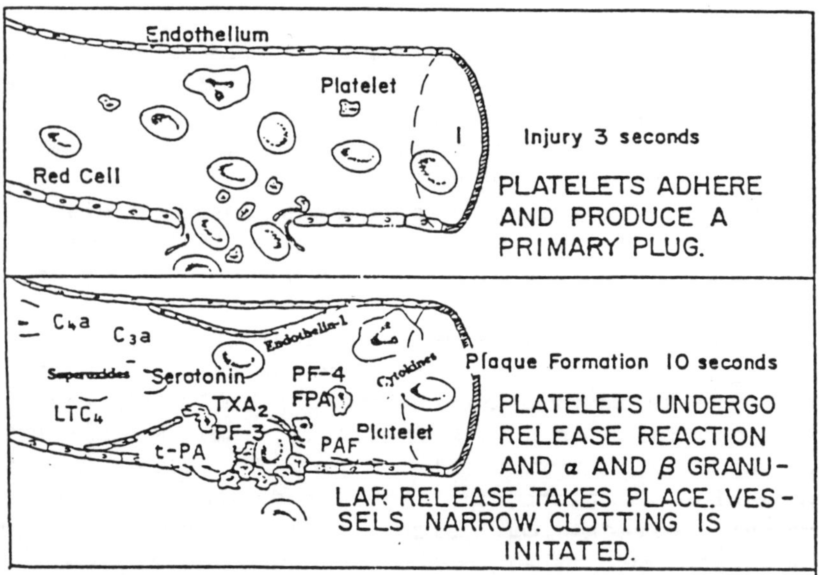

Venous insufficiency, blood plasma related disorders, fibrinolytic deficit and an imbalance of the regulatory proteins result in the activation of the coagulation system. Post-surgical trauma, inflammation and sepsis also lead to the activation of the coagulation process leading to venous thrombosis. The primary process in venous thrombosis is the generation of thrombin. Thus, drugs targeting the coagulation protease activation are useful in the treatment of venous disorders.

Advances in biotechnology and separation techniques have also contributed to the development of newer antithrombotic drugs [10, 15, 25]. Drugs and devices which have been or are being developed based on newer concepts can be classified into the following groups as listed below.

I. Heparin related drugs

1. Low molecular weight heparins.
2. Medium molecular weight heparins.
3. High molecular weight heparins.
4. Chemically modified heparins.
5. Dermatans.
6. Heparans.
7. Semisynthetic heparin conjugates.
8. Chemical synthesized antithrombotic oligosaccharides.
9. Sulfated dextrans.
10. Synthetic hypersulfated compounds.
11. Polyanionic agents.
12. Marine polysaccharides.

II. Antiplatelet drugs

1. Ticlopidine and related antiplatelet drugs.
2. Pletaal and related phosphodiesterase inhibitors.

3. Prostanoid modulators.
4. Eicosanoids and related drugs.
5. -3 fatty acids and fish oil related products.
6. Antibodies targeting membrane glycoproteins.
7. Peptide and proteins modulating platelet function.

III. Endothelial lining modulators

1. Nucleic acid derivatives.
2. Sulfomucopolysaccharides mixtures.
3. DDAVP and related peptides.
4. Growth factor related peptides.
5. Proteins digests.
6. Vitamins.

IV. Viscosity modulators

1. Synthetic and natural polymers.
2. Pentoxifylline.
3. Venoms (defibrinating agents).
4. Polyelectrolytes.

V. Biotechnology based proteins

1. t-PA and mutants.
2. Hirudin, mutants and fragments.
3. Protein C and protein S.
4. Thrombomodulin.
5. Thrombomodulin-thrombin complex.
6. Antithrombin III.
7. Antithrombin III-Heparin complex.
8. Recombinant heparin cofactor II.
9. Thrombomodulin.

10. Glycoprotein targeting proteins and peptides.

VI. Physical and mechanical devices

1. Angioplasty and atherectomy.
2. Stents.
3. Sequential compression devices.
4. Endothelial seeding.
5. Sound waves.
6. Lasers.
7. Hemodilution.

VII. Newer drug delivery systems and formulations

1. Oral.
2. Transdermal.
3. Sustained release.
4. Target specific antithrombotic drugs (antibody directed).
5. Catheters and devices capable of targeted drug delivery.

VIII. Polytherapy of thrombotic disorders

1. Heparin/antiplatelet drugs
2. Coumadin/antiplatelet drugs.
3. Thrombolytic agents/heparin.
4. Thrombolytic agents/antiplatelet drugs.
5. Recombinant drug conjugates.
6. Hirudin/antithrombotic agents.
7. Hirudin/glycoprotein targeting antibodies.

It can be appreciated from the above survey that the antithrombotic drugs represent a wide spectrum of natural, synthetic, semi-synthetic and biotechnology produced agents with marked differences in chemical composition, physicochemical properties, biochemical actions and pharmacologic effects. The use of physical means to treat a thrombotic disorder and an advanced means of drug delivery add to the expanding nature of this area. The endogenous action of the antithrombotic drugs are remarkably complex. It is no longer valid to assume that an antithrombotic drug must produce anticoagulant action in blood as the classical heparin and oral anticoagulants. Many of the drugs listed in various categories do not produce any alteration of blood clotting parameters, yet they are effective therapeutic agents because of their interactions with the various elements of the vascular and other blood elements. Another perspective is that several of these agents require endogenous transformation to become active products. Therefore, it becomes important to rely on the pharmacodynamic actions of these agents rather than on their in vitro characteristics to assess potency or efficacy of a product. The hematologic modulation plays a key role in the mediation of the antithrombotic actions of these drugs involving red cells, white cells, platelets and blood proteins.

The development of low molecular weight heparin has added a new dimension to the clinical management of venous thrombosis. These agents have revolutionized the prophylaxis of post-surgical thrombosis. More recently these drugs have been used for the treatment of arterial thrombosis. In particular, their relative effects on platelets are minimal in comparison to heparin. Thus, these agents are of value in platelet compromised patients. In addition to the basic low molecular weight heparins several other heparin related antithrombotic agents are being developed. For example, various molecular forms of heparin have been chemically modified to obtain derivatives with high affinity to the endothelial lining. These agents are useful in the treatment of vascular disorders and in providing support therapy following angioplasty and atherectomy. Dermatans, heparans and chondroitin sulfates are known to produce antithrombotic actions; however, even though they are related to heparin, they do not significantly alter the coagulation parameters.

These agents are now being used for the treatment and prevention of venous thrombosis. High antithrombin III affinity oligosaccharides which have been chemically synthesized have also been found to be antithrombotic in experimental animal models. More recently, the chemically synthesized pentasaccharide has been used in a Phase I clinical trial. This agent has been found to show extended half-life.

For the management of arterial thrombosis and atherosclerosis, the interest in conventional antiplatelet drugs such as aspirin has grown. Never drugs acting on platelets and endothelium are also being developed. Defibrotide, a polydeoxy-ribonucleotide derivative, has been established as an antithrombotic and vascular facilitory agent producing its effects via endothelium and platelet function modulation. Pentoxifylline, ticlopidine, pletaal and other synthetic analogues of prostanoids are being tested for their efficacy in various arterial disorders. Recently a thromboxane receptor inhibitor was tested in human volunteers. Various newer antiplatelet agents have also been developed.

Specific modulators of blood viscosity, representing a wide range of chemical and natural drugs, are being developed. Heparins, defibrotide and many antiplatelet drugs are known to modulate blood viscosity. The rheologic effects of a drug may be direct or indirect. The direct acting drugs produce a reduction of viscosity by physical effects such as dilution or modification of red cell structure. The indirect acting drugs produce their action by reducing fibrinogen or releasing certain endogenous substances which can reduce blood viscosity. Hemodilution and cytophoresis is also used as a means to reduce blood viscosity.

Through recombinant technology it is now possible to obtain cost effective antithrombotic proteins such as hirudin, t-PA, protein C, protein S, thrombomodulin and antithrombin III. Many of these proteins are in clinical use, showing great promise. Hybrodoma technology has enabled the production of complexes such as thrombomodulin - thrombin, antithrombinIII-heparin fragments and heparin cofactor II-dermatans. Monoclonal antibody techniques have been used to prepare target specific antithrombotic and

thrombolytic drugs. Major advances have been made in the development of glycoprotein targeting proteins and peptides. These agents can be used for both the therapeutic and diagnostic purposes.
One of the major break-throughs anti thrombotic drug therapy achieved through biotechnology has been the development of specifically designed mutant proteins. These agents are not acted upon by natural endogenous inhibitors and thus can be used in cases where the native drug would not be effective. Several mutant forms of t-PA are now being experimentally evaluated. These forms exhibit an extended half-life and are resistant to the actions of plasminogen activator inhibitors. In addition to these developments, by using monoclonal antibodies it is possible to make agents more target specific. The introduction of hirudin for specific anticoagulant purposes has added a new dimension to the arena of surgical anticoagulation and the management of cardiovascular disorders. This agent does not appear to alter platelet function, and thus the bleeding as associated with heparin is not seen. Due to the potency of hirudin, however, the use of this agent in prophylaxis, arterial and venous thrombosis is questionable. Currently there are several ongoing clinical trials in progress to address this issue. Concerns over the inhibition of the thrombin regulated bio-pathways by hirudin has been expressed and needs to be investigated. Such processes and the regulating actions of proteins C and thrombin mediated hemostasis are addressed.

Different physical and mechanical devices such as angioplasty, sequential compression devices and magnetic resonance to modulate the vasculature are in use clinically. One of the major developments in this area is the use of laser probes. Several approaches combining laser with surgical and pharmacologic agents have also been investigated. More recently, atherectomy is also used to remove coronary clots. Hemodilution has also been used in the management of thrombotic disorders.

With a clearer understanding of the multicomponent pathogenesis of thrombosis and the patient's own predisposing factors, the original concept of monotherapy is no longer considered valid. In the past venous thrombosis has been treated with heparin and/or coumadin and arterial thrombosis has been treated with aspirin. The triggering factors for either venous or arterial thrombosis may involve more than one pathologic component each of which may differ from patient to patient. Thus, beside the use of more specifically targeted drugs, combination therapy has been recommended. This form of therapy has added a new concept in the overall management of thrombotic disorders.

The concept of polytherapy in the management of complicated thrombotic disorders is being seen more and more as the most effective treatment. Due to synergistic and other potentially harmful effects caused by drug interactions, the simultaneous use of various drugs/devices requires careful investigation. Certain therapeutic combinations are currently being optimized for high-risk patients. The recently published data on the efficacy of streptokinase in myocardial infarction in patients who were pre-treated with aspirin is an excellent example of the clinical implications of drug synergism. In several studies it has been demonstrated that the mortality rate is reduced with combination streptokinase/aspirin therapy in patients with myocardial infarction. Similarly, heparin is also known to augment the therapeutic action of several agents. Treatment protocols are currently based on the individual hemostatic profiles of each patient. The effect of age plays an important role in the pharmacologic response of a drug in the patient. Objective considerations are also being given to this entity to optimize therapy. Treatment protocols are currently based on the individual hemostatic profiles of each patient. The effect of age plays an important role in the pharmacologic response of a drug in the patient. Objective considerations are also being given to optimize therapy in the elderly patient where thrombotic disorders are much more prevalent.

Antithrombotic drugs produce their clinical effects via different mechanisms targeted against single or multiple components of hemostasis. Their therapeutic effects can be produced through multicomponent actions not necessarily related to antithrombin III mediated pathways as with heparin, but through the cellular/non-cellular elements of blood and vasculature. Unlike coumadin and heparin, the monitoring of some of the newer drugs is difficult due to the limitations of the current laboratory methods. Moreover, their true therapeutic and toxic actions may not be quantitatable by any one given method. This situation is further complicated when more than one drug is used for treatment. Thus, the safety/efficacy issues with newer drugs are only assessed in well-defined clinical trials.

Furthermore, there is debate as to the value of any laboratory monitoring of these newer agents. For example, thrombolytic treatment is often given without any laboratory evaluation. In most of the laboratory assays, blood is used for the overall evaluation of the effect of antithrombotic drugs. However, if a new drug does not produce any effect on blood then monitoring of blood related parameters may be useless. Bleeding complications, ineffective treatment and possible harmful effects from drug interactions could be overlooked if this becomes an acceptable practice. In certain cases it may not be necessary to monitor drugs, such as with low molecular weight heparins when they are used as prophylactic agents. However, drugs that have therapeutic actions and mechanisms requiring endogenous cofactors from the patient,s own physiologic system, such as therapy in stroke requiring ATIII, warrant monitoring. Carefully designed clinical trials are, however, needed to demonstrate the relevance of ex vivo monitoring of a drug with its pharmacologic effects.

The currently used methods such as PT, APTT, TT and Heptest^{R} are inadequate for the monitoring of the clinical effects of the newly introduced antithrombotic agents, as well as for low dose coumadin and low dose heparin. New methods are thus urgently needed; however, one must consider the relevance of assayed parameters to the true pharmacologic efficacy. In certain cases absolute drug levels measured by chemical, physical or immunologic methods may not correlate with the observed pharmacologic actions. The antithrombotic actions of newer drugs target non-blood sites which are not monitorable by measuring plasma parameters. Thus, the overall evaluation of patients own hemostatic process may be a more useful parameter than the actual quantitation of the drug.

The introduction of new methods based on immunologic principles in which specific products of hemostatic activation or inhibition are measurable may be of value in assessing the endogenous effects of these newer antithrombotic drugs. For example, the quantitation of fibrinopeptide A, D-dimer and thrombin-antithrombin complexes can be used for the monitoring of drugs against venous thrombosis. Antiplatelet and endothelial modulatory drugs can be monitored by quantitating platelet release products (platelet factor 4 and ß thromboglobulin), eicosanoids (thromboxane B_2 and 6-keto-$PGF_{1\alpha}$) and endothelial release products (t-PA, ACE). Thrombolytic agents have been monitored utilizing the immunologic methods for fibrinogen/fibrin related products and cytokines such as TNF.

In view of the complex mechanisms of action of antithrombotic drugs, it should remain clear that while monitoring of the actions of any antithrombotic drug is an integral component in the management of patients with thrombotic disorders. Universal methods to assess the effects of antithrombotic drugs are not available. A multiparametric laboratory profile of individual drugs should be developed for large scale clinical trials. Applicable methods can then be chosen for each form of therapy [25, 26] This, however, will require additional clinical trials to determine the relevance of the laboratory methods with the therapeutic index of each drug.

The developments in antithrombotic therapy have warranted a revision of our educational and training programs both at the level of the physician and of the allied health personnel. Equally well, cost considerations will play a major role in the development and use of newer antithrombotic drugs. Despite these issues, it is projected that our current clinical practices for the management of thrombotic and atherosclerotic disorders will undergo major transitions in the near future.

Regulatory agencies such as the European Commission, United States FDA and pharmacopeial organizations will, therefore, face many challenges in developing mechanisms to approve these new drugs in consistency with the high standards set for the established drugs. One important consideration is to organize all of the antithrombotic drugs and devices under one umbrella. The establishment of the division of antithrombotic drugs at WHO, Geneva, is, therefore, warranted to centralize the internationalization of newer drugs. Thus, for regulatory consistency, all antithrombotic drugs, regardless of their origin (natural, synthetic or recombinant) and devices would be best regulated by this dedicated division of the World Health Organization.

REFERENCES

1. FAREED J. Development of heparin fractions. Some overlooked considerations. Semin Thromb Hemostas 11(2), 227-236, 1985.

2. FAREED J. Heparin, its fractions, fragments and derivatives. Semin Thromb Hemostas 11(1), 1-9, 1985.

3. FAREED J. New methods in hemostatic testing. In: Fareed J (Ed). Perspectives in hemostasis. New-York, Pergamon Press, pp 310-348, 1981.

4. FAREED J, BAKER WH, HAYES A, WALENGA JM. Molecular markers of hemostatic activation in established atherosclerosis. Semin Thromb Hemostas 12(2), 102-109, 1986.

5. FAREED J, BAKER WH, WALENGA JM, MESSMORE HL. Molecular markers of pathophysiological activation of hemostasis: Current perspectives and future trends. In: Ulutin,

ON and Vinazzer H (Eds). Thrombosis and hemorrhagic diseases. Istanbul, Turkey, Gozlem Matbaachk Koll. Sto., pp 83-88, 1986.

6. FAREED J, BICK RL, SQUILLACI G, WALENGA JM, BERMES EWJr. Molecular markers of hemostatic disorders. Implications in the diagnosis and therapeutic management of thrombotic and bleeding disorders. Clin Chem 29(9), 1641-1658, 1983.

7. FAREED J, KUMAR A, WALENGA JM, EMANUELE RM, WILLIAMSON K, HOPPENSTEADT D. Antithrombotic actions and pharmacokinetics of heparin fragments. Nouv Rev Fr Hematol 26, 267-275, 1984.

8. FAREED J, MESSMORE HL, BERMES EWJr. New perspectives in coagulation testing. Clin Chem 26(10), 1380-1891, 1980.

9. FAREED J, MESSMORE HL, WALENGA JM, BERMES EWJr. Laboratory evaluation of antithrombin III: A critical overview of currently available methods for antithrombin III measurements. Semin Thromb Hemostas 8(4), 288-301, 1983.

10. FAREED J, WALENGA J, BREDDIN K, CAEN JP. Newer avenues in antithrombotic therapy. Semin Thromb Hemostas 15(1&2), 1989.

11. FAREED J, WALENGA JM. Biochemical and pharmacological considerations in the development of heparin and its depolymerized derivatives. Med J Australia 144, 21-30, 1986.

12. FAREED J, WALENGA JM. Current trends in hemostatic testing. Semin Thromb Hemostas 9(4), 379-391, 1983.

13. FAREED J, WALENGA JM, BICK RL, MESSMORE HL. Low molecular weight markers of hemostatic defects: impact of automation on the

quantitation of hemostatic disorders. Semin Thromb Hemostas 9(4), 354-378, 1983.

14. HULL R, HIRSH J. Long term anticoagulant therapy in patients with venous thrombosis. Arch Int Med, 143, 2061-2063, 1983.

15. ISIS-2 (Second International Study of Infarct Survival). Collaborative Group. Randomized trial of intravenous streptokinase, oral aspirin both or neither among 17,187 cases of suspected acute myocardial infarction. Lancet 13, 349-360, 1988.

16. LAGERSTEDT CI, FAGHER B, OLSSON C, OQVIST BW. Need for long-term anticoagulant treatment in symptomatic calf vein thrombosis. Lancet 515-518, 1985.

17. MARKWARDT F. Pharmacological approaches to thrombin regulation. Ann NY Acad Sci USA 485, 204-214, 1986.

18. MARKWARDT F. Pharmacology of hirudin: One hundred years after the first report of the anticoagulant agent. Biomed Biochim Acta 44, 1007-1013, 1985.

19. MARKWARDT F, FINK E, KAISER B, KLOCKING HP, NOWAK G, RICHTER M, STURZEBECHER J. Pharmacological survey of recombinant hirudin. Pharmazie 43, 202-207, 1988.

20. MESSMORE HL, WALENGA JM, FAREED J. Molecular markers of platelet activation. Semin Thromb Hemostas 10(4), 264-269, 1984.

21. PETITTI DB, STROM B, MELMON K. Duration of warfarin anticoagulant therapy and the probabilities of recurrent thromboembolism and hemorrhage. Am J Med 81, 255-259, 1986.

22. SUAREZ CR, FAREED J, TOMICH P. Neonatal and natural hemostasis: Value of molecular markers in the assessment of hemostastic

status. Semin Thromb Hemostas 10(4), 208-284, 1984.

23. SUMMARIA L, CAPRINI JA, McMILLAN R, SANDESARA J, AXELROD CA, MUELLER ME, VAGHER JP, WALENGA J, FAREED J. Relationship between post-surgical fibrinolytic parameters and deep vein thrombosis in surgical patients treated with compression devices. Amer Surgeon 54(3), 156-160, 1988.

24. ULUTIN ON, FAREED J, KUMAR A, WALENGA JM, HOPPENSTEADT D. Pharmacologic profiling of the action of defibrotide in animal models of hemostatic and thrombotic disorders. In: Ulutin ON and Vinazzer H (Eds). Thrombosis and hemorrhagic diseases. Istanbul, Turkey. Gozlem Matbaachk Koll. Sto., pp 101-110, 1986.

25. WALENGA JM, FAREED J, HOPPENSTEADT D, EMANUELE RM. Laboratory monitoring of heparin: Old vs. new methods. CRC Critical Review in Lab Sci 22(4), 386-389, 1986.

26. WALENGA JM, FAREED J, MESSMORE HL. Newer avenues in the monitoring of antithrombotic therapy: The role of automation. Semin Thromb Hemostas 9(4), 346-354, 1983.

2

Antithrombotic drugs

F. Azougagh Oualane, F. Doutremepuich

Thromboembolic diseases are major cause of global mortality. Thrombosis genesis can be induced by endothelial injury, hyperviscosity and fibrinolysis decrease. The anatomic origin of thrombosis disorders differs according to diverse types of pathophysiology.

The aim is of antithrombotic therapy is to antagonize factors involved in this genesis. It is intented for preventing thrombogenic risk factors. These factors are hyperlipemia, hypercholesterolemia, arterial hypertension, smoking associated to arterial thrombosis or stasis of venous blood after surgery, abnormalities of certain coagulation factors and the physiological inhibitors such as genetic deficiencies of C and S proteins and antithrombin III (ATIII) associated to venous thrombosis.

The most effective methods to prevent and abate thrombotic diseases are the use of anticoagulant and antiplatelet therapies.

2. Anticoagulant therapy

Anticoagulant drugs may be divided on three families:

- drugs that inhibit indirectly the coagulation factors via antithrombin III (AT III) or heparin cofactor II (HC II).
- drugs that inhibit directly coagulation factors.

- drugs that act on synthesis of plasmatic serine protease.

2.1 Drugs that inhibit indirectly the coagulation factors

2.1.1 Heparins

Heparin is an anticoagulant drug discovered by Mac Lean in 1916. The first clinical trial was done in 1936. The mechanism of its anticoagulant activity was only understood in 1970.

Unfractionnated heparin (UFH) is mucopolysaccharide chains of various length that range from 5000 to 30000 daltons. It is extracted from beef liver or pork intestines.

The basic structure of heparin is constituted by alternating glucosamine and uronic acid (D-glucuronic acid or L-iduronic acid). Heparin is considered as a mixture of polysaccharide chains of variable length and of variable degree of heterogeneity. The minimal binding site region is a pentasaccharidic sequence (DEFGH). It countains a nonsulfated D-glucuronic acid (E) and trisulfated glucosamine unit carrying an unique 3-O-sulfate group (molecular weight: 2500 daltons).

Heparin is constituted by two fractions following its action with AT-III:

- with high affinity for AT-III and is about one third.
- with low affinity for AT-III and is about two third.

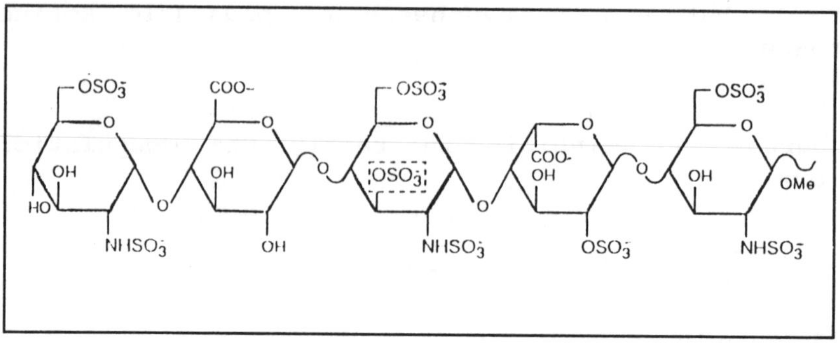

Figure 1: Pentasaccharide sequence, minimal sequence of heparin wich interact with AT-III

Heparin possesses numerous activities. The most important is anticoagulant activity. This activity is largely associated with the plasma protein AT-III.

AT-III forms complexes with the coagulation proteins (thrombin and factor Xa) leading to inhibit their enzymatic activities. This complexation which is associated with a conformational transition of AT-III is normaly a slow process. By forming a strong equimolar complex with AT-III, heparin potents AT-III activity [33].

Heparin acts on platelets and vascular endothelium.

It inhibits platelet aggregation induced by collagen [5]; and binds to endothelial cells and provokes substances release as heparin like products such as heparan sulfate, dermatan sulfate. It may provoke an increase in tissular plasminogen activator (t-PA) release [41, 42].

Heparin can be administered by either intravenous or subcutaneous ways, but can not be administered by oral one.

Heparin is indicated in prophylactic and curative treatment of venous and arterial thrombosis, in pulmonary embolism and in acute phase myocardial infarctus it is also used in the extra-corporeal circulation (ECC) and hemodialysis.

The monotoring of biological activities of heparin requires platelet count, dosage of anti-Xa activity and Activated Partial Thromboplastin Time (APTT). In case of overdosage, heparin is neutralized by protamine.

Heparin effectiveness is influenced by concentration of platelet factor 4 (PF4) [31] released in plasma and by circulatory level of lipoprotein.

Thus, heparin is not a perfect anticoagulant owing to its short half-life in the circulating blood. A loading dose is insufficient to ensure the anticoagulation, so a maintaining dose is needed to keep its effect for several hours. In addition, a draw back of its usage consists of hemorragic and thrombopenic risks. Heparin is contra- indicated in cases of hemorrhagic diseases, arterial hypertension and hepatic insufficiency.

In attempt to palliate these disadvantages, UFH has been replaced by low molecular weight heparin (LMWH).

2.1.2 Low molecular weight heparins (LMWH)

LMWH are obtained from heparin through different ways of depolymerization and fractionation [29]. Their ways molecular weight generally ranges between 4000 and 6000 d. Like heparin, LMWH are heterogeneous in composition and are composed by two fractions: one with low affinity for AT-III (about 75%) and one with high affinity for ATIII (about 25%).

In vitro and ex vivo dosages of anti-factor Xa and anti-factor IIa activities have shown that the anti-factor Xa activity is higher in LMWH, whereas the anti-factor IIa activity is low [8].

Like UFH, LMWH act on endothelial cells and provoke t-PA release [41, 42], but have low effect on platelets and are less hemorrhagic.

Actually, LMWH are used in curative and prophylaxis treatments of venous thrombosis, pulmonary embolism and in hemodialysis [14].

Biological monotoring involves only platelet count and dosage of anti-Xa activity.

2.1.3 Dermatan Sulfate

Dermatan Sulfate (DS) is a glycosamino- glycan extracted from intestinal mucous of pork. Its molecular weight is about 19000 daltons.

DS accelerates thrombin inhibition by interacting with (HCII) [39]. In contrast with heparin, DS does not inhibit factor Xa, and is virtually inactive in vitro as anticoagulant in conventional clotting assays. It has been showed that DS has anticoagulant activity. It is also effective as antithrombotic agent with little effect on bleeding when used at antithrombotic levels. Its anticoagulant activity is related to the degree of sulfatation.

In comparison to heparin, DS causes a relatively weak prolongation of clotting time. Despite the fact that these compounds are weak anticoagulants, they are potent inhibitors of the intrinsic pathway for thrombin generation [35].

As antithrombotic agent, DS has been shown to be as effective as heparin, but with a lower risk of bleeding complications.

2.1.4 Pentosan Polysulfate

Pentosan Polysulfate (PPS) is a synthetic heparinoïd used as an antithrombotic. Its molecular weight is about 6000 daltons.

It acts principally on factor Xa and inhibits essentially intrinsic coagulation. Its mechanism of action is not well understood. Some authors think that PPS acts through AT-III pathway by AT-III [36], but others affirm that HCII is required for its action [34].

PPS has anticoagulant and antifibrinolytic properties in clinical man and in animal [22].

It involves thrombopenia by reducing platelets aggregation. It improves heamodynamic conditions by decreasing blood viscosity.

It is used in man for the prophylaxis of thrombo-embolic diseases and it is administered by intramuscular and intravenous ways.

2.2 drugs that inhibit directly coagulation factors

2.2.1 Natural hirudin

Hirudin discovered in 1884 by Haycrafft is produced in the salivary gland of the medicinal leeches (Hirudo Medicinalis) [18]. Up to the discovery of heparin, several years later, this was the only way to prevent blood from clotting.

It is a small protein with a molecular weight of 7000 daltons. The sequence is 65 amino acids long. The amino acid composition of hirudin is characterized by a remarkably high content of acidic amino acids, a sulfated residue on tyrosine-63 as well as by the absence of arginine, methionine and tryptophane.

Hirudin inhibits thrombin selectively [30]. From kinetic studies it was proposed that the binding of hirudin to thrombin involves at least two steps. The initial interaction is diffusion controlled and involves an ionic interaction. In a second step, this complex rearanges to form a tighter complex in which hirudin is also bound at the active site [9].

Hirudin forms with thrombin equimolar complexes. All proteolytic functions of the enzyme are blocked.

Thus, hirudin prevents not only fibrinogen clotting but also further thrombin-catalysed hemostatic reactions such as thrombin-induced platelet reaction.

2.2.2 Recombinant hirudin

As native hirudin has to be isolated from medicinalis leeches, a number of difficulties arose.

Under these circumstances based on genetic engineering.

Recombinant-hirudin can now be produced in different biological systems such as bacteria (Escherichia coli) or yeast cells (Saccharomyces cervisiae). These recombinant products were expressed as desulfato-hirudin and showed the same configuration [37]. The most studied is CGP39393 obtained by yeast (Laboratorie Ciba Geigy).

The clinical indications are post-operative prophylaxis against deep vein thrombosis and pulmonary embolism, prevention of reocclusion after anticoagulant administration during cardiovascular bypass surgery.

2.2.3 Hirudin fragments

At present, hirudin fragments may be produced by chemical synthesis in basing on carboxyl-terminal sequence, which is implicated in the interaction between thrombin and hirudin and is responsable of antithrombin properties of hirudin. The main polypeptides effective as antithrombin products are BG8865 and MDL28,050.

BG8865 is a sulfated dodecapeptide [20]. It is constitued from residue 53 to residue 64:
[**NH_2-Asn-Gly-Asp-Phe-Glu-Ile-Pro-Glu-Glu-Tyr(SO^{3-})-Leu- COOH**].

Mao and al. have shown that the synthetical dodecapeptide MDL28,050 is the minimal and functional sequence required to bind to α-thrombin and so to inhibit coagulation [26]. It is constituted from residue 55 to residue 65:
[**Suc-Tyr-Glu-Pro-Ile-Pro-Glu-Glu-Ala-Cha-D-Gl-OH**]
(Suc: Succinyl and Cha: ß-cyclohexyl-alanine)

This peptide is stabilized and protected against degradation by the presence of an acyl group at the N-terminal end, two proline and D-amino acid at the C-terminal end.

Recombinant hirudins and synthetized fragments are effective antithrombotic drugs in inducing thrombosis by stasis, arterial thrombosis, (DIC), coronary occlusion and in reocclusion after thrombolysis. In addition, these hirudins have some advantages compared to heparins. They possess exclusive antithrombin activity independently of cofactor (AT-III and HCII). This activity is not inhibited by PF4. However, the inconvenient of their use is the non-existence of antidote in the case of hemorrhage.

2.2.4 Hirulog peptides

Hirulog peptides represent a novel family of bivalent inhibitors of thrombin [5, 27]. Inactivation of α-thrombin is obtained by the binding at its catalytic site and the fibrin(ogen) recognition exosite simultaneously. These products are constituted by the amino acid (53-64) COOH- terminal domain of hirudin [28]. This extremity is constituted by the sequence Arg-Pro which prevents thrombin cleavage of hirulog sequence $(Gly)_4$ and is responsable for its high affinity to thrombin.

Hirulog-1 is a peptide of 20 amino-acids, synthetized by using the protein hirudin as a model : [**D-Phe-Pro-Arg-Pro-$(Gly)_4$desulfo-hirudin$^{53-64}$**].
The amino acid D-Phe was found to increase the inhibitory activity of hirulog peptide. X-ray cristallography studies demonstrate that hirulog-1 binds to both the anion exosite and the catalytic site of thrombin.

Some studies indicate that hirulog-1 has potent anticoagulant properties for the treatment of disorders associated with thrombus formation in human [40].

2.3 Drugs which interfere with the synthesis of plasmatic serine protease.

2.3.1 Vitamin K

Vitamin K (VK) represents a group of liposoluble substances which derive from a 2-methyl-1,4-naphtoquinone nucleus. They participate essentially to the activation process of some factors of coagulation known as "vitamin K dependant" such as prothrombin (II), proconvertin (VII), antihemophilic B, factor (IX), Stuart factor (X), and C and S proteins.

At this site, VK accumulates some glutamic residues in order to allow the fixation of the protein on the membrane phospholipids by Ca^{++} bridges. These residues must be converted to gamma-carboxyglutamic acid. Thus, VK acts as a cofactor of hepatic carboxylase. This participation is effected during the enzymatic reactions of the post-transductional phase of synthesis of VK dependent proteins.

At the same time, the structure and the definitive function of factors of coagulation are obtained by the formation of disulfur bridges and the glycosylation of proteins.

2.3.2 Vitamin-K Antagonists

The antivitamin-K (AVK) are divided in two main groups according to their chemical structures:

1. the coumarine group (warfarin, acenocoumarol...).
2. the indanedione group (phenindione, bromindione...).

The AVK drugs have similar structure than VK, this conferes a same mode of action: AVK and VK compete on the enzymatic activation sites of epoxyde reductase [6]. The AVK drugs inhibit the enzyme activity and block the VK cycle and the gamma-carboxylation [19]. This blockage prolong the prothrombin time and blood related coagulation tests.

The precursors of VK dependant factors or PIVKA (proteins induced in VK absence or in presence of AVK) are accumulated in the hepatocytes secreted in the circulation. Although they do not have any procoagulant activity, they can have an inhibitory effect by their competitive action with homologue active proteins.

These oral drugs are almost exclusively used because of their effect on blood coagulation [6].

They decrease successively the level of proconvertin (VII), antihemophilic B (IX), Stuart (X) and prothrombin (II) factors. About C-protein, a physiological inhibitor of coagulation factors (VIII, V), its level may reach 0.25 U/ml (normal level: 0.65-1.45 U/ml) in chronic treatment: this parameter must be taken in consideration in treatment under monotoring in order to prevent thrombosis due to quantitative deficit of C-protein.

The AVK are usually prescribed for chronic treatment. During this period some other drugs may be given as adjuvants or for other purpose, this drugs may disturb the anticoagulant treatment by a slight change in the chemotherapeutic index of AVK. Any antiaggregant drug (salicylates, ticlopidine, dipyridamole, phenylbutazone, indomethacin..) increases the hemorrhagic tendency and the effect of AVK if they are used simultaneously.

A.V.K are indicated as preventing agents in case of arterial or venous thrombosis [19]. They may be indicated in such case as treatment and prevention of venous thrombosis concomitly with heparin: deep phlebits, pulmonar embolism, diseases jointly thrombosis: congenital or acquired deficit of AT-III, myocardiacal infarction and aorto- coronary bypass.

In some cases AVK treatment is absolutely contraindicated as in case of pregnancy, hepatic or renal deficiency, gastric ulcer, severe arterial hypertension and hemopathies with hemostatic troubles.

AVK is not contraindicated in case of feeding although they pass in the mother milk: hypocoagulability of neonate is weak.

Some precautions must be taken in case of recent cerebrovascular accidents, biliary insufficiency and chirugical interventions.

Due to individual reactions, dose must be adapted with monotoring of biological tests. Generally, AVK is given daily.

Biological monitoring of treatment with AVK is carried out with APTT, PT (Prothrombin Time and INR or International Normalized Ratio which is:

INR = (patient time/reference time)^{ISI}

ISI: Indice of International Sensibility

Therapeutic zones in INR were defined by Loeliger in evidence with the importance of anticoagulation wanted.

- Pre- and post-operative anticoagulation: pelvis operations: 2.0-3.0; other surgical operations: 1.5-2.5.
- Prophylaxis of venous primitive or secondary thrombosis : 2.0-3.0.
- Pulmonary embolism, during phlebitis evolution and in case of relapsing phlebitis: 2.0-4.0.
- Arterial prophylaxis, artificial cardiac valve: 3.0-4.5.

AVK are largely used in human clinic because they are irreplaceable in the treatment of some cases. Such treatment need an intensive monotoring, an accurate and adapted biological control.

3. ANTIPLATELETS

The activation of platelets secondary to vascular injury initiates a serie of changes within platelets. This promotes the release reactions. The α-granules and dense bodies release their contents. The adenosine diphosphate (ADP) released by the dense bodies mediates the adhesion of other platelets at the site of injury. ADP and thromboxane A_2 (TxA_2) are critical in the induction of platelet aggregation which leads to formation of platelet or hemostatic plug.

Antiplatelet medications produce their effects in a great extent on a platelet activation by inhibiting prostaglandin (PG) metabolism, or by inhibiting some platelet receptors or lastly by inhibition release of intraplatelet contents [23]. These medications include aspirin (ASA), ticlopidine and dipyridamole, which are used to prevent and to decrease the arterial forms of thrombosis.

At present, a new way of research is under investigation. It is the use of monoclonal antibody directed against the $GPII_b/III_a$ receptor of platelet [8-10].

3.1 Aspirin

The cyclooxygenase plays an important role in the conversion of arachidonic acid into the cyclic endoperoxides PGG_2 and PGH_2. This enzyme may be blocked by anti-inflammatory drugs such as aspirin. Acetylsalicylic acid (Aspirin) is a weak acid. At present, it is obtained by acetylation of salicylic acid by acetic anhydride. It inhibits cyclo-oxygenase irreversibly by acetylating it.

- In platelets, the acetylation inhibits irreversibly the formation of TxA_2 and this effect persists for the life of the platelets (8 at 10 days) because platelets are unable to synthetize new enzyme molecules to replace those that have been inactivated for ever the life. Platelet function is fully restored only when new platelets enter the circulation, although about 10% of affected platelets will have restoration of near-normal function.
- In endothelial cells, the acetylation of cyclo-oxygenase leads to inhibition of prostacyclin synthesis. However, in contrast with platelets, this inhibition is not permanent. This can be explained by the fact, that these cells can synthetize the enzyme.

Whereas, aspirin inhibits only secondary aggregation related to release reaction, it has little effect on ADP-induced aggregation as shown in rat and is totally inactive on PG endoperoxide- or TxA_2-induced platelet aggregation.

Aspirin increases bleeding time [3].

It is indicated as antiplatelet drug in number cases: coronary disease, valvulopathy, arteriopathy and brain ischemia accident

At present, four posologies are used:

- < 100 mg/kg
- 100 to 200 mg/kg
- 200 to 500 mg/kg
- > 500 mg/kg

3.2 Ticlopidine (Ticlid[R])

Ticlopidine,5-(2-chrobenzyl)-4,5,6,7-tetra dydrothieno[3,2,-c)] pyridine hydrochloride (53-32c) is a potent, long acting inhibitor of platelet aggregation [2]. It inhibits platelet aggregation induced by ADP, collagen, thrombin, arachidonic acid, adrenaline and prostaglandin endopyroxides or TxA_2, in man and in a wide range of animal species [4], but this effect may be overcome at high agonist concentrations.

Some studies carried out in rat have shown that the inhibitor effect of ticlopidine is directed against ADP-induced aggregation. It has no effect on cyclooxygenase or thromboxane synthetase [21]. It is neither a powerful inhibitor of phosphodiesterase nor of adenosine uptake, nor a stimulant of adenylate cyclase in platelet [2, 4, 7].

The exact target of this inhibition is not yet well defined. It has been shown that ticlopidine inhibits the binding of fibrinogen to its receptor $GPII_b/III_a$.

Slight but significant inhibition of ADP-induced aggregation was obtained 24 to 48 hours after the beginning of the treatment. The maximum is reached between the 3th and 6th day and persists more than three days after therapy interruption. This effect is dose-dependent.

The $GPII_b/III_a$ complex binds adhesive proteins by a specific sequence of amino-acids. Synthetic analogues of this binding sequence are potent inhibitors of the action of these proteins in the aggregation mechanism, such as some fibrinogen degradation products. Ticlopidine is a potent inhibitor of platelet aggregation. It acts through the inhibition of the binding of adhesive proteins to $GPII_b/III_a$ complex by a mechanism that is still unsolved.

It inhibits primary phase aggregation induced by ADP and adrenaline [15] in human platelets, and ADP-induced aggregation of prostaglandin endoperoxide - induced aggregation of rat platelets [2].

The studies demonstrate that ticlopidine administration resulted in irreversible and selective changes in certain enzyme activity and function of platelets, suggesting a unique mechanism of action of ticlopidine. The central action of ticlopidine is on platelet membrane adenylate cyclase activity. Platelet C-AMP phosphodiesterase activity was not significantly affected by ticlopidine treatment.

Ticlopidine treatment elevated basal adenylate cyclase activity in platelet membrane fraction and this effect was markedly amplified when Mg divalent cation removed by EGTA. Ticlopidine also elevated the PGE_1-stimulated adenylate cyclase activity but it failed to enhance the enzyme activity stimulated by adenosin or sodium fluoride.

Ticlopidine is indicated in some situations. It prevents peripheral arterial ischemia, brain ischemia accident and platelet alterations in cardiopulmonary bypass (CPB).

However, it presents a number of side effects like hemorrhagic risk and thrombocytopenia.

Ticlopidine prolongs the bleeding time in man [15] and in animals. This effect does not always the parallel inhibition of aggregation by ADP. The maximal antiaggregant activity appears after 3-5 days.

It has no or minimal influence on all coagulation tests and on fibrinolysis. Thus, the increase in the bleeding time is presumably due to its effects on platelets and perhaps on the endothelial cells. Lastly, several authors have claimed that ticlopidine increases the deformability of red cells and diminishes the blood viscosity in animals and in patients suffering from vascular diseases.

These properties are presumably relevant to the reported clinical efficacy of ticlopidine in the following situations: ECC in cardiac surgery and in haemodialysis, aorto-coronary by-pass and thrombosis of the central retinal vein.

Extensive clinical trials are in progress to assess its value in other conditions.

3.3 Dipyridamole (Persantin^{R})

Dipyridamole is a pyrimido-pyrimidine. It exerts its antiplatelet activity by increasing C-AMP levels vasodilatator and inhibitor of platelet aggregation, thus, suppressing platelet ADP necessary for platelet aggregation. Dipyridamole inhibits also endothelial cells uptake of adenosine, an important nucleotide precursor. It increases the coronary flow increasing blood irrigation and the supply of oxygen to heart. It also increases platelet half-life which is shortened in patients with prosthetic heart valves.

Dipyridamole is rarely used alone. Combined with aspirin, it has been used to prevent the extension of peripheral vascular diseases. It is also used combined with AVK and enhances their effect in coronary patients with artificial valve [32].

Dipyridamole alone at therapeutic doses does not prolong bleeding time or increase bleeding during cardiopulmonary bypass (CPB) operations.

3.4 Platelet anti-receptors antibodies

Platelet membrane glycoprotein (GP) II_b/III_a complex plays a major role in platelet aggregation and it is a representant of integrins family involved in the functions of vascular cells. When platelets are activated by ADP or other agonists, the binding site of fibrinogen is exposed on the $GPII_b/III_a$ complex.

Blockage of the platelet fibrinogen receptor, the glycoprotein $GPII_b/III_a$, might be of higher chemical benefit in arterial thrombosis than aspirin. Recently, it has been shown in vitro, that monoclonal antibodies directed against specific epitopes on the $GPII_b/III_a$ complex can completely block platelet fibrinogen binding and aggregation induced by ADP [12].

A murine monoclonal antibody 7E3 is chimeric antibody directed against the $GPII_b/III_a$ complex [10]. It is reconstructed by the variable part of mouse light chain coupleted to the human kappa constant part and by the variable part of mouse heavy chain coupled to C_1 domain of human IgG_1. This product binds to human platelet $GPII_b/III_a$ complex with high affinity preventing the adhesive interaction of fibrinogen or von Willebrand factor [11, 12].

This product has been tested in different models of arterial thrombosis in dogs.

4. Conclusion

UFH and AVK have been for long time the most used anticoagulant drugs. Heparin has been the choice drug to treat thromboembolic diseases. But the development of LMWH have added a new dimension to the managment of venous thrombosis and have shown their effectiveness in some clinical situations. At present, some synthetic antithrombotic drugs such as new heparin derivatives, hirudin fragments, hirulogs and antibodies directed against $GPII_b/III_a$ complex will be developed for various indications and will play an important role in the managment on the disorder.

REFERENCES

1. AGNELLI G, COSMI B, DI FILIPPO. A randomised, double blind-placebo controlled trial of dermatan sulfate for prevention of deep vein thrombosis in hip fracture. Thromb Haemost 67, 203-208, 1992.

2. ASHIDA S, ABIKO Y. Inhibition of platelet aggregation by a new agent, ticlopidine. Thromb Heamost 40, 542-550, 1979.

3. BEAUMONT JL, CAEN JP, BERNARD J. Action hémorragique de l'acide acétylsalicylique au cours des maladies du sang. Bull Soc Méd Hôp Paris 71, 1087, 1985.

4. BONNE C, MARTIN B, REGNAULT F. Potentiation of antiaggregating prostaglandins by ticlopidine. Thromb Haemost 46, Abst 67, 1981.

5. BOURDON P, JABLONSKI JA, CHAO BH, MARAGANORE JM. Structure-function relation-ships of hirulog peptide interactions with thrombin. FEBS Lett 294, 163-166, 1991.

6. BRUNO J, YANG D, TAYLOR LA, LEAMSTER G. Role of platelet cAMP and prostaglandin synthesis in platelet aggregation inhibition by ticlopidine hydrochloride. Thromb Heamost 46, Abst 194, 66, 1981.

7. CADE JF, BUCHANAN MR, BONEU B, OKLEFORD P. A comparison of the antithrombotic and heamorrhagic effects of low molecular weight heparin fractions: The influence of the method of preparation. Thromb Res 35, 613-625, 1984.

8. CHANG JY. The functionnal domain of hirudin a thrombin-specific inhibitor. FEBS Lett 25, 4622-4628, 1986.

9. COLLER BS. A new murine monoclonal antibody reports an activation-dependent change in the conformation and/or microenvironnement of the platelet $GPII_b/III_a$ complex. J Clin Invest 76, 101, 1985.

10. COLLER BS, FOLTS JD, SCUDDER LE, SMITH SR. Antithrombotic effect of a monoclonal antibody to the platelet glycoprotein II_b/III_a receptor in an experimental animal model. Blood 68, 783-786, 1986.

11. COLLER BS, PEERSCHKE EI, SCUDDER LE, SULLIVAN CA. A murine monoclonal antibody that completely blocks the binding of fibrinogen to platelet produces a thrombasthenic-like state in normal platelets and binds to glycoproteins II_b and/or III_a. J Clin Invest 72, 325, 1983.

12. CZAPEK EE, KWAAN HC, SZCZECINSKI M. The effect of sulfated polysaccharide on ATIII. J Lab Clin Med 95, 783-790, 1980.

13. ELLIS DJ, ROE RL, BRUNO JJ, CRAUSTON BJ, McSPADDEN MM. The effect of ticlopidine hydrochloride on bleeding time and platelet function in man. (ABST). Thromb Heamost 46, 1973, 1981.

14. HARKER LA, SLICHTER SJ. Studies of platelets and fibrinogen kinetics in patients with prosthetic valves. N Engl J Med 283, 1302-1305, 1970.

15. HARVEY RP, DEGRYSE E, STEFANI L, SCHAMBER F, CAZENAVE JP, COURTNEY M, TOLSTOSHEV P, LECOCQ JP. Cloning and expression of cDNA coding for the anticoagulant hirudin from the bloodsucking leech. Proc Natl Acad Sci USA 83, 1084-1088, 1986.

16. HAYCRAFT JB. On the action of a secretion abtained from the medicinal leech on the coagulation of the blood. Proc R Soc Lond 36, 478-487, 1884.

17. HEMKER HC, FRANK HLL. The mechanism of action of oral anticoagulants and its consequences for the practice of oral anticoagulation. Heamostasis 15, 203-270, 1985.

18. JAKUBOWSKI JA, MARAGANORE JM. Inhibition of coagulation and thrombin-induced platelets activities by a synthetic dodecapeptide modeled on the carboxy-terminus of hirudin. Blood 75, 399-406, 1990.

19. KLÖCKING HP, MARKWARDT F. Pentosan polysulfate-induced release of plasminogen activator. Heamostasis 6, 370-374, 1977.

20. LECOMPTE TH, KHER A, GAILLARD JL, SAMAMA M. Pharmacologie des agents antiplaquettaires J des Mal Vasculaires 8, 3, 1983.

21. LEE H, PATON RC, RUAN C, CAEN JP. The in vitro effect of ticlopidine on fibrinogen and factor VIII binding to human platelets. Thromb Heamost 46, 590-592, 1981.

22. LINDAHL U. Biosynthesis of heparin and heparan sulfate. Upsal. J Med Sci 82, 78-79, 1977.

23. MAO SJT, YATES MT, OWEN TJ, KRSTENANSKY JL. Interaction of hirudin with thrombin: Identification of a minimal binding domain that inhibits clotting activity. Biochemistry 27, 8170-8173, 1988.

24. MARAGANORE JM, BOURDON P, JABLONSKI JA. Design and characterisation of hirulogs: A novel class of bivalent peptide inhibitors of thrombin. Biochemistry 29, 7095-7101, 1990.

25. MARAGANORE JM, CHAO BH, JOSEPH ML, et al. Anticoagulant activity of synthetic hirudin peptides. J Biol Chem 264, 8692-8698, 1989.

26. MARDIGUIAN J. Methods of preparation of low molecular weight heparins. Low Molecular Weight Heparins in Clinical Practice. Marcel DEKKER Edit NEW-YORK, 7-12, 1992.

27. MARKWARDT F. Hirudin as an inhibitor of thrombin. Methods Enzymol 19, 924-932, 1970.

28. BRECKENBRIDGE AM. Oral anticoagulant drugs. Sem Heamatol 15, 19-26, 1978.

29. DOUTREMEPUICH C, LALANNE MC, DOUTREMEPUICH F, PUYAL C. Low molecular weight heparins today: Pharmacological considerations. In: Low Molecular Weight Heparins in Clinical Practice (C. DOUTREMEPUICH (Eds)). Marcel DEKKER, NEW-YORK, pp 85-96 1992.

30. JOHNSON M, HEYWOOD JB. Possible mode of action of ticlopidine: A novel inhibitor of platelet aggregation. Thromb Heamost 42, 367, 1979.

31. NATH N, NIEWIAROWSKI S, JOIST JH. Platelet factor 4-antiheparin protein releasable from platelets: Purification and properties. J Lab Clin Med 82, 754-768, 1973.

32. TOPOL EJ, SCARPACE DG, PALABRICA TM, SUTOR RJ, FOX IH, MARAGANORE JM. Hirulog, a direct thrombin inhibitor peptide, instead of heparin for routine coronary angioplasty: pilot experience. Circulation (Supplement II), 84, Abstract 2354, 1991.

33. RAJAH SM, CROW MJ, AHMAD R, WATSON DA. The effect of dipyridamole on platelet function. Correlation with blood levels in man. Br J Clin Pharmacol 4, 129-133, 1977.

34. ROSENBERG RD, DAMUS PS. The purification and mechanism of action of human antithrombin-heparin cofactor. J Biol Chem 248, 6490-6505, 1973.

35. SCULLY MF, KAKKAR VV. Identification of heparin cofactor II as the principal plasma cofactor for the antithrombin activity of pentosan polysulfate (SP54). Thromb Res 36, 187-194, 1984.

36. SIE P, OFOSU F, FERNANDEZ F, BUCHANAU MR, PETITOU M, BONNEU B. Respective role of antithrombin III and heparin cofactor II in the in vitro anticoagulant effect of heparin and of various sulphated polysaccharides. Br J Haematol 64, J 707-714, 1986.

37. SORIA C, SORIA J, RYCKEWAERT JJ, HOLMER E, CAEN JP. Anticoagulant activities of pentosane polysulfate: comparison with standard heparin and a fraction of low molecular weight heparin. Thromb Res 19, 455-463, 1980.

38. TALBOT MD, AMBLER J, BUTLER KD, FINDLAY VS, PETERS RF, TWEED MF, WALLIS RB. Recombinant desulfato-hirudin (CGP39393) anticoagulant and antithrombotic properties in vivo. Thromb Haemost 61, 77-80, 1989.

39. THOMAS DP, MARTON RE, BARROWCLIFFE TW, MULLOY B, JOHNSON EA. Antifactor Xa activity of heparan sulfate. , 14, 501-506, 1979.

40. TOLLEFSEN DM, PETSKA CA, MONAFO WJ. Activation of heparin cofactor II by dermatan sulfate. J Biol Chem 258, 6713, 1983

41. VAIREL EG. Heparins and fibrinolysis.In: Low Molecular Weight Heparins in Clinical Practice (C. DOUTREMEPUICH (Eds)). Marcel DEKKER, NEW-YORK, pp 51- 61, 1992.

42. VAIREL EG, BROUTY-BOYE H, TOULEMONDE F, DOUTREMEPUICH C. Rôle de l'activité fibrinolytique indirecte des héparines et de composés voisins dans la prophylaxie des thromboses. Ann Pharma Franç 41, 339-353, 1983.

3

Heparin and non-heparin glycosaminoglycans : future perspectives for future applications

P. Bianchini

Two main development lines distinguish these last 50 years:

- the study of proteoglycans and their physiopathologic role [10, 11, 24, 41].
- the study of glycosaminoglycans, the polysaccharidic part of proteoglycan molecules, and their pharmacological and therapeutical importance [17, 27, 30, 32, 36].

It is odd that the study on proteoglycans has always been focused on both cellular component and extracellular connective tissue matrix, whereas that on glycosaminoglycans has been focused mainly on blood biochemistry.

Proteoheparan sulfates are located on cell surfaces and play a role in cell growth and differentiation [38], in cell attachment [40], in matrix formation [31, 49], in lipoproteinolipase binding [43].

Other proteoglycans of endothelial cell surface are involved in blood coagulation by means of thrombomodulin system [28].

The most investigated proteoglycan is, with no doubt, heparan sulfate, while the glycosaminoglycan which aroused the greatest interest among researchers is certainly heparin.

It is most surprising that proteoglycans were discovered only in 1954 by Shatton and Schubert [42] whereas the study of glycosaminoglycans is much older. In effect heparin was discovered in 1918 [26] and for many years considered no more than an anticoagulant drug.

Only 25 years after, in 1943, Hahn [21] discovered a new activity of heparin, lipoproteinolipase releasing activity.

This discovery opened a new chapter in heparin field and led researchers to the separation of anticoagulant and antilipaemic activities, through chemical modifications of heparin molecules: for instance, the heparides [45] an the so-called heparinoids were obtained.

Table I: In vitro and ex vivo characteristics of international heparin standard (WHO III), commercial heparin, dextran sulphate (DEXT-S), mucopolysaccharide polysulphate (MPS-PS), pentosan polysulphate (P-PS), heparamin, dermatan and heparan.
(LPL-RU = lipoprotein lipase releasing units).

Sample	MW kDa	IN VITRO		EX VIVO	
		USP/ mg	APTT U/ mg	LPL RU/ mg	APTT U/ mg
WHO III	13,0	173,4	173,4	35,31	20,98
HEPARIN	14,0	157,5	182,5	32,96	18,47
DEXT-S	3,5	0,2	0,9	0,86	0,29
MPS-PS	4,7	17,9	26,2	47,23	5,20
P-PS	2,9	11,1	16,7	14,00	4,90
HEPARAMIN	8,5+4,5	17,7	5,6	0,45	0,35
DERMATAN	27,5	4,1	3,7	0,67	0,68
HEPARAN	20,8	3,1	5,3	1,13	1,11

Table I reports some in vitro and ex vivo characteristics of semisyntethic heparinoids in comparison with heparin and naturally occurring heparinoids (dermatan-heparan).

The separation of the different biological characteristics of heparin is a general problem.

One kind of separation takes into account the heterogeneity of this molecular population [33, 34], where it is possible, for instance, to single out the molecules bearing the sequence of affinity for ATIII by centrifugation [29] or by ATIII affinity chromatography [25].

Other methods utilize gel filtration chromatography to separate heparin fractions of different molecular weights [22] and different biological activities [4].

Only a third of heparin molecules have ATIII-affinity [1], therefore it is clear that not all biological effects are ATIII dependent, but it is likely that the no-affinity molecules are involved in other mechanisms.

One has to consider that ATIII is a member of the serpin superfamily, which comprises various proteins like, for instance, Heparin Cofactor II, C_1-INH, α_2-antiplasmin, Plasminogen Inhibitor, Antitrypsin, α_1-antichymotrypsin.

Heparin can bind itself to these proteins and to other proteins such as fibronectin [44] or heparin-binding (fibroblast) growth factors [7].

In these last 10 years the demonstration that the antithrombotic activity of heparin could be dissociated from its anticoagulant action played an important role [5, 6].

In effect anticoagulant in vitro tests like APTT or anti-Xa, cannot predict the antithrombotic activity of heparin or heparin related compounds, even if one of the first hypotheses held selective inhibition of factor Xa responsible for antithrombotic activity.

Nevertheless the general opinion on the importance of AXa inhibition induced by ATIII in presence of particular sequences in heparin molecule, stimulated researches in the field of heparin structure.

The results of these studies are probably the most important contribution to the knowledge of the active site of heparin (pentasaccharide) [8] and to the comprehension of the structure-activity relationship.

In the aforesaid period many researchers focused their attention on heparin naturally occurring fractions and chemically or enzymatically degraded fragments in order to obtain coumpounds safer than unfractionated heparin.

The main target was to obtain a drug having low anticoagulant activity and high antithrombotic effect and to dissociate the antithrombotic action from the haemorrhagic side-effects [35].

In effect the antithrombotic activity as well as the bleeding effect are multifactorial phenomena involving many plasmatic and cellular components.

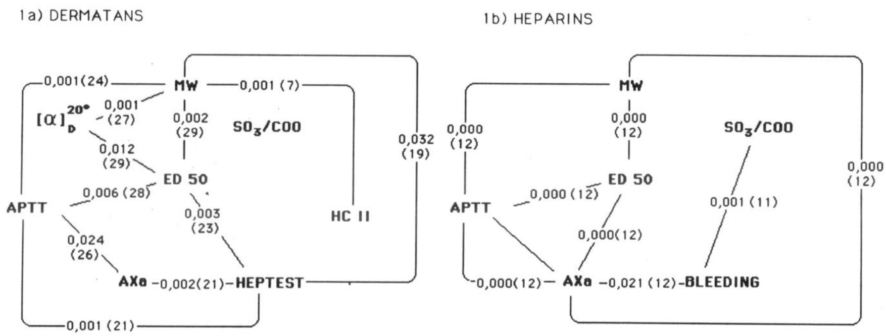

Figure 1:

1a) Dermatans : correlation between antithrombotic effect (ED 50) and physicochemical and in vitro biological parameters.

1b) Heparins: correlation between anti thrombotic effect (ED 50), bleeding and physicochemical and in vitro biological parameters.

Between the different parameters the significance of the Spearman correlation and, in brackets, the number of paired observations are indicated.

GAGs interfer with thrombogenesis: they affect both plasmatic and cellular components.
As example, a few correlations among some physico-chemical and in vitro biological parameters of dermatans and heparins have been examinated and reported in Fig 1a,b.

The reported data show that some parameters directly correlate with the antithrombotic in vivo activity (ED50) [39] while other parameters are correlated only indirectly. Anyway "correlation" it is only a mathematic concept which does not indicate a cause-effect relationship but only a statistical probability between two effects.

The development of thrombi is a dynamic equilibrium between thrombogenesis and thrombolysis: to this balance participate a cascade of events where thrombin generation and activation play a key role [19].

This cascade of events may be triggered by inflammatory and immunological processes by means of the activation of the complement system and leukocytes.

The involvement of cellular components is a less dramatic, but not less important aspect of thrombogenesis.

During inflammatory or immunological processes activated polymorphonuclears (PMN) release toxic oxygen radicals [2] and proteolytic enzymes that contribute to the thrombotic disease [18].

Moreover PMN adhesion to endothelial cells is another fundamental event of inflammatory process [23] mediated by to distinct molecular mechanisms, like GMP 140 heparin- binding glycoprotein [20], or Lectin Adhesion Molecule-1 (LECAM-1) [47].

Also platelet aggregation is induced by PMN exposed to chemotactic agents [14].

As reported in Figure 2 heparin and heparin fragments reduce superoxide anion generation depending on the doses.

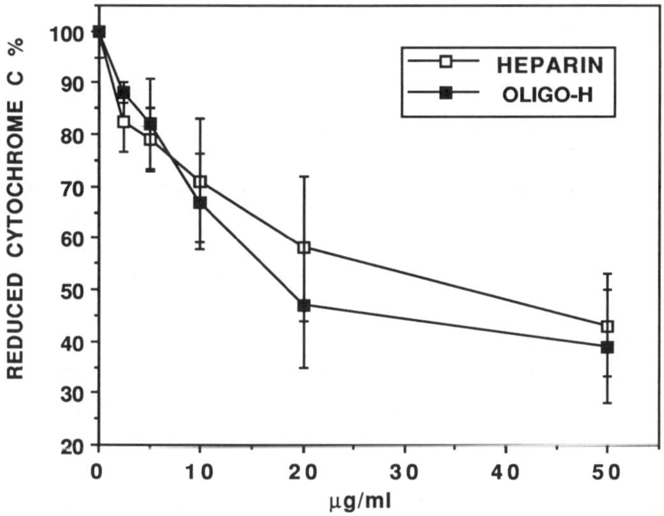

Figure 2: Superoxide anion production inhibition measured as cytochrome C reduction.
Cultured PMN ($5x10^6$ cells/ml) were stimulated by 100 nM of N-formyl-Met-Leu-Phe (f-MLP) in presence of heparin and oligo-heparin fragment (2 kD).

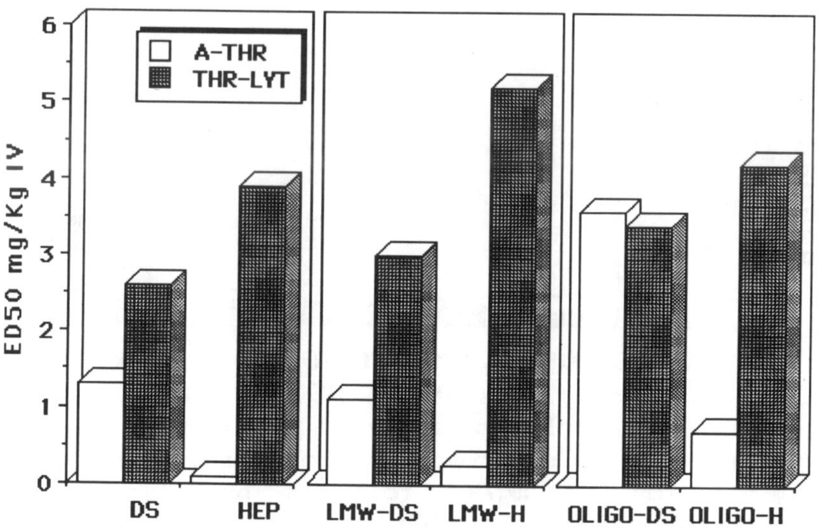

Figure 3: Comparison between antithrombotic and thrombolytic effect of Dermatans and Heparins in rats.

Antithrombotic activity was evaluated by vena cava ligature thrombosis model [25] injecting samples 10 min before vena cava ligature: thrombi were withdrawn 2 hours later.

Thrombolytic activity was evaluated by the same method injecting samples 2 hours after ligature : thrombi were extracted 6 hours after treatment.

Moreover heparins inhibit PMN adhesion to cultured bovine aorta endothelial cell [13].

Heparin, dermatan and their fragments inhibit also platelet aggregation and platelet calcium movement induced by activated PMN [3].

A part from the mechanisms of thrombogenesis, the thrombolytic event, which initiate just after fibrin-m polymerization, have to be taken into account.

The activity of GAGs, as thrombolytic agents, has not yet been clarified.

Our pharmacological experiments show an impressive thrombolytic effect when heparins and dermatans are administered intravenously in rats by bolus (Figure 3).

The activity of continuous infusion of dermatans in comparison with urokinase is reported in Figure 4.

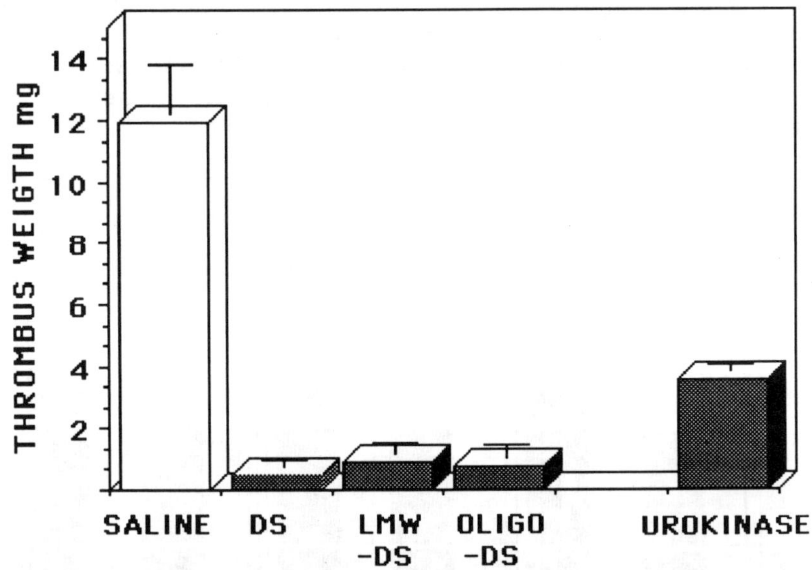

Figure 4: Thrombolytic activity of Dermatans. Rats were treated 2 hours after thrombosis induction with a bolus iv of 2.5 mg/Kg followed by a continuous infusion of 1.25 mg/ Kg/h/6h.

At the same experimental conditions a group of rats was treated with a bolus of 2500 U./kg Urokinase followed by infusion of 1250 U./Kg/h/6h.

As from these data it is evident that the examined compounds, administered at equigravimetric doses, induce different activities. Heparins resulted less thrombolytic than dermatans but more effective in the prevention of thrombosis.

For instance, dermatan is 13 times less active than heparin as antithrombotic agent, but 1.5 times more active than heparin as thrombolytic agent. The low thrombolytic activity of heparins in comparison with their antithrombotic activity, can explain the conflicting results reported as thrombolytic.

Thrombolysis induced by dermatans can be related to the stimulation of tPA release and inhibition of PAI release, as it has been observed in humans after subcutaneous and intramuscular administration [15]. These compounds are pratically devoid of anticoagulant and bleeding actions and can be proposed as potential drugs for the therapy of thrombosis.

While the possibility to produce heparins having low-anticoagulant and high antithrombotic activity is well demonstrated, there is a different situation regarding the dissociation between antithrombotic and haemorrhagic effects (bleeding). Many mechanisms are responsible for bleeding, as for instance the primary haemostasis involving vessel walls smooth muscle cells contraction and platelet aggregation, the hemocoagulation cascade and fibrinolysis.

It is therefore evident that some compounds can provoke bleeding, acting on primary haemostasis without any effect on haemocoagulation or fibrinolytic systems.

Heparin itself injected intravenously in rats induces an increase in tail transection bleeding time at dosages not yet active on APTT and A-Xa (Figure 5a, b): the same situation is much more evident when the drug is administered subcutaneously (Figure 5c, d) [37].

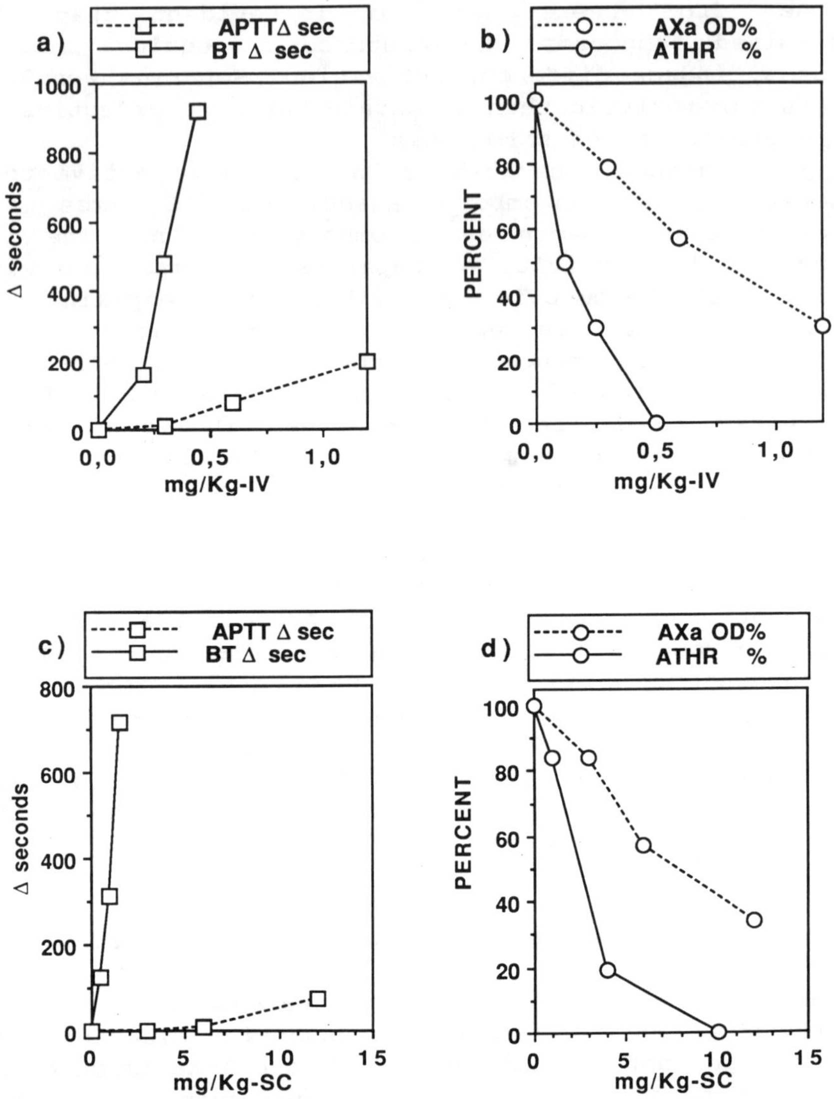

Figure 5: Dissociation between bleeding effect and anticoagulant activity of heparin after iv (a) and sc (c) administration.

Dissociation between antithrombotic and Anti-Xa activity after iv (b) and sc (d) administration.

Comparing the different activities, the dose-related events appear to be in sequence: bleeding effect, antithrombotic activity, A-Xa (ex vivo) and APTT (ex vivo).

These last two parameters indicate the heparin action on plasma proteins of coagulation cascade, whereas it is likely that the first two events indicate heparin action also on cellular components.

According to recent papers heparin and heparin very low fragments produce bleeding because they contain a disaccharide having a sulfate group at C-6 position: this particular structure should be responsible for heparins competition against ATP on myosin [16].

We also demonstrated, in agreement with Dietrich's observation, that heparins having different molecular weights are competitive inhibitors of muscle cells myosin ATPase.

Heparin is likely to interact, despite the presence of ATP, on the catalytic site of ATPase [46].

In skin scarification bleeding test [9] ATP is able to inhibit the haemorrhagic effect of locally administered heparin.

On tail transection bleeding test we observed that the haemorrhagic effect induced by intravenous injection of heparin or heparin fragments is inhibited by local application of ATP and that the inhibition is inversely correlated to the molecular weight, as Figure 6 shows.

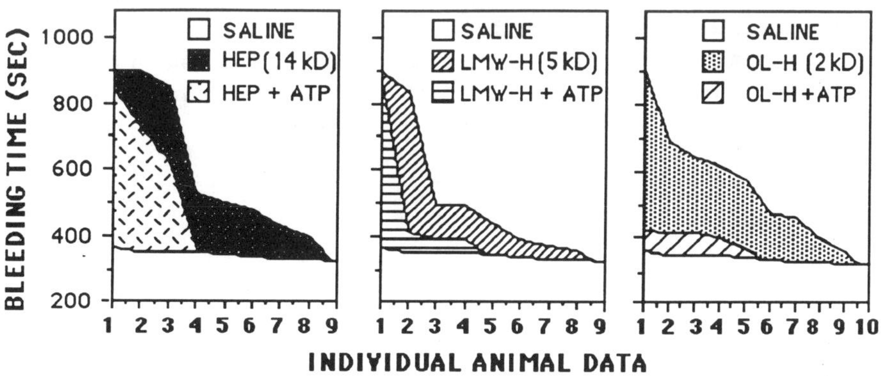

Figure 6: Bleeding effect of three different molecular weight heparins (0.5 mg/Kg iv) in presence and in absence of TAP.

Tail transection bleeding model in rats [12].

Only some provocative examples of the GAGs related problems have been reported in this paper.

Another topic that have to be considered is the interaction of heparins with growth factors like the members of HBGFs family.

These fibroblast growth factors are involved in many functions, as neurotropic and angiogenetic modulators in early development, embryogenesis and organogenesis [48].

The mechanism of secretion of HPGFs is still unknown, as the mechanisms of interaction with the extracellular matrix.

We do not know if heparin or heparin fragments in their interactions with this kind of molecules have stimulatory or inhibitory effects.

In some cases fragments can compete with the GAG molecules causing a reversion of the activity, and GAG molecules can compete with the proteoglycans in the same way.

Many problems have not yet been solved in the last 50 years.

We know the constitutive disaccharides of many glycosaminoglycans, the ATIII binding sequence of heparin. But we do not know the complete sequence of heparin and other GAGs and the meaning of their "heterogeneity".

This heterogeneity could be the molecular basis for enzymic and cellular modulation.

The field of cellular modulation of GAGs is still open and it is clear that the number of problems is increasing as rapidly as our knowledge.

REFERENCES

1. ANDERSON LO, BARROWCLIFFE TW, HOLMER E, JOHNSON EA, SIMS GEC. Anticoagulant properties of heparin fractionated by

affinity chromatography on matrix bound antithrombin III and by gel fraction. Thromb Res 9, 575-581, 1976.

2. BABIOR BM. Oxidants from phagocytes : agents of defense and destruction. Blood 64, 959, 1984.

3. BAZZONI G, BELTRAN NUNEZ A, BIANCHINI P, MASCELLANI G, DEJANA E, DEL MASCHIO A. Modulation of human polymorphonuclear leukocyte function by heparin and dermatan sulfate (In press).

4. BIANCHINI P, OSIMA B, PARMA B. Lack of correlation of some pharmacological activities of heparin with in vitro and in vivo tests. In : Ricci G et al. (Eds). Therapeutic selectivity and risk/benefit assessment of hypolipidemic drugs. Raven Press New York, pp 195-199, 1982.

5. BIANCHINI P, OSIMA B, PARMA B, NADER HB, DIETRICH CP. Lack of correlation between in vitro and in vivo antithrombotic activity of heparin fractions and related compounds. Heparan sulfate as an antithrombotic agent in vivo. Thromb Res 40, 597-607, 1985.

6. BIANCHINI P, OSIMA B, PARMA B. Antithrombotic activity of low molecular weight heparins and commercial heparins. VIIIth Int Congr on Thromb. Istanbul. Abst. 313, June 4-7, 1984.

7. BURGESS WH, MACIAG T. The heparin-binding (fibroblast) growth factor family of proteins. Ann Rev Biochem 58, 575-606, 1989.

8. CHOAY J, PETITOU M, LORMEAU JC, SINAY P, CASU B, GATTI G. Structure-activity relationship in heparin : a synthetic pentasaccharide with high affinity for Antithrombin III and eliciting high anti-factor Xa activity. Biochem Biophys Res Commun 116, 492-499, 1983.

9. CRUZ WO, DIETRICH CP. Antihemostatic effect of heparin counteracted by adenosine triphosphate. Proc Soc Exp Biol Med 126, 420-426, 1967.

10. CULP LA, LATERRA J, LARK M, BEYTH RJ, TOBEY SL. Heparan sulfate proteoglycan as mediators of some adhesive responses and cytoskeletal reorganization of cells on fibronectin matrices: independent versus cooperative functions. In: Functions of the proteoglycans. Ciba Foundation Symposia, Wiley New York, 124, 158-186, 1986.

11. CULP LA, MUGNAI G, LEWANDOWSKA K, VALLEN EA, KOSIR MA, HOUMIEL KL. Heparan sulfate proteoglycans of Ras-transformed 3T3 or neuroblastoma cells. Ann NY Acad Sci USA 556, 194-216, 1989.

12. DEJANA E, VILLA S, DE GAETANO G. Bleeding time in rats: a comparison of different experimental conditions. Thromb Haemost 48, 108-111, 1982.

13. DEL MASCHIO A, BAZZONI G, BIANCHINI P, PARMA B, OSIMA B, DEJANA E. Effects of unfractionated and very-low molecular weight heparin and dermatan sulfate on polymorphonuclear leukocyte (PMN) responses. Thromb Haemost 65, Abst. 1971, 1991.

14. DEL MASCHIO A, EVANGELISTA V, RAJTAR G, CHEN ZM, CERLETTI C, DE GAETANO G. Platelet activation by polymorphonuclear leukocytes exposed to chemotactic agents. Am J Physiol 258, H870, 1990.

15. DI PERRI - Personal communication.

16. DIETRICH CP, IVARNE LS, TERSARIOL ILS, DA SILVA RG, BIANCHINI P, NADER HB. Dependence of the C-6 sulfate of the glucosamine moiety and 1->4 glycosidic linkage of heparin disaccharides for production of hemorrhage:

reversal of the antihemostatic activity of heparin and their fragments by adenosine triphosphate and myosin. Semin Thromb Haemostas 17 Suppl. 1, 65-73, 1991.

17. DUCLOS JP. L'héparine. Fabrication, structure, propriétés, analyses. Masson, Paris, p 414, 1984.

18. ERNST E, HAMMERSCHMIDT DE, BAGGE U, MATRAI A, DORMANDY JA. Leukocytes and the risk of ischemic diseases. JAMA 257, 2318, 1987

19. FENTON II JW. Thrombin. Ann NY Acad Sci USA 485, 5-15, 1986.

20. GENG JG, BEVILACQUA MP, MOORE KL, Mc INTYRE TM, PRESCOTT SM, KIM JM, BLISS GA, ZIMMERMAN GA, McEVER RP. Rapid neutrophil adhesion to activated endothelium mediated by GMP-140. Nature 343, 757, 1990.

21. HAHN GF. Abolishment of alimentary lipemia following injection of heparin. Science 98, 19-20, 1943.

22. HALL M, RICKETTS CR, MICHAEL SE. The potency of heparin fractions obtained by gel filtration. J Pharm Pharmacol 21, 626-628, 1969.

23. HARLAN J. Leukocyte-endothelial interactions. Blood 65, 513, 1985.

24. HASCALL VC, HASCALL GK. Proteoglycans. In : Hay ED (Ed). Cell biology of extracellular matrix. Plenum. New-York, pp 39-63, 1986.

25. HOOK M, BJORK I, HOPWOOD J, LINDAHL U. Anticoagulant activity of heparin : separation of high-activity and low-activity heparin species by affinity chromatography on immobilized antithrombin. FEBS Lett 66, 90-93, 1976.

26. HOWELL WH, HOLT E. Two new factors in blood coagulation; heparin and pro-antithrombin. Ann J Physiol 47, 325-341, 1918.

27. KAKKAR VV, THOMAS DP. Heparin. Chemistry and clinical usage. Academic Press London, p 376, 1976.

28. KJELLEN L, LINDAHL U. Proteoglycans : structures and interactions. Ann Rev Biochem 60, 443-475, 1991.

29. LAM LH, SILBERT JE, ROSENBERG RD. The separation of active and inactive forms of heparin. Biochem Biophys Res Commun 69, 570-577, 1976.

30. LANE DA, LINDAHL U. Heparin : Chemical and biological properties, clinical applications. E. Arnold, London, p 623, 1989.

31. LARK MW, CULP LA. Turnover of heparan sulfate proteoglycan from substratum adhesion sites of murine fibroblast. J Biol Chem 259, 212-217, 1984.

32. Mc DUFFIE NM. Heparin : Structure, cellular function and clinical applications. Academic Press N.Y., p 387, 1979.

33. NADER HB, Mc DUFFIE NM, DIETRICH CP. Heparin fractionation by electrofocusing : presence of 21 components of different molecular weights. Biochem Biophys Res Commun 57, 488-493, 1974.

34. NADER HB, TAKAHASHI HK, GUIMARAES JA, DIETRICH CP, BIANCHINI P, OSIMA B. Heterogeneity of heparin : characterization of one hundred components with different anticoagulant activities by a combination of electrophoretic and affinity chromatography methods. Int J Biol Macromol 3, 356-360, 1981.

35. OFOSU FA. Antithrombotic mechanisms of heparin and related compounds. In : Lane DA & Lindahl U (Eds). Heparin-Chemical and biological properties, clinical applications, pp 433-454, 1989.

36. OFOSU FA, DANISHEFSKI I, HIRSH J. Heparin and related polysaccharides. Structure and activities. Ann NY Acad Sci USA 556, 501, 1989.

37. PARMA B, BIANCHINI P, OSIMA B. Bleeding and antithrombotic effects of a low molecular weight heparin (LMW/OP 2123). Thromb Res Suppl. VI, Abst. 188, 1986.

38. PIEPKORN M, FLECKMAN P, CARNEY H, LINKER A. Glycosaminoglycan synthesis by proliferating and differentiated human keratinocytes in culture. J Invest Derm 88, 215-219, 1987.

39. REYERS I, MUSSONI L, DONATI MB, DE GAETANO G. Failure of aspirin at different doses to modify experimental thrombosis in rats. Thromb Res 18, 669-674, 1980.

40. ROLLINS BJ, CATHCART MK, CULP LA. Fibronectin-proteoglycan binding as the molecular basis for fibroblast adhesion to extracellular matrices. In : Horowitz (Ed). The glycoconjugates. Academic New-York, Vol. III, pp 289-329, 1982.

41. ROTHENBERG ME, AUSTEN KF. Influence of fibroblast environment on the structure of mast cell proteoglycans. Ann NY Acad Sci USA 556, 233-244, 1989.

42. SHATTON J, SCHUBERT M. Isolation of a mucoprotein from cartilage. J Biol Chem 211, 565-573, 1954.

43. SHIMADA K, GILL PJ, SILBERT JE, DOUGLAS WHJ, FANBERG BL. Involvement of cell surface heparan sulfate in the binding of lipoprotein

lipase to cultured bovine endothelial cells. J Clin Invest 68, 995-1002, 1981.

44. VAHERI A, VARTIO T, SALONEN EM, HEDMAN K, DE PETRO G, BARLATI S. Conditional interaction of fibronectin. In : Egbring R & Klingemann HG (Eds). Factor XIII and fibronectin. Mariourg-Lahn, pp 195-202, 1983.

45. VELLUZ L, NOMINE G, MATHIEU G. Recherches sur l'héparine. Les héparides antilipémiques. Bull Soc Chim Biol 41, 415-435, 1959.

46. VOLPI N, BERGONZINI GL, PARMA B, BIANCHINI P, BOLOGNANI L. Heparins, myosin and haemostasis: role of vasal muscular component in bleeding effect. Thromb Haemorrh Disorders (In press).

47. WAYNE SMITH C, KISHIMOTO TK, ABBASS O, HUGHES B, ROTHLEIN R, McINTYRE LV, BUTCHER E, ANDERSON DC. Chemotactic factors regulate Lectin Adhesion Molecule 1 (LECAM-1)-dependent neutrophil adhesion to cytokine-stimulated endothelial cells in vitro. J Clin Invest 87, 609, 1991.

48. WILSON H, MACIAG B, MACIAG T. The heparin-binding (fibroblast) growth factor family of proteins. Ann Rev Biochem 58, 575-606, 1989.

49. WOODS A, COUCHMAN JR, HOOK M. Heparan sulfate proteoglycan of rat embryo fibroblast. J Biol Chem 260, 10872-10879, 1985.

4

Antithrombotic activity of heparin and its derivatives: reliable and other putative mechanisms

M. Sarret

For 50 years, heparin has been the drug most widely used in the prophylaxis and treatment of thromboembolic disorders, particularly DVT and pulmonary or systemic embolism although cardiologists also largely used the drug as adjunctive therapy in patients with myocardial infarction or unstable angina [101, 146, 159]. In most Western countries, the low molecular weight heparins (LMWH) are now preferred [56, 91, 192].

Curioulsy enough, the increasing wide clinical use of heparin in prophylaxis and treatment of thromboembolic disorders was not supported, at least until the mid-seventies, by a corresponding increase in basic knowledge regarding both the nature of heparin molecules and the precise correlation between their molecular structure and their biological activity.

The suggestion that the binding of heparin to AT III -its plasma cofactor- induces an increasing reaction with thrombin (and other clotting proteinases) and leads to the formation of an inactive complex of the two proteins is presently at the basis of the current concepts of the mechanism of anticoagulant activity of heparin [2, 165], even if more recently, a second plasma heparin-dependent inhibitor of thrombin, heparin cofactor II was identified [187].

Only during the last decade, as a result of the analysis of the specific ATIII-binding heparin region and the successful chemical synthesis of a particular sequence - a unique pentasaccharide containing a critical 3-O - sulfated glucosamine - the precise structural requirement ascribed to the main anticoagulant mechanism of heparin molecules have been elucidated [20, 40, 116]

However, assuming that the anticoagulant activity of heparin and LMWH is chiefly related to their ability to activate AT III, and bearing in mind that this activity accounts for only one third of their molecules, there are grounds for speculation that most of their molecular structure may contribute to interactions with other biological systems and much more remains to be elucidated to clearly identify the complete mechanisms of antithrombotic activity of heparin.

1. Anticoagulant/antithrombotic meaning

Before considering some of these mechanisms, it is important to distinguish between the terms of "anticoagulant" and "antithrombotic" although there may exist a certain relationship between them. The anticoagulant effect is related to in vitro tests and reflects the capacity of the drug to prolong plasma coagulation time (e.g. APTT assay, pharmacopoeial assays) or to potentiate inhibition of coagulation factors such as factor Xa or factor IIa (thrombin). This in vitro activity, or potency, is expressed in Units (U) reffering to available standards.

The antithrombotic activity refers to the in vivo ability of heparin and derivatives to inhibit thrombus formation in experimental or clinical situation exposing to the risk of developing thrombosis.

The purpose of this review is to briefly present the so-called "classical anticoagulant mechanism" of heparin and its derivatives and to focus on some of the possible mechanisms not directly related to their "specific" capacity for binding to AT III, that may contribute to their antithrombotic effectiveness; in particular we will examine the role of heparin and its fragments in relation to some of the blood and endothelial cell functions. All these heparin properties are largely related to its molecular structure.

2. From heparin low molecular weight heparins

2.1 Heparin structure

Heparin is a heterogeneous mixture of sulfated polysaccharide chains belonging to the glycosaminoglycan family naturally present in several organs and tissues. These polysaccharide chains may be structurally considered as linear anionic polyelectrolytes [100].

A major problem with the determination of heparin structure is due to the fact that it cannot be ascribed to a unique sequence of carbohydrate residues.

The structure of mammalian heparin is largely accounted for by an alternate sequence of uronic acid and hexosamine units. The major constituents of the glycosaminoglycan chains are the acid L-iduronic 2-O-sulfate and the aminosugar D-glucosamine N-sulfate 6-O sulfate, linked 1,4.

Although typical heparin chains largely consist of regular segments with a relatively constant pattern of sulfate constituents, these chains are interrupted by heterogeneous segments containing undersulfated (and less frequently oversulfated) disaccharide units where the uronic acid may also be D-glucuronic acid and the glucosamine may be N-acetylated [34, 35].

The active site for the binding to AT III has been identified among these irregular sites and consists of a specific pentasaccharide sequences where an atypical glucosamine N-6 trisulfate unit is present [36, 40, 116, 117]. The chemical synthesis of this natural pentasaccharide has been achieved [42, 175] (Figure 1).

Various saccharide sequences are unevenly distributed in heparin chains. These chains have different lengths (4-6 units in the shorter chains and up to 100 in the longer ones) with a molecular weight (MW) range of 1.500 to 50.000 daltons.

Heparin fractions obtained from standard heparin by various chemical and physical techniques [124] demonstrated that anticoagulant activity mainly reflecting the antithrombin activity and expressed in coagulation tests (e.g. the United States Pharmacopoeia - USP units - or activated partial thromboplastin time "APTT") was proportional to their molecular weight : the higher the molecular weight, the higher the activity, whereas the factor Xa inhibitory activity underwent practically no change following a reduction in molecular weight [6, 93, 112]. On this basis, fractionation or fragmentation of heparin (i.e. LMW heparins) have therefore been proposed as a means of obtaining safer and more efficient antithrombotics (varying in MW from 2000 to 8000 daltons) with more specific chemical and biological characteristics in comparison to conventional unfractionated heparin. Apart from their MW, heparin chains can also be characterized by their anionic charge density, their stereochemical configuration, the variable functional groups of their basic structural units or their specific antithrombin binding region. It has been suggested that the activities of heparin may depend on their great conformational flexibility and on their exact matching with protein or cell surface active sites [37, 99, 100].

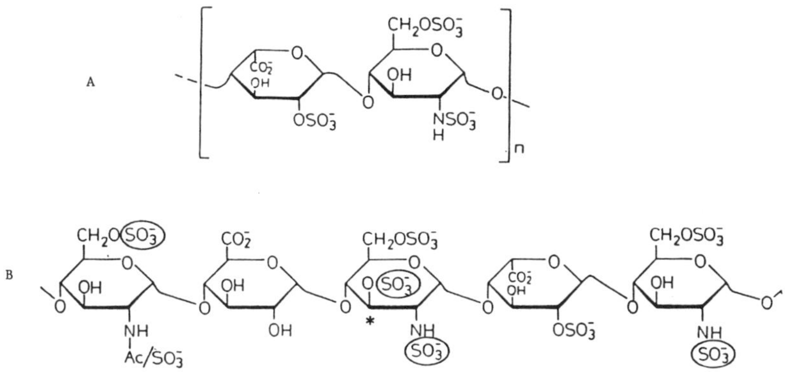

Figure 1: Heparin structure: major components

A : Trisulfated disaccharide units

B : Pentasaccharide sequence. The circled sulfate groups proposed to be essential for high-affinity binding to antithrombin.

As schematically illustrated in Figure 2 the strong negative charges of heparin molecules in fact allow numerous interactions (binding, hindering, activation, inhibition, displacement) with positively charged proteins such as plasma coagulation and anticoagulation factors, growth factors, PF 4, lipoproteins, etc.

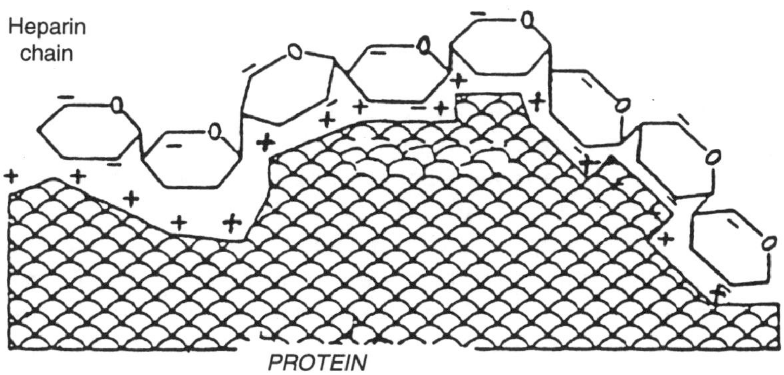

Figure 2: Schematic representation of interactions between the negative charges of heparin chains and the positive charges of a basic protein.

Table I: Main bilogical activities of heparin and heparin fractions

Hypocoagulation/antithrombotic
Lipoprotein lipase activation
Fibrinolysis activation
Cellular immunologic system modulation
Defense mechanism activation
Complement system inhibition
Angiogenesis modulation
Antimetastasis
Growth factors inhibition
Growth and tissue repair modulation

When it interacts with proteins, heparin induces a facilitating conformational change in these proteins that may be necessary for the expression or enhancement of their activities [99, 109].

These particular structural features may explain the impressive list of biological activities which has been identified for heparin, in addition to its anticoagulation effect (Table I).

2.2 "Classical" anticoagulant mechanism

As expected from its ability to complex with, and change the properties of proteins, heparin can modify the activity of many enzymes. The best-known property of heparin as an enzyme inhibitor is its anticoagulant activity. This activity mainly reflects its ability to accelerate through a particular site of their molecules - a pentasaccharide sequence - the formation of a molecular complex between the physiological coagulation inhibitor AT III and serine proteases of the coagulation system, e.g. thrombin and factor Xa, thus enhancing the overall inhibition rate of the AT III reaction against coagulation factors [20, 51, 165].

This interaction between heparin chains and AT III was originally considered to be related to the anticoagulant activity of heparin molecules.

AT III affinity chromatography techniques provided a useful system to distinghish between "active" heparin i.e heparin fractions with high affinity (HA) for AT III from "inactive" heparin i.e. heparin fractions with low affinity (LA) for AT III.

So, according to their affinity for AT III, commercial heparins can be fractionated into two distinct fractions: the HA fractions making up approximatively one-third by weight of the starting material and containing the critical pentasaccharide sequence for the specific antithrombin-binding region, and the low-affinity (LA) fraction almost devoid of this specific binding sequence.

The HA chains are responsible for the in vitro anticoagulant activity and account for 30 per cent of the activity of the starting material while the LA chains only have low activity [6, 96, 107, 132].

Secondly from in vitro observations, it was shown that a shortening of the heparin chains with a consequent lowering of their MW, led to a decreased effect on clotting assays such as APTT while their original level of factor Xa inhibiting activity was maintained [5, 6, 93, 112, 184].

In other words, AT III-mediated anti-Xa activity is still amplified by smaller oligosaccharides (down to the pentasaccharide) but only octadecasaccharides and longer fragments can activate AT III against thrombin [41].

By the end of the seventies the idea was thus emerging that it might be possible to fractionate heparin into low molecular weight fractions endowed with biological properties differing from those of standard heparin, thereafter reffered to as "unfractionated heparin" or "conventional heparin".

Moreover, on the basis of the generally accepted hypothesis that factor Xa inhibition might be the expression of antithrombotic activity (since being common to both intrinsic and extrinsic pathways, it is a key factor in coagulation) whereas thrombin inhibition is the expression of anticoagulant activity, it seemed logical to consider the low molecular weight heparins (LMWH) - also referred to as heparin derivatives - as potential antithrombotics with a reduced risk of hemorrhage [29, 95]. In fact, it has been argued that heparin fragments might exhibit an antithrombotic effect by virtue of their undiminished in vitro anti-Xa function while their decreased influence on overall coagulation would lead to fewer hemorrhagic consequences.

However, important discrepancies have rapidly been observed between the in-vitro and ex-vivo blood levels of LMW heparins measured as anti-Xa activity [14, 147]. Furthermore, the lack of correlation between their apparent plasmatic activity and their antithrombotic efficacy would suggest that their anti-Xa activity is only a partial expression of their therapeutic potential and that other properties of their molecules may contribute to their antithrombotic efficacy [26, 108].

As often it happens, the initial hypothesis on the biological selective action of the heparin fragments has been phased out by another property that was neither foreseen from in vitro studies. Surprinsingly, it was observed that after subcutaneous injection, their biovailability - measured as biological activity - was nearly 90-100 %. In contrast, biovailability was only partial (25-30 %) for heparin [52, 78]. Furthermore, the initial mechanism of their antithrombotic activity mainly based on anti-Xa effect has since been superseded by newer concepts.

Recent biochemical studies have demonstrated that heparin and its LMW derivatives exert their antithrombotic effects primarily through their ability to accelerate inhibition of thrombin generation. It has been argued that the inhibition of thrombin participating in the activation of cofactors factor V and factor VIII (feedback loop) is the prime anticoagulant action of heparin molecules [18, 148].

Whatever the relative importance of heparin ability to either inhibit factor Xa or thrombin generation, these activities are always AT III-dependent.

Interesting experimental data obtained from normal and from anti-AT III-antibodies animal have shown that heparin and heparin fractions are able to inhibit, at the same extent, the thrombus formation both in control and in ATIII-depleted animals [152].

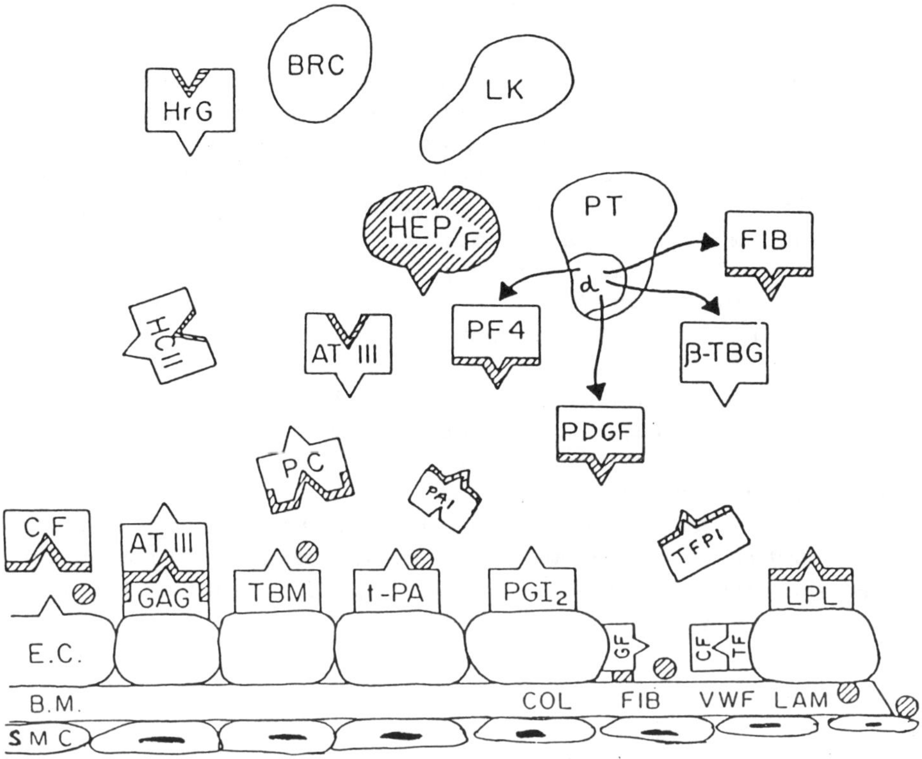

Figure 3: Some heparin interactions with endothelium/blood cells.

SMC	Smooth muscle cell	FIB	Fibronectin
BM	Basement membrane	LAM	Laminin
EC	Endothelial cell	COL	Collagen
TBM	Thrombomodulin	GF	Growth factor
CF	Clotting factor	PGI2	Prostacyclin
BRC	Blood red cell	PT	Platelet
VWF	Von Willebrandt	LK	Leukocyte
GAG	Glycosaminoglycan	TF	Tissue factor
PF4	Platelets factor4	ATIII	Antithrombin III
TFPI	Tissue factor pathway inhibitor		
t-PA	Tissue plasminogen activator		
PAI	Tissue plasminogen inhibitor		
H-r-G	Histidin-rich-glycoprotein		
PDGF	Platelet derivated growth factor		
LPL	Lipoprotein Lipase		
HC II	Heparin cofactor II		
β-TBG	Beta-thromboglobulin		

These results give grounds to suggest that the antithrombotic effect of heparin molecules is not entirely AT III-dependent and that other properties may contribute to their antithrombotic efficacy.

We must also keep in mind that activation of blood coagulation leading to excessive thrombin generation and therefore to thrombosis can be partially or totally controlled by various natural inhibitory mechanisms such as serine protease inhibitors, endothelial surface binding inhibitors, the extrinsic pathway inhibitor (EPI), the endothelial fibrinolytic system or the hepatic inactivation.

As schematically illustrated in Figure 3, inactivation heparin molecules may interfere with several of these natural protective mechanisms. In the following two sections, we shall expand on those aspects. The first section examines the heparin interactions with some endothelial cell functions; the second part concerns the heparin activities in relation with blood components.

3. Antithrombotic mechanims: heparin/ derivatives and endothelium functions

The concept that the vessel wall could be only an inert vascular "blood container" has now become obsolete. During the past two decades, convincing data have illustrated its role as functional organ and its involvement among other numerous functions, in the regulation of the hemostatic system.

The vascular endothelium is able to prevent or promote activation of the coagulation system, but under normal physiological conditions the endothelial vessel wall appears to be naturally thromboresistant [138]. This thromboresistance is mainly ascribed to the continuous luminal endothelial cell layer which provides a barrier between the circulating blood and the subendothelium structures and is promoted by a complex system of physico-biological functions which is able to synthesize, secrete or bind various pro- or anti- coagulant factors.

Noxious influences due to trauma or pathological states may induce injury and subsequent loss of the vessel wall integrity with subsequent alteration of the natural antithrombotic function and exposure of highly reactive subendothelial structures intended to assume the hemostatic response; platelet adhesion and aggregation, binding and activation of coagulation factors.

Heparin interferes with many of these functions and it has been observed that over than ten known endothelial cell-damaging agents can be blocked by heparin administration [138].

3.1 Endothelial heparin like molecules

The possibility that glycosaminoglycan (GAG) sequences present in proteoglycans that compose constituting part of the endothelial cell glycocalix may be responsible for the non-thrombogenicity of the endothelium has generated extensive investigation [122].

This concept appears to be supported by the demonstration that endothelial cells synthetize sulfated glycosaminoglycans (mainly heparan sulfate).

These "heparin-like molecules" degraded by heparinase and other GAG-specific enzymes, originate solely from the endothelial cells and possess anticoagulant properties. These endogenous heparin-like substances contain a small though significant population of active chain heparin-like binding sites for AT III capable of accelerating thrombin-antithrombin interaction by means of a mechanism similar to that of exogenous conventional heparin [84]. Binding sites for both thrombin and AT III exist on the luminal surface of endothelial cells as well as the subendothelial matrix.

It has been argued that endothelial cells of the microcirculation contains GAG that mediate AT III and thrombin binding in order to catalyze thrombin inhibition. In contrast, aortic endothelial cells might neutralizing thrombin through heparin-like binding sites, the endothelial inactivation occurring in presence of plasmatic AT III. However, it must be kept in mind that the types of glycosaminoglycans and their "functional density" may significantly vary in vascular tissues (cerebral, retinal) and that the microcirculation may provides a more potent glycosamynoglycan dependent anticoagulation than the macrocirculation.

Heparin, as well as LMWH, enhances in a dependent manner the synthesis of heparan sulfate by endothelial cells [139]. It is interesting to note that heparin specifically affects the synthesis of heparan sulfate in endothelial cells and not in another cell line also derived from the vessel wall (smoth muscle cells).

After injury of the endothelial lining cells, the endothelium offers its highly reactive surface and in this situation AT III can also bind largely to heparan sulfate located in the basement membrane of the intimal smooth muscle cells for the purpose of inactivating clotting proteases [84].

The extent to which heparan-bound AT III contributes to the antithrombogenic properties of the deendothelialized intimal surface is presumably of positive nature. Circulating heparin may assist in promoting the biological functions of endogenous glycosaminoglycans enhancing the binding of thrombin to AT III, reducing the risk of thrombus formation.

3.2 Electronegativity

One of the causes of the non-thrombogenicity of the vascular endothelium to circulating blood cells or proteins has been ascribed to the strong lining cells electronegative charges produced and maintained by dynamic forces and metabolic processes which originate a repellent effect. The normal intima has a negative charge (- 160 mV) and a thrombus could form when endothelium charges become electropositive (+ 260 mV). It has been shown that the injection of heparin restores a normal electronegativity after injury [89, 139, 170, 176].

Endothelium electronegativity has been confirmed by the identification of anionic sites on the luminal surface of capillary endothelial cells in mice [174]. The surface density of endothelial anionic sites is lower in venules than in arterioles and capillaries. These sites are located in specific microdomains (fenestral diaphragms) and are apparently composed of heparin and/or heparan sulfate. These anionic sites may be charge-depleted by cationic substances (protamine, cationized ferritin), depriving the endothelial surface devoid of these sites and thus allowing thrombus formation. In experimental hypercholesterolemic animals with early or advanced endothelial lesions, the binding sites for cationized ferritin are drastically reduced indicating a progressive loss of surface anionic sites and negative charge. The decrease of the endothelial negative charges has been associated with an increased adhesion of polymorphonuclear leukocytes resulting in inflammatory effects and a thrombogenic state.

Furthermore, the normal electronegativity of the endothelial cells allows a charge-based barrier to the passage of macromolecules between the intravascular compartment and the interstitial space (e.g. low-density lipoproteins-LDL-). Surface anionic charges have an important regulatory role in the binding and internalization of proteins. It has been observed that depletion of the surface anionic sites of baboon aortic smooth muscle cells resulted in a marked increase in the binding and internalization of albumin. These results suggest that cellular endocytosis is regulated by cell surface anionic charge distribution [63, 122].

By virtue of its sulfate and carboxyl groups and its ability to reach an extremely extended configuration in aqueous solution, heparin may expose the totality of its negatively charged goups conferring a high negative charge density to the endothelium surface and facilitating strong interactions with cationic proteins. Interstingly that these properties of heparin as a polyelectrolyte are not shared by other glycasaminoglycans.

Heparin (fragments) which are taken up by and concentrated in the endothelium would increase the negative potential of the damaged vessels, maintaining the normal negative endothelial surface charge and thus preventing thrombosis.

3.3 Endothelial injury

Endothelium injury which is the requesite initial event leading to a thrombogenic state has been defined as any insult that disrupts not only the continuous luminal endothelial cells layer but also their normal function without visible evidence of morphologic endothelial abnormality. As shown in Table II endothelial injury of dysfunction may be caused by large variety of factors [138].

Different experimental models, such as electrical stimulation of vessel wall, injection of irritating agents, laser-induced damage, stasis, damage of cultured endothelial cells by free radicals can be used to induce endothelial cells injury and subsequent thrombus formation for in vivo models. In all these experimental situations, heparin and LMW heparins - mainly after intravenous administration - minimize the extension of vascular endothelium injury as shown by electron microscopic study or as measured by endothelial cell viability and release of breakdown metabolic markers [89, 92, 171, 188].

While this direct protective activity on vascular cells is not fully elucidated, however it persists longer than does the active "anticoagulant" activity.

Table II: Noxious factors for endothelial cells dysfunction and injury

Physical injury
- thermal injury
- radiation
- electric current
- osmotic changes
- vascular catheters
- contrast media

Mechanical injury
- trauma
- rheological/hemodynamic effects/stasis

Ischemic injury
- vascular occlusion
- anoxia
- shock

Biochemical injury
- inflammatory processes
- viral infection/bacteria
- endotoxins
- activated leukocyte mediator release
- complement system
- immune complexes, interleukins
- serum sickness
- stress and catecholamines
- malignant diseases, tumor cells
- necortic tissue
- metabolic defects (homocystinemia)
- blood lipids (VLDL)
- activated platelet mediator release
- toxins
- various drugs
- oxygen free radicals
- inhibition of detoxifying capacity

3.4 Endothelial cell binding

Heparin molecules are taken up by and concentrated in the endothelium. It has been argued that heparin concentration in the endothelium after IV administration is much greater than in the blood, indicating specific uptake (receptors) in the endothelium [88]. LMW heparins retain the same ability as standard heparin to bind to endothelium [72].

The direct effects of heparin on endothelial cells (EC) have been investigated in vitro and in vivo on thrombin binding to normal and deendothelialized aorta. Heparin inhibits thrombin binding to, or displace bound thrombin from the normal vascular endothelium [81, 82]; on a model of deendothelialized aorta, heparin is able to inhibit thrombin binding by the exposed subendothelium. This effect is observed within the therapeutic concentration range since the IC 50 is less than 2 U/ml. It is intersting to note that hirudin of specific thrombin inhibitors are without effect on this model [83].

Data obtained in vitro on human umbilical or adrenal vein endothelial cells are quite different but particularly informative about molecular glycosaminoglycan cell binding mechanisms. These in vitro data clearly show that heparin-endothelium affinity is directly related to the molecular weight, charge density (degree of sulfation) and AT III affinity of heparin. These binding sites are not specific for heparins and the interactions are mostly electostatic [15, 17, 90, 190, 191].

Binding of heparin, a saturable phenomenon, is associated with endocytosis; about 35% of indissociably bound heparin is internalized by EC, where it is subsequently depolymerized into low MW fragments in the lysosomes. These fragments exhibit a low antiprotease activity characterized by a higher ratio of anti-Xa/anti-IIa activity (Figure 4).

High molecular weight heparin (HMWH) preferentially binds to endothelial surface cell; its anticoagulant properties is pratically neutralized.
Binding of heparin is accompagnied by endocytosis. After internalization, heparin chains are depolymerized into low MW fragments which exhibit a greater AXa activity than anti-IIa activity.

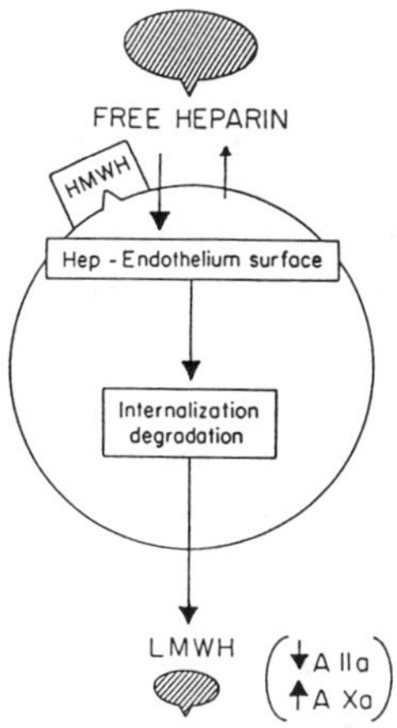

Figure 4: Heparin kinetics in endothelial cell

Although the exact role of binding of heparin molecules to EC is not elucidated, it could represent a positive contribution to the antithrombogenic nature of endothelium. Furthermore, in view of the relatively high affinity of heparin fragments for EC at concentrations not far from therapeutic levels, and also in view of the in vivo importance of the endothelial surface (high endothelial mass to blood volume ratio), it may be assumed that the binding of heparin molecules to EC could significantly contribute not only to the non-thrombo- genicity of endothelium but also to the pharmacokinetics of heparin molecules.

3.5 Endothelial cell heparin binding: implication for pharmacokinetics

Unexpectedly, subcutaneous administration of LMW heparins induces a longer life time of their biological effect as compared with unfractionated heparin when measured in terms of anti-Xa activity or as total glycosaminoglycan levels.

The anti-Xa activity is logically higher but also longer as compared with antifactor IIa activity [10, 22, 52].

The longer plasma half life time of LMW heparin anti-Xa activity as compared with unfractionated heparin has been ascribed to the poor efficiency of the saturable clearance mechanism, (cellular pool), which would be compatible with their low endothelium affinity.

Preferential endothelial cell binding of high MW heparin chains, which possess greater anti-IIa activity, might also contribute to the discrepancy between in vitro and in vivo anticoagulant activities.

In this respect, ex vivo differences between the diseappearance of the anti-Xa and anti-IIa activities of unfractionated heparin [54] might be ascribed to the remaining LMW heparin fractions (which possess mainly anti-Xa activity) in the circulation after binding of the high MW heparin molecule chains. It was also shown that renal inactivation of anticoagulant heparin activity is less marked for anti-Xa than for APTT activity, and that the heparin fractions appear to be a poor substrate for renal lysosomal inactivation [127].

We must keep in mind that the better bioaviability of LMW heparins is evident mainly after subcutaneous administration or with low or medium therapeutic intravenous doses. A preferential endothelial cell binding and renal lysosomal inactivation of high MW heparin chains may contribute to the increased bioavailability of heparin fragments.

3.6 Arterial smooth muscle cells

If current concepts of the etiology of arterial thrombosis have focused on the primary role of pathologic vascular damage, the proliferative "response-to-injury" has also been considered as the initial event in atherogenesis [166]. Furthermore, histopathological studies indicate that the great majority of acute myocardial infarctions occurs with coronary artery lesions on which occluding thrombus superimposed on disrupted atherosclerotic plaques [97]. It was also observed that intimal hyperplasia at the anastomatic sites of venous and prosthetic grafts is a pivotal factor affecting the outcome of these grafts [181]. The straight relationship between atherosclerosis and thrombosis is regulated by complex interactions among blood components and endothelium [172].

The smooth muscle cells (SMC) located in the intima and media of the arterial vessel wall and embedded in a highly organized extracellular matrix, in addition to contractibility, have the capacity to proliferate, migrate and synthesize various components of extracellular matrix.

The proliferation of smooth muscle cells that are components of arteries, provides a normal repair process following important vessel wall damage; uncontrolled regulatory mechanisms following injury lead to abnormal of SMC growth and accumulation of the matrix proteins within the intimal tissues inducing subsequent intimal thickenings and, together with accumulation of platelets, fibrin, lipids and white blood cells, may play a major role in the development of the atherosclerotic plaques.

Arterial smooth muscle cells occur in at least two distinct states referred to as synthetic and contractile phenotypes. The former (synthetic phenotype) predominates in growing organism and provides the cellular proliferation and the production of extracellular matrix components. The latter (contractile phenotype) is present in the adult organism; these muscle-like cells which contract in response to stimuli can return to a synthetic phenotype and this process appears to be fundamental in the early events in atherogenesis.

This phenotype shift leading to cell proliferation is regulated by several matrix components, (e.g. adhesive proteins such as fibronectin, vitronectin, thrombospondin or laminin) or by various polypeptide mitogens such as platelet-derived growth factor (PDGF), fibroblast growth factor (FGF), epidermal growth factor (EGF) interleukin, (IL1 or insulin-like growth factor); inhibitors such as transforming growth factor ß have opposite actions. It has also been proposed that the regulation of differentiated properties and proliferation of SMC could be under the control of the basement membrane of the endothelium.

This barrier normally helps the cells to maintain a contractile state. If injured, the plasma membrane may interact with growth promoting factors and induce a transition from the contractile to the synthetic phenotype [185].

In many of these complex processes contributing to atherogenesis, numerous investigations have emphasized the role of heparin and derivatives in the regulation of SMC proliferation [62, 185].

Within the past decade it has been observed that heparin administration could prevent hyperplasia of the vessel wall media occurring after injury of the intima by balloon catetherization in a rodent model [44, 45, 59, 76, 149].

Low molecular weight heparins also reduce both mitosis and proliferation of intimal SMC after balloon angioplaty of a fibromuscular plaque [50, 145, 199].

Further studies have demonstrated that endothelial cells produce a heparin-like inhibitor of smooth muscle cells proliferation [30, 69].

It has been suggested that the normal function of heparin species present within the arterial wall is to maintain medial SMC in quiescent proliferation state by opposing the action of mitogens and that heparin and heparan sulfate in the basement membrane of endothelial and SMC inhibit the modulation of SMC from a contractile to a synthetic phenotype [39].

Heparin not only binds to endothelial cells as referred before, but also binds to smooth muscle cells and is ingested by endocytosis [33, 87, 162]. It has been observed that SMC treated with heparin are arrested in the G0/G1 phase of the growth cycle. This growth inhibition has been attributed either to the ability of this anionic mucopolysaccharide to complex with platelet-derived mitogens thus decreasing their availability or activity or to direct antiproliferative effects after binding to specific sites on the cell surface [32, 163].

Heparin has also been reported to modulate the secretion of several proteins by cultured SMC including collagen or thrombospondin - an extracellular matrix glycoprotein involved in the entrance into the S phase of the cell cycle. The stimulation of SMC proliferation with the mitogen PDGF induces the synthesis of thrombospondin. Heparin inhibits the effect of thrombospondin on mitogenesis as well as its incorporation in the extra- cellular matrix [121, 186].

Heparin potentiates the activity of the inhibitor transforming growth factor ß, thus contributing to down regulate SMC proliferation [129].

The antiproliferative activity of the heparin molecule depends on oligosaccharide size and charge but not on anticoagulant activity, the critical structure being a pentasaccharide fragment [31, 200].

To summerize, these various activities of heparin and sulfated polysaccharides on SMC proliferation suggest their important contribution to the prevention of the atherosclerotic process and thereby to the prevention of thrombogenic states. Unfortunatly, the clinical efficacy of heparin and LMW heparins in the prevention of late restenosis after angioplasty is still controversial.

3.7 Lipoprotein lipase activity

At endothelial cell level, heparin has another important property, which may be indirectly related with the non-thrombogenicity of endothelium. In fact, heparin exerts a lipolytic effect on circulating triglycerides by releasing lipoprotein (LPL) from the capillary endothelium.

This activity results in the degradation of triglyceride-rich lipoproteins with a splitting off of free fatty acid (FFA), glycerides and remnants in the circulating blood [150].

A high lipemia enhances the atherosclerotic process and both the agglutination and aggregation of red blood cells as well as the aggregation of platelets on injured endothelium [73].

Heparin (and related glycosaminoglycans) by inducing triglyceride lipolysis, may therefore be beneficial in counteracting the atherosclerotic process and consequently in decreasing the risk of thrombosis. On the other hand, the stimulation of lipolysis may have a harmful effect in cardiopathic patients during

anticoagulant treatment with conventional heparin since the related increase of circulation FFA might induce further arrhythmias [182].
Contradictory data have been reported concerning LMW heparin-induced LPL activity. Most reports reveal a lower lipolytic activity (measured as overall LPL or hepatic LPL levels) for LMWH as compared with heparin following a single IV or SC administration, without any increase in plasmatic FFA. Other studies report that the amount of hepatic lipase released with LMW heparins is significantly higher than with standard heparin [77, 86, 153]. This latter point could be interesting because it has been suggested that the release of hepatic triglyceride lipases after the administration of glycosaminoglycans may indirectly contribute to their in vivo anti-Xa activity by inhibiting thrombin generation [13, 198]. Furthermore, whereas the total lipoprotein lipase release results correlated with the charge density of heparin molecules, the hepatic lipase release rate did not [140, 154].

In conclusion, heparin fragments may promote a lower lipoprotein lipase release, with fewer effects on circulating FFA, than heparin. This may be considered an advantage over conventional heparin in cardiopathic patients.

3.8 Extrinsic tissue factor pathway inhibitor (TFPI).

This glycoprotein inhibitor, initially discribed as an inactivating moiety for the tissue factor coagulant activity (anti-convertin) is receiving renewed recognition as a possible important endothelial contributor to haemostatic and thrombotic regulation [160].

Haemostasis is initiated via the extrinsic pathway when after tissue injury there is exposure of blood to tissue factor (TF), either through damage to the vascular vessel wall, e.g. by cytokines such as interleukin 1 and tumor necrosis factor or by generation of TF on the surface of blood mononuclear cells resulting in the formation of a factor VIIa-TF complex. This complex proteolytically activates factors IX and X. The formation of this procoagulant complex is therefore a potent trigger of the coagulation cascade.

The plasma system contains a Ca^{2+} -dependent inhibitor of thromboplastin factor VII that requires factor Xa for its function [25].

This inhibitor, officially named Tissue Factor Pathway Inhibitor (TFPI) was previously termed Extrinsic Pathway Inhibitor (EPI) or Lipoprotein-Associated Coagulation Inhibitor (LACI). The inhibition of TF/Factor VII enzymatic activity mediated by a factor Xa-TFPI complex is believed to be a major regulator of coagulation via the extrinsic pathway during hemostasis, competitively restricting further interaction of substrate factors X and IX with the TF/FVIIa complex [169]. Direct inhibition of FXa by TFPI was also reported [142].

TFPI contains three Kunitz - type inhibitory domains and is found at least in three different pools. More than 50% or TFPI plasma activity is an fact associated with plasma lipoproteins (mainly VLDL and LDL); 5-10% are sequestered within platelets. The third pool or "heparin - releasable EPI" seems to be the endothelial lining cells. It was shown that a bolus intravenous injection of heparin raises several fold plasma TFPI levels - this effect is dose dependent on the circulating heparin through the vascular bed suggesting release of TFPI from the vascular wall. Thus the major amount of the total intravascular pool of this inhibitor appears to be bound to the vascular endothelium possibly by attachment to the glycosaminoglycans on the luminal surface [9, 46].

Furthermore, several cultured cell types are able to synthetize TFPI but vascular endothelium is believed to serve as a major site for synthesis of human TFPI in vivo. The evidence for a role of TFPI as a natural anticoagulant is now well documented and it was recently shown that recombinant TFPI may protect against DIC induced by infusion of crude thromboplastin in rabbits [53] or prevent arterial reocclusion after thrombolysis in dogs [80].

Interestingly enough the TFPI released into the blood stream by exogenous heparin is a more powerful coagulation inhibitor than is recombinant TFPI [115]. Intravenous low molecular weight heparin appear to possess the same ability as the parent drug to increase EPI level [141]. The exact mechanism of TFPI action is not yet elucidated, but there are reasons to postulate that heparin and its derivatives contribute to the natural anticoagulant properties of endothelium by activating the release of this physiological inhibitor from its endothelial pool.

3.9 Thrombomodulin/Protein C/Protein S System

The thrombomodulin/protein C/protein S system provides another important process for the control of coagulation [43, 67].

The presence of plasmatic thrombin induces the capillary endothelial cells to express a membrane associated glycoprotein, thrombomodulin, that binds thrombin through two sites, one of which is provided by a chondroitin sulfate-like GAG moiety. The binding of thrombin to thrombomodulin changes thrombin's substrate specificity from a procoagulant to an anticoagulant via the protein C pathway [68, 180].

Human protein C (PC) is the zymogen of a vitamin K-dependent plasma serine protease: when activated by the thrombin - thrombomodulin complex on endothelial cells; activated protein C in turn functions as an anticoagulant by proteolyticaly degrading factor Va and VIIIa and thereby limits the generation of thrombin. Protein S is a cofactor in these reactions [179].

Heparin interacts with the protein C system in at least two distinct ways [47].

First, the activation of PC can be blocked by administering low doses of heparin. This inhibiting action on thrombin occurs either before thrombin is bound to the endothelial cell-associated thrombomodulin or after the thrombin has formed a complex with the thrombomodulin. Secondly, heparin, at relatively high levels (5 μg/ml); stimulates the own unique inhibitor of activated protein C (Figure 5).

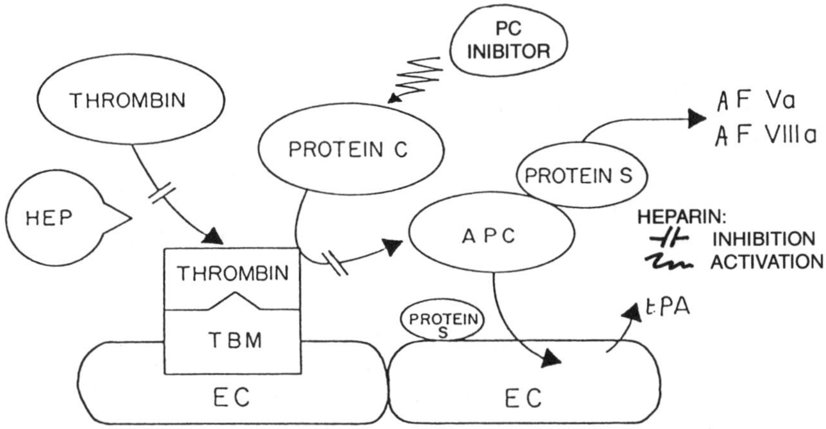

Figure 5: Thrombomodulin / Protein C and heparin interactions. Heparin inhibits:

a) the complex formation between thrombin and thrombomodulin (TMB) or endothelial cells (EC)

b) the activation of protein C (APC). Conversely, heparin activates the inhibitor of protein C.

The activation of protein C inhibitor, obtained with heparin and other related sulphated polysaccharides, seems related to the MW and to some sulphate groups [104].

It would seem reasonable to hypothesise that heparin fragments with a lower MW, and which therefore affect thrombin to a lesser extent, may either produce less effect on the thrombin-thrombomodulin complex or cause a lower level of protein C inhibitor activation, thus preserving the natural anticoagulant activity of this enzyme.

Conversely, it has been reported that heparin alone or related GAG do neither displace thrombin from its endothelial cell receptor nor do they interfere with the functions of the thrombomodulin/thrombin complex, such that during therapy the initiation of the protein C pathway would not be affected [156]. Whether these opposite findings may correlate with the physiological regulatory mechanisms remains to be established, although in this thrombomodulin/protein C system, exogenous heparins may weaken this natural antithrombotic process.

3.10 Prostacyclin

Endothelial cells are the most important source of prostacyclin (PGI_2) an extremely fast acting metabolite of arachidonic acid. PGI_2 is a potent vasodilator and the strongest known inhibitor of platelet aggregation. Among the various factors that regulate PGI_2 synthesis, clotting factors such as thrombin and FXa have an important role since stimulate PGI_2 released by activation of endothelial cells. Endothelial cells can also use platelet endoperoxides for their own PGI_2 synthesis suggesting that the endothelial antithrombotic properties is amplified by activated platelets [155]. The effects of heparin on PGI_2 activities have been scarcely studied.

In vitro studies have shown that heparin impedes the inhibitory effect of PGI_2 on platelet aggregation [44]. This anti-inhibitory action is less marked for heparin fragments [128, 135]. Once again, the extent to which in vitro observation using citrated plasma reflects in vivo events is not clear. In fact, in vitro evidence itself argues against a direct heparin - PGI_2 interaction; heparin, by intensifying platelet aggregation, reduces the antiaggregatory effect of PGI_2 [19]. Furthermore, haparin or LMWH bound to endothelial cells specifically steps up thrombin-stimulated PGI_2 production [16].

It may be presumed that in vivo, heparin or LMW heparins do not impede the direct production of PGI_2 by the endothelial cells.

3.11 Fibrinolytic system

The fibrinolytic system acting both against fibrin deposition and for its destruction on both vessel wall and extravascular compartments provides an important protection against thrombosis. The key substance of this system is plasminogen which, when activated, releases plasmin, which in turn dissolves fibrin. This activation is mainly ascribed to the serine referred as tissue plasminogen activator (t-PA). This ubiquitous serine protease is also synthetized by endothelial cells as well as its (own) inhibitor, the plasminogen activator inhibitor (PAI) [119, 164].

Although association between heparin and fibrinolysis was already considered since the late fourties, many controversies [126] have been raised on the role of heparin and its derivatives upon the fibrinolytic system. It has been successively suggested that heparin could be fibrinolytic either by a direct or an indirect process. The indirect activity could be related to heparin ability to prevent the enlargement of a thrombotic process by virtue of its anticoagulant activity thus permitting natural endogenous fibrinolysis to produce clot dissolution and recanalisation more easily.

The direct fibrinolytic property of heparin was revived when heparin, heparin fractions and a semisynthetic polysaccharide were shown to in vitro shorten, euglobin lysis time (ELT). Further in vitro studies have shown that the magnitude of fibrinolysis activation calculating from the shortening of ELT depends partly on the molecular weight of heparins. LMWH having no bearing on this test and on the degree of sulfation [70]. It is believed that heparin molecules may facilitate the release of t-PA from endothelial cells [125, 151].

From in vitro studies there is now agreement that t-PA induced plasminogenolysis measured as chromogenic activity of the resulting plasmin is stimulated by concentration of heparin within the therapeutic range. In addition, unfractionated heparin as well as LMWH enhance the plasminogenolytic activity of urokinase plasminogen activator (U-PA) and pro-urokinase [178, 196].

Experimental data obtained in animal models about effects of heparin fragments and other GAG on fibrinolysis are consistent with an enhancement of the fibrinolytic system.

In a rabbit jugular vein model, it was shown that heparin, and more particularly LMW heparin, contribute to a greater degree of rt-PA induced thrombolysis as detected by means of a reduction of trapped radiolabelled fibrin in the clot; on the same model, both epsilon-aminocrapoic acid and aprotinin, impair fibrinolytic enhancement due to heparin and LMWH [21, 57, 189].

In clinical studies carried out both on healthy volunteers or in patients, heparin and LMW heparins have repeatedely been repeted to enhance or to unaffect fibrinolysis [126].

These discrepancies can be ascribed to the measured parameters, to the principle and method used for the evaluation (t-PA activity or t-PA antigen), to the route of administration (subcutaneous or intravenous) or to the doses (level, single or repeated bolus). Natural circadian variations of fibrinolytic components can also account for enhanced activity. Two published studies with opposite results regarding identical drugs (unfractionated heparin and a LMWH) illustrate this conflicting situation. In the "negative" study [65] the tested drugs were administered subcutaneously in a single low dose; in the "positive" study [4] the active doses (higher for the LMWH than for standard heparin) were given intravenously. Furthermore, if the tested parameters were identical (t-PA), the methodology was quite different - measure of t-PA activity was linked with positive results, t-PA antigen with negative one. From these results, it was concluded that unfractionated and LMWH have a pronounced influence on fibrinolysis activity only when given intravenously and that for LMWH the required doses must be higher than unfractionated heparin one. These findings have not necessarily been verified since studies claiming enhancement of heparin - induced fibrinolytic activity involve measurement of t-PA activity rather than antigen. Furthermore, in most of these studies heparin was given as a single dose. Intevestingly, an enhancement of tPA antigen level has been evidenced after repeated heparin administration over periods ranging from 3-5 days [8].

The responses to venous occlusion measured by ELT have been in some studies considered as enhanced by heparin and LMWH through studies not affected since the modifications could be within the diurnal range of variation.

The vasopressin analogue dDAVP induces a marked increase in plasma level of t-PA [24]. This dDAVP capacity, used for the investigation of patients with deficient fibrinolysis, is increased with standard heparin and even more with LMWH [3, 173].

Heparin is largely used as adjuvant therapy with thrombolytic agents in patients suffering acute myocardial infarction. Most of the studies in which heparin is considered as an effective therapy because it accelerates the rate and the delay of reperfusion, do not distinguish between a direct fibrinolytic activity and the antithrombotic affect which prevents further deposition of fibrin therefore allowing physiological and therapeutical fibrinolysis to process the coronary clot. However, some data argue in favor of a direct interference of heparin with the fibrinolytic system: it has been suggested that heparin potentiates the thrombolytic effects of pro-uPA via the inhibition of thrombin-induced cleavage of the activator. It is believed that thrombin bound in the fibrin mesh of the colt becomes exposed after fibrinolytic therapy, thus degrading the thrombolytic agent and bringing about coagulation [75]. Such effects are prevented by heparin.

In conclusion, numerous findings support the enhancing ability of heparin on physiological fibrinolysis but neither the clinical relevance nor the molecular mechanism of identity of this potentiation have been clearly established.

4. Heparin (fragment) interactions with blood constituents

4.1 Hemorheology

Hemorheology which is related to the "deformation and flow properties of cellular and plasmatic components of blood with the rheological properties of the vessel structure" [48] is essential for homeostasis. Thrombosis and hemostasis occur locally in flowing blood as a dynamic interaction between blood and the vessel wall in the presence of various coagulation proteins [120]. Blood stasis, one of the three components of the so called "Virchow's triad" is facilitated by increasing blood viscosity.

The main event in coagulation is the thrombin-catalyzed conversion of fibrinogen (a soluble protein) into fibrin, an insoluble polymeric network.

This conversion is beleived to be the major mechanism by which fibrinogen contributes as a risk factor to a thrombotic event.

Furthermore, an increase in plasma fibrinogen concentration increases both plasma viscosity and erythocyte or platelet aggregation. Reduction in plasma fibrinogen is therefore a logical procedure to improve the flowing properties of blood.

By using an ex vivo perfusion chamber model, it was observed that fibrin deposition on a thrombogenic surface (exposed subendothelium from everted rabbit aorta) was prevalent at low shear rates and only minimal at high shear rate and was inhibited by heparinized blood in a dose-dependent manner.

Platelet deposition or platelet release (thrombin) were reduced by high dose-heparin only at low or intermediate shear rates but not at high shear rates [98].

Similar results were observed on heparin-coated surfaces (heparinized arterio-venous shunts implated in dogs) since in low wall shear rate segments. FXa and thrombin inhibitory capacities were equivalent whereas in high wall shear rate, thrombin inhibitory capacity was decreased [7]. These results clearly indicate that heparin-ATIII-mediated inhibition of the serine proteases is dependent on the wall shear rate. More extensively, they might explain why heparin is more active as an antithrombotic agent in a venous system (low shear rate) that in arterial system (high shear rate).

Recent clinical trials and epidemiological observations indicate that elevated plasma fibrinogen as well as fibrinopeptide-A (FPA) levels are strongly correlated with an increased frequency of angina episodes, myocardial infarction and stroke and represent an independant risk factor for cardiovascular diseases [66].

Heparin has been shown to lower fibrinogen and FPA levels following intravenous, subcutaneous and intrapulmonary administrations [102].

The significance of fibrinogen reduction by heparin may be relevant to cardiovascular thromboembolic disorders and atherosclerosis as recently emphasized in the Framingham Heart Study [103].

Interesting studies have shown that in the absence of thrombin, the fibrinogen molecules aggregate and gel to form what is known as fibrinogenin, a formation that may be inhibited by certain heparin preparations or by some LMW heparins [49]. It is likely that a decrease in surface viscoelasticity rigidity may contribute to preventing thrombosis, but plasma proteins other than fibrinogen and other plasma constituents may also affect surface hemorheological values.

4.2 Heparin and platelet functions

Extensive interactions of blood constituents with the functional machinery of the vessel wall surface appear to be essential for maintaining a balanced homeostasis in the circulatory system. It has been suggested that adhesion, aggregation and activation of blood cells (mainly platelet and leukocytes) on endothelium may induce changes in endothelial functions that would affect hemostasis and thrombogenesis.

4.2.1 Platelet adhesion

Platelets strongly adhere to the subendothelium structure by attachement to collagen of surface adhesive proteins exposed after endothelial cells injury; thereafter, they undergo activation and subsequent recruitment to form rapidly enlarging thrombi.

The process of adhesion which involves the diffuse transport of platelets to the reactive surface and the interactions of their glycoproteins receptors with subendothelial structures is strongly reduced mainly by LMWH shown in ex vivo studies on bovine extracellular matrix [105].

These experiments can be related to the non thrombogenecity of laser-damaged micro vessels observed after treatment with heparin and LMW heparins. In this model adhesion and subsequent aggregation to injured vessels were inhibited in a dose-dependent manner by heparins and this antithrombotic effect lasted far longer than the ex vivo measurable effect on coagulation.

4.2.2 Platelet aggregation

The relationship of heparin with platelet function is less clear than is its action on clotting proteins. Conflicting data are obtained from different in vitro systems, and this is even more the case when in vitro and in vivo observations are correlated [195].

Several authors report that addition of heparin to platelets in vitro causes platelet aggregation in approximately 75% of the platelet-rich human plasmas (PRP) tested [23, 61, 168], while others observe either no effect [11, 85, 128, 197] or an inhibition of platelet aggregation [12, 133].

Almost all in vitro studies concur in reporting an increase in the rate of aggregation induced by various aggregant agents (ADP, arachidonic acid, PAF, adrenaline, collagen) following the addition of heparin [128].

In equivalent experimental conditions or in ex-vivo studies, heparin fragments prove generally less active than conventional heparin [23, 118, 128, 136, 168, 197], but some differences have been observed between the various LMW heparins tested [85].

Also the heparin-induced platelet aggregation mechanism is not yet fully understood, the enhancement of platelet reactivity appears to be linked with the molecular weight of the heparin molecules [94, 130, 168], while the availability of fibrinogen receptors on the platelet surface has been related to the degree of sulfation of the heparin molecules [177]. While it is difficult to establish any correlation between in vitro and in vivo phenomena, the occurence of thrombocytopenia during extended heparin therapy cannot be denied and it was argued that enhancement of platelet aggregation by heparin may be the predominant factor in inducing mild (non-immune) thrombocytopenia in patients under heparin treatment [74]. The lack of reactivity of heparin fragments with platelets gives grounds for assuming that the use of LMWH would be safer. The lower level of platelet activation obtained with heparin fractions should be relevant in the treatment of arterial thrombosis. Experimental data obtained on a canine model of coronary thrombosis (induced by an anodal current) have demonstrated that a LMWH displays a higher antithrombotic activity than unfractionated heparin when administered by the SC route and that this antithrombotic efficacy is not related to plasma anti-Xa activity [134].

4.2.3 Platelet release

The platelet release reaction occuring during adhesion and aggregation at sites of vascular injury gives rise to the secretion from their α granules of proteins including platelet factor 4 (PF4), ß thromboglobulin (ßTG) and platelet-derived growth factor (PDGF).

PF4 was first noted as an antiheparin factor; although PF4 is not a very basic protein it shows a high binding affinity with heparin which becomes no longer active as an anticoagulant [194].

On the other hand, when heparin is injected intravenously, a large amount of PF4 is released into the circulation. This PF4, known as the heparin-mobilizable pool of PF4, does not directly originate from platelets but from the endothelium after its release from activated platelets and binding to endothelial cells [27, 38].

This pool of PF4 (observed only after IV administration, not after SC injection), is dependent upon the type of heparin used. Like heparin binding to PF4, heparin-induced PF4 release is a function of the size and charge density of the heparin molecules; LMW heparins do not cause the plasma PF4 rebound observed with conventional heparin [143]. PF4 interacts with the glycosaminoglycans of the endothelial cells and strongly binds with heparin and heparin sulfate, and to a lesser extent with dermatan sulphate [55]. PF4 interferes with the binding of ATIII to the endothelial heparin-like molecules [28], decreasing the enhancement of the antithrombotic activity of ATIII.

It was observed that heparin induces a greater PF4 release in diabetic or atherosclerotic patients than in the healthy population. These patients present an increased risk of thrombotic phenomena.

Accordingly this been suggested that PF4 secreted from the platelets and absorbed onto the endothelium play a role in thrombogenesis by masking the efficacy of the heparin-like molecules [144]. It has further been speculated that heparin may exert an antithrombotic activity since, by displacing endothelium-bound PF4, it may also re-establish the anticoagulant properties of the heparin-like molecules within the endothelial surface, which were previously blockded by bound PF4 [28, 55, 143, 144].

Based on this hypothesis, LMW heparins ought to be less efficient as antithrombotic agents than heparin, but the contrary has been demonstrated.

Since the exact biological importance of PF4 in the bloodstream (before or after binding to endothelial cells) is not established, PF4 may be considered as an in vitro anti-heparin factor.

4.3 Interactions with leukocytes

Interactions between neutrophil granulocytes and endothelial cells (EC) are a normal physiological phenomenon since there exists an equilibrium between the free circulating pool and the margined pool in contact with EC. However, like platelets, blood leukocytes may be involved in thrombus generation [79]. It was shown that during venous stasis leukocytes adhere to the luminal surface through specific endothelial cells (Endothelial Leukocytes Adhesion Molecule: ELAM) and that neutrophil activation may lead to their aggregation and to the release of potentially cytotoxic products e.g. granule proteases and oxygen-derived free radicals. Monocytes/ Macrophages express tissue factor when stimulated by endotoxin, IL 1, TNF or PGDF thereby giving rise to thrombi production [60].

Such enzymatic activities and release of unstable radicals may cause tissue damage amplifying both the inflammatory process and chronic vascular injury.

Heparin prevents in vitro phagocytosis and adherence of polymorphonuclear (PMN) and decreases granulocyte activation thus preventing enzyme release and free radical liberation thereby leukocyte-mediated vascular damage [1, 106]. Heparin binds to, and is internalized by, human monocytes [137] modulating their procoagulant activities and secretory phenotypes. These effects are partially inhibited by histidine-rich glycoprotein [113].

Studies using scanning and/or transmission electroscopy have revealed that heparin and the derivatives administered by IV route inhibit leukocyte adhesion and migration through the endothelium in a rabbit stasis model [183]. In an experimental venous thrombosis model, it has also been reported that heparin and LMW heparin enhance the number of circulating leukocytes (mainly the PMN) and the total count of leukocytes (mononuclear sales into the thrombi) [58]. These apparent contradictory results and the mechanism of this heparin property remain to be elucidated.

Heparin inactivates proteinase release from PMN such as elastase-like enzyme and inhibits neutrophil-derived cathepsin G induced platelet activation [71, 161, 193]. These findings may have important pathophysiological bearings since leukocytes play a major role in the inflammatory reaction. It is now recognized that thrombosis and inflammation responses have common multicellular processes being biochemically linked as part of overall mechanims of host defense [123].

It is tempting to speculate that the well recognized anti-inflammatory properties of heparin might be in part explained by the inactivation of mediators release by PMN by the inhibition of neutrophil free radical production or neutrophil chemotaxis and thereby might be synergistic with its antithrombotic activities.

4.4 Histidine-rich glycoprotein

The expression of the biological effects of exogenous (or endogenous) heparin molecules in vivo may be restricted by binding to various neutralizing proteins. In addition to PF4, a second major heparin-neutralizing protein, histidine-rich glycoprotein, has been identified [110, 114].

This plasma protein, largely present in blood, inhibits the anticoagulant effect of heparin in plasma in the presence of divalent cations. It appears however that the lower affinity of this protein, as compared with PF4, with endogenous heparin-like molecules such as heparin sulfate makes it difficult to predict its exact role in controlling the heparin compounds in vivo [112].

On the basis of experimental data it has been suggested that LMW heparins may be expected to be more resistant to neutralization by histidine-rich glycoprotein (and PF4) than commercial heparin [110]. This would also explain the prolonged plasmatic anticoagulant activities of these compounds as compared with those of heparin.

4.5 Other plasma / Extracellular matrix proteins

Due to the strongly anionic nature of heparin and its great flexible conformation, protein binding to heparin is quite a common property. In many instances, the physiological significance of these interactions is well established (as discussed in this presentation).

Other proteins found in plasma and/or in the extracellular matrix have also been documented to bind to heparin (e.g. fibronectin, vitronectin, thrombospondin, laminin, collagen), but in some cases the practical and biological significance of these interactions is uncertain so they will not be discussed further here; among these proteins; mention will be made only for vitronectin (named also S-protein), which acts as an adhesive and a spreading factor and exerts, as histidine-rich glycoprotein, an heparin-neutralizing activity [157]. More particularly, this heparin-neutralizing activity of vitronectin is expressed in the glycosaminoglycan -catalyzed inhibition of thrombin and F-Xa by AT-III.

Neutralization is achieved with high and low molecular weight heparin fractions. Unlike histidine-rich glycoprotein, vitronectin and at a lesser degree PF4 readily neutralize vessel wall-derived heparan sulfate [158] and it has been argued that these finding might be related to an important modulation of the anticoagulant heparin-like activities proposed to be expressed at the luminal side of endothelial cells [155].

5. Conclusion

While a considerable knowledge concerning heparin interactions with blood components and endothelium has been acquired over the last few years, we still have a long way to go before we arrive at a full comprehension of the complex in vivo antithrombotic properties of heparin.

Endogenous transformations of heparin (fractions/fragments) may result in the generation of lower MW fragments capable of producting antithrombotic effects via various mechanisms.

Table III: Heparin/fragments antithrombotic activity. Some putative positive (+) and negative (-) contributing factors

	Unfractionated Heparin	LMW Heparins
ENDOTHELIUM FACTORS		
Negative surface charge	+	+
Heparin-like molecules	+	+
Endothelial binding	+	(+)
Neutralization clotting factors	+	(+)
Fibrinolysis	+	+
Thrombomodulin/ protein C system	-	(-)
Lipoprotein lipase	+	(+)
SUBENDOTHELIUM FACTORS		
SMC proliferation	+	+
Fibronectin	+	+
Thrombospondin	+	?
Vitronectin	+	

Owing to their particularly flexible molecular structure skeleton, heparin molecules present a great capacity to form complexes with a number of proteins and cell components. Their antithrombotic activity may thus be ascribed to the cumulative actions of their components down-or upregulating various antithrombotic or prothrombotic processes (as summarized in Table III and IV), the final result being basically beneficial with respect to their antithrombotic action.

Table IV: Heparin/fragments antithrombotic activity. Some positive (+) and negative (-) contributing factors

Blood components	Unfractionared heparin	LMW heparins
Clotting factors		
Thrombin (FIIa)	+	(+)
Thrombin generation	+	+
Factor Xa	+	+
Anticoagulant proteins		
AT III	+	+
HC II	+	0
TFPI	+	+
PC	-	-
Fibrinogen	+	+
Platelet		
Adhesivity	+	+
Aggregation	-	(-)
PF4	-	(-)
Histidine-rich-glycoprotein	-	(-)
Leukocyte		
Aggregation	-	?
Adhesivity	+	+
Red blood cell	?	?

It is still difficult, however, to appraise the role of each factor and also to establish whether a single mechanism may be more important or as efficient than combined mechanisms in the prevention of thrombosis.

REFERENCES

1. ABBATE R, GORI AM, MODESTI PA, ATTANASIO M, MARTINI F, COLELLA A, GIUSTI B, CECIONI I, NERI SERNERI GG. Heparin, monocytes and procoagulant activity. Haemostasis 20(1), 98-100, 1990.

2. ABILDGAARD U. Highly purified antithrombin III with heparin cofactor activity prepared by disc gel electrophoresis. Scand J Clin Lab Invest 21, 89-91, 1968.

3. AGNELLI G, LEVI M, COSMI B, TEN CATE JW, NENCI G. Additive effect of dDAVP and standard heparin in increasing : plasma t-PA. Thromb Haemost 61, 507, 1989.

4. AGNELLI GC, BORM J, COSMI B, LEVI M, TEN CATE JW. Effect of standard heparin and a low molecular weight heparin (Kabi 2165) on fibrinolysis. Thromb Haemost 60, 311, 1988.

5. ANDERSSON LO, BARROWCLIFFE TW, HOLMER E, JOHNSON EA, SODERSTROM G. Molecular weight dependency of the heparin potentiated inhibition of thrombin and activated factor X. Effect of heparin neutralization in plasma. Thromb Res 15, 531-541, 1979.

6. ANDERSSON LO, BARROWCLIFFE TW, HOLMER E, JOHNSON EA, SIMS GEC. Anticoagulant properties of heparin fractionated by affinity chromatography on matrix bound antithrombin III by gel filtration. Thromb Res 9, 575, 1976.

7. ARNANDER C, PASCHE B, KODOMA K, RASMUSON A, OLSSON P. Influence of high and low wall shear rates on the inhibition of factor Xa and thrombin at surfaces coated with immobilized heparin. Artificial Organs 13, 521, 1989.

8. ARNESEN H, ENGEBRETSEN LF, UGLAND OM, SELJE FLOT I, KIERULF P. Increased fibrinolytic activity after surgery induced by low dose heparin. Thromb Res 45, 553, 1987.

9. BAJAJ MS, KUPPUSWAMY MN, SAITO H, SPITZER SG, BAJAJ SP. Cultured normal human hepatocytes do not synthesize lipoprotein-associated coagulation inhibitor. Evidence that endothelium is the principal site of its synthesis. Proc Natl Acad Sci USA 87, 8869, 1990.

10. BARA L, BILLAUD E, GRAMOND G, KHER A, SAMAMA M. Comparative pharmacokinetics of a low molecular weight heparin (PK10169) and unfractionated heparin after intravenous and subcutaneous administration. Thromb Res 39, 631-639, 1985.

11. BARIADAS MA, MIKHAILIDIS DP et al. Comparison of the platelet pro-aggregatory effect of conventional unfractionated heparins and a low molecular weight heparin fraction (CY 222). Brit J Haematol 67, 451-457, 1987.

12. BARRETT PA, BUTLER KD, MORLEY J, PAGE CP, PAUL W, WHITE AM. Inhibition by heparin of platelet accumulation in vivo. Thromb Haemost 51, 366-370, 1984.

13. BARROWCLIFFE TW, GRAY E, KERRY PJ, GUTTERRIDGE JMC. Triglyceride rich lipoproteins are responsable for thrombin generation induced by lipid peroxides. Thromb Haemost 52, 7-10, 1984.

14. BARROWCLIFFE TW, MERTON RE, HAVERCROFT SJ. Low affinity heparin potentiates the action of high affinity heparin in oligosaccharides. Thromb Res 34, 125, 1984.

15. BARZU T, MOHLO P, TOBELEM G. Binding and endocytosis of heparin by human endothelial cells in culture. Biochim Biophys Acta 845, 196-203, 1985.

16. BARZU T, MOLHO P, CARION R, TOBELEM G, CAEN JP. Heparin binding to endothelial cells potentiates thrombin-stimulated PGI_2 stimulation. Thromb Haemost 58, Abst 41, 1987.

17. BARZU T, VAN RIJN JLML, PETITOU M, MOLHO P, TOBELEM G, CAEN JP. Endothelial binding sites for heparin. Biochem J 238, 847-854, 1986.

18. BEGUIN S, LINDHOUT T, HEMKER HC. The mode of action of heparin in plasma. Thromb Haemost 60, 457, 1988.

19. BERTELE U, RONCAGLIONI MC, DONATI MB, DE GAETANO G. Heparin counteracts the antiaggregating effect of prostacyclin by potentiating platelet aggregation. Thromb Haemost 49, 81-83, 1983.

20. BJORK I, OLSON ST, SHORE JD. Molecular mechanisms of the accelerating effect of heparin on the reactions between antithrombin and clotting proteinases. In : Lane DA & Lindhal U (Eds). Heparin, chemical and biological properties, clinical applications. Edward Arnold, London, pp 229, 1989.

21. BONEU B, BUCHANAN MR, CADE JF, VAN RYN J, FERNANDEZ FF, OFOSU FA, HIRCH J. Effect of heparin, its low molecular weight fractions and other glycosaminoglycans on thrombus growth in vivo. Thromb Res 40, 81-89, 1985.

22. BONEU B, CARANOBE C, CADROY Y, DOL F, GABAEG AM, DUPOUY D, SIE P. Pharmacokinetic studies of standard unfractionated heparin, and low molecular weight heparins in the rabbit. Semin Thromb Hemostas 14, 18-27, 1988.

23. BRACE LD, FAREED J. Heparin-induced platelet aggregation : dose/response relationships for a low molecular weight heparin derivative (PK 10169) and its subfractions. Thromb Res 42, 769-782, 1986.

24. BROMMER EJ, BARRETT-BERGSHOEFF MM, ALLEN RA,SCGICHT I, BERTINA RM, SCHALEKAMP MA. The use of desmopressin acetate (dDAVP) as a test of the fibrinolytic capacity of patients. Analysis of responders and non responders. Thromb Haemost 48, 156-161, 1982.

25. BROZE GJ, WARREN LA, NOVOTNY WF, HIGUCHI DA, GIRARD TJ, MILETICH JP. The lipoprotein-associated coagulation inhibitor that inhibits the factor VII-tissue factor complex also inhibits factor Xa : insight into its possible mechanism of action. Blood 71, 335-343, 1988.

26. BUCHANAN MR, BONEU B, OFOSU F, HIRSH J. The relative importance of thrombin inhibition and factor Xa inhibition to antithrombotic effects of heparin. Blood 65, 198-201, 1985.

27. BUSCH C, DAWES J, PEPPER DS, WATERSON A. Binding of platelet factor 4 to cultured human endothelial cells. Thromb Res 9, 129-137, 1980.

28. BUSCH C, DAWES J, PEPPER DS, WASTESON A. Binding of platelet 4 to cultured human

umbilical vein endothelial cells. Thromb Res 19, 129, 1980.

29. CARTER CJ, KELTON JG, HIRSH J, GENT M. Relationship between antithrombotic and anticoagulant effects of low molecular weight heparin. Thromb Res 21, 169, 1981.

30. CASTELLOT JJ Jr, ADDONIZIO ML, ROSENBERG R, KARNOVSKY MJ. Cultured endothelial cells produce a heparinlike inhibitor of smooth muscle cell growth. J Cell Biol 90, 372, 1981.

31. CASTELLOT JJ Jr, BEELER DL, ROSENBERG RD, KARNOVSKY MJ. Structural determinants of the capacity of heparin to inhibit the proliferation of vascular smooth muscle cells. J Cell Physiol 120, 315, 1984.

32. CASTELLOT JJ Jr, PUKAC LA, CALEB BL, WRIGHT TC Jr, KARNOVSKY MJ. Heparin selectively inhibits a protein kinase C-dependent mechanism of cell cycle progression in calf aortic smooth muscle cells. J Cell Biol 109, 3147, 1989.

33. CASTELLOT JJ Jr, WONG K, HERMAN B, HOOVER RL, ALBERTINI DF, WRIGHT TC, CALEB BL, KARNOVSKY MJ. Binding and internalization of heparin by vascular smooth muscle cells. J Cell Physiol 124, 13-20, 1985.

34. CASU B. Methods of structural analysis. In : Lane DA, Lindhal U (Eds). Heparin, chemical and biological properties, clinical applications. Edward Arnold, London, p 25, 1989.

35. CASU B. Structure and biological activity of heparin. Advances in carbohydrate chemistry and biochemistry, 43, 51, 1985.

36. CASU B, ORESTE P, TORRI G, ZOPPETI G, CHOAY J, LORMEAU JC, PETITOU M, SINAY P. The

structure of heparin olisaccharides with high anti-factor Xa activity containing the minimal antithrombin III binding sequence. Biochem J 197, 599-609, 1981.

37. CASU B, PETITOU M, PROVASOLI M, SINAY P. Conformational flexibility : a new concept for explaining binding and biological properties of D-uronic acid containing glycosaminoglycans. TIBS 13, 221, 1988.

38. CELLA G, COLBY SI, TAYLOR AD, McCRACKEN L, PARISI AF, SASAHARA AA. Platelet factor 4 (PF4) and heparin-released platelet factor 4 (HR PF4) in patients with cardiovascular disorders. Thromb Res 29, 499-509, 1983.

39. CHAMLEY-CAMPBELL JH, CAMPBELL GR. What controls smooth muscle phenotype ? Atherosclerosis 40, 347, 1981.

40. CHOAY J, LORMEAU JC, PETITOU M, SINAIJ P, FAREED J. Structural studies on a biologically active hexasaccharide obtained from heparin. Ann NY Acad Sci USA 370, 644, 1981.

41. CHOAY J, PETITOU M. The chemistry of heparin: a way to understand its mode of action. Med J Austr Heparin (Suppl.) 144, HS7, 1986.

42. CHOAY J, PETITOU M, LORMEAU JC, SINAY P, CASU B, GATTI G. Structure-activity relationships in heparin : a synthetic pentasaccharide with high affinity for antithrombin III and eliciting high anti-factor Xa activity. Biochem Biophys Res Commun 116, 492-499, 1980.

43. CLOUSE LK, COMP PC. The regulation of hemostasis. The protein C system. N Engl J Med 314, 1298, 1986.

44. CLOWES AW, CLOWES MM. Kinetics of cellular proliferation after arterial injury. IV.

Heparin inhibits rat smoth muscle mitogenesis and migration. Circ Res 58, 839, 1986.

45. CLOWES AW, KARNOVSKY MJ. Suppression by heparin of smooth muscle cell proliferation in injured arteries. Nature 265, 625, 1977.

46. COLBURN P, BUONASSISI V. Identification of an endothelial cell product as an inhibitor of tissue factor activity. In vitro. Cell Dev Biol 24, 1133, 1988.

47. COMP PC. Heparin-protein C interaction. Nouv. Rev Fr Hematol 26, 239-242, 1984.

48. COPLEY AL. Fluid mechanic and biorheology. Thromb Res 57, 315, 1990.

49. COPLEY AL, KING RG. A survey of surface hemorheological experiments on the inhibition of fibrinogen formation employing surface layers of fibrinogen systems with heparin and other substances. Thromb Res 35, 237, 1984.

50. CURRIER JW, POW TK, HAUDENSCHILD CC, MINIHAN AC, FAXON DP. Low molecular weight heparin (Enoxaparin) reduces restenosis after iliac angioplasty in the hypercholesterolemic rabbit. J. Am Coll Cardiol 17(6), (Suppl. B), 118B-125B, 1991.

51. DANIELSSON A, RAUB E, LINDAHL U, BJORK I. Role of ternary complexes, in which heparin binds both antithrombin and proteinase, in the acceleration of the reactions between antithrombin and thrombin of factor Xa. J Biol Chem 261, 15467, 1986.

52. DAWES J, PROWSE CV, PEPPER DS. Absorption of heparin, L.M.W. heparin and SP 54 after subcutaneous injection, assessed by competitive binding assay. Thromb Res 44, 683-693, 1986.

53. DAY KC, HOFFMAN LC, PALMIER MO, KRETZMER KK, HUANG MD, PYLA EY, spokas e, BROZE GJ, WARREN TG, WUN TC. Recombinant lipoprotein-associated coagulation inhibitor inhibits tissue thromboplastin-induce intravascular coagulation in the rabbit. Blood 76, 1538-45, 1990.

54. DE SWART CAM, NIJMYER B, ROELOFS JMM, SIXMA JJ. Kinetics of intravenously administred heparin in normal humans. Blood 60, 1251-1258, 1982.

55. DENTON J, LANE DA, THUNBERG L, SLATER AM, LINDAHL U. Binding of platelet factor 4 to heparin oligosaccharides. Biochem J 209, 455, 1983.

56. DOUTREMEPUICH C. Low molecular weight heparins in clinical practice. Dekker M (Ed). New-York, 1992.

57. DOUTREMEPUICH C, DEHARO E, DOUTREMEPUICH F, LALANNE MC, TOULEMONDE F. Kinetic study of tPA release induced by heparin and heparin fragment. Thromb Res 58, 615, 1989.

58. DOUTREMEPUICH C, TOULEMONDE F, DE SEZE O, PEREIRA F, ANNE MC, DOUTREMEPUICH F. Influence of heparin and low molecular weight heparin fraction on the leukocytes in an experimental venous thrombosis model. J Leukocyte Biol 42, 628-631, 1987.

59. EDELMAN ER, ADAMS DH, KARNOVSKY MJ. Effect of controlled adventitial heparin delivery on smooth muscle cell proliferation following endothelial injury. Proc Natl Acad Sci USA 87, 3773, 1990.

60. EDWARDS RL, RICKLES FR. The role of monocyte tissue factor in the immune response. In : Pick E (Ed). Lymphokine reports. New-York, Academic Press, vol 1, p 181, 1980.

61. EIKA C. Anticoagulant and platelet aggregating activities of heparin. Thromb Res 2, 349-360, 1973.

62. ENGELBERG H. Heparin and the atherotic process. Pharmacol Rev 86, 91, 1984.

63. ENGELBERG H. Heparin and the prevention of atherosclerosis. In : Engelberg H (Ed). Basic research and clinical application. Wiley-liss, New York, 1990.

64. ENGELBERG H. Heparin, non heparin glycosaminoglycans and heparinoids : an overview of their application in atherosclerosis. Semin Thromb Hemostas 17, 5-8, 1991.

65. ERIKSON E, WOLLTER IM, CHRISTENSON E, STIGENDAL L, RISBERG B. Heparin and fibrinolysis. Comparison of subcutaneous administration of unfractionated and low molecular weight heparin. Thromb Haemost 59, 284, 1988.

66. ERNT E. Fibrinogen an independent risk factor for cardiovascular disease. Biol Med J 303, 596, 1991.

67. ESMON CT. The regulation of natural anticoagulant pathways. Science 235, 1348, 1987.

68. ESMON CT, ESMON NL, HARRIS KW. Complex formation between thrombin and thrombomodulin inhibits both thrombin-catalyzed fibrin formation and factor V activation. J Biol Chem 257, 7944, 1982.

69. FAGER G, HANSSON GK, OTTOSSON P, DAHLLOF B, BONDJERS G. Human arterial smooth muscle cells in culture : effects of platelet-derived growth factor and heparin on growth in vitro. Exp Cell Res 176, 319, 1988.

70. FAREED J, WALENGA J, HOPPENSTEADT D, MESSMORE HL. Studies on the profibrinolytic actions of heparin and its fractions. Semin Thromb Haemostas 11, 199, 1985.

71. FERRER P, RENESTO P, CHIGNARD M. Inhibition by heparin of platelet activation induced by human neutrophil-derived Cathepsin G. Am Rev Resp Dis 141(4), A108, 1990.

72. GENSINI GF, FORTINI A, LOMBARDI A, PESCIULLESI E, PIERONI C, SERNERI GG. Binding of low-molecular weight heparin to aortic endothelium in rabbits. Haemostasis 14, 446-472, 1984.

73. GOROG P, SHAFI S. Increased accumulation of lipoprotein and cholesterol in re-endothelialized artery after laser damage. Atherosclerosis 57, 33, 1985.

74. GREEN D. Heparin - induced thrombocytopenia. The Med. J. Australia, 144, HS 37, 1986.

75. GULBA DC, FISHER K, REIL GH, DANIEL WG, LICHTIEN PR. Potentiation of the thrombolytic efficacy of single-chain urokinase (pro-urokinase) by heparin. Thromb Haemost 60, 350, 1988.

76. GUYTON JR, ROSENBERG RD, CLOWES AW, KARNOVSKY MJ. Inhibition of rat arterial smooth muscle cell proliferation by heparin. In vivo studies with anticoagulant and non anticoagulant heparin. Circ Res 46, 625-633, 1980.

77. HARENBERG J, GNASCO A, DE VRIES JX, ZIMMERMANN R, AUGUSTIN D. Anticoagulant and lipolytic effects of a low molecular weight heparin fraction. Thromb Res 39, 683-692, 1985.

78. HARENBERG J, WUERZNER B, ZIMMERMANN R, SHETTLER G. Bioavailability and

antagonization of the low molecular weight heparin CY 216 in man. Thromb Res 44, 549-554, 1986.

79. HARLAN JM. Leucocytes-endothelial interactions. Blood 65, 513, 1985.

80. HASKEL EJ, TORR SR, DAY KC. Prevention of arterial reocclusion after thrombolysis with recombinant LACI. Circulation 84, 821, 1991.

81. HATTON MWC, DEJANA E, CAZENAVE JP, REGOECZI E, MUSTARD JF. Heparin inhibits thrombin binding to rabbit thoracic aorta endothelium. J Lab Clin Med 96, 861, 1980.

82. HATTON MWC, MOAR SL. Comparative behaviour of thrombin and an inactive derivative, FPR-thrombin, towards rabbit vascular endothelium : heparin liberates FPR-thrombin from the endothelium in vivo. Circulation Res 67, 221, 1990.

83. HATTON MWC, MOAR SL. Comparison of the effects of heparin and hirudin on thrombin binding to the normal and the de-endothelialized rabbit aorta in vivo. Thromb Haemost 66, 208, 1991.

84. HATTON MWC, MOAR SL, RICHARDSON M. On the interaction of rabbit antithrombin III with the luminal surface of the normal and deendothelialized rabbit thoracic aorta in vitro. Blood 67, 878, 1986.

85. HEINRICH D, GOERG T, SCHULTZ M. Effects on unfractionated and fractionated heparin on platelet function. Haemostasis 18(3), 48-54, 1988.

86. HERAIHI Z, LUTZ O, FREY A, BACH AC. In vivo and in vitro release of lipoprotein lipase and hepatic lipase by low molecular weight heparin. Arch Int Pharmacodyn 297, 286, 1986.

87. HERBERT JM, MAFFRAND JP. Heparin interactions with cultured human vascular endothelial and smooth muscle cells : incidence on vascular smooth muscle cell proliferation. J Cell Physiol 138, 424, 1989.

88. HIEBERT LM, JAQUES LB. Heparin uptake on endothelium. Artery 2, 26, 1976.

89. HIEBERT LM, LIU JM. Protective action of polyelectrolytes on endothelium. Semin Thromb Hemostas 17, 42, 1991.

90. HIEBERT LM, McDUFFIE N. The internalization and release of heparins by cultured endothelial cells : the process is cell source, heparin source time and concentration dependent. Artery 17, 107, 1990.

91. HIRSH J, LEVINE MN. Low molecular weight heparin. Blood 79, 1, 1992.

92. HLADOVEC J. The effect of heparin on endothelial stability. Thromb Res 35, 347, 1984.

93. HOLMER E, KURACHI K, SODERSTROM G. The molecular weight dependence of the rate enhancing effect of heparin on the inhibition of thrombin, FXa, FIXa, FXIa, FXIIa and kallikrein by antithrombin. Biochem J 193, 395, 1981.

94. HOLMER E, LINDAHL U, BACKSTROM G, THUNBERG L, SANDBERG H, SODERSTROM G, ANDERSON LO. Anticoagulant activities and effects on platelets of a heparin fragment with high affinity for antithrombin. Thromb Res 18, 861-869, 1980.

95. HOLMER E, MATTSSON C, NILSSON S. Anticoagulant and antithrombotic effects of heparin and low molecular weight heparin fragments in rabbits. Thromb Res 25, 475, 1982.

96. HOOK M, BJORK I, HOPWOOD J, LINDAHL U. Anticoagulant activity of heparin : separation of high-activity and low-activity heparin species by affinity chromatography on immobilized antithrombin. FEBS Lett 66, 90, 1976.

97. HORIE T, SEKIGUCHI M, HIROSAIVA K. Coronary thrombosis in pathogenesis of acute myocardial infarction : histopathological study of coronary arteries in 108 necropsied cases using serial section. Br Heart J 40, 153, 1978.

98. INAVEN W, BAUMGARTNER HR, BOMBELLI T, HAEBERLI A, STRAUB PW. Dose - and share rate - dependent effects of heparin on thrombogenesis induced by rabbit aorta subendothelium exposed to flowing human blood. Arterosclerosis 10, 607, 1990.

99. JAQUES LB. Heparin : a unique misunderstood drug. Trends in Pharm Sci 3, 289-291, 1982.

100. JAQUES LB. Heparins. Anionic polyelectrolyte drugs. Pharmacological Reviews, 31, 99, 1979.

101. KAKKAR VV, HEDGES AR. Use of heparin as a prophylactic agent against venous thromboembolism. In : Lane DA, Lindhal U (Eds).Heparin chemical and biological properties, clinical applications. Edward Arnold, London, p 455, 1989.

102. KANABROCKI EL, SOTHEM RB, BREMMER WF et al. Heparin lowers plasma fibrinogen and fibrinopeptide A levels. Its relevance to cardiovascular disease (In press).

103. KANNEL WB, WOLF PA, CASTELLI WP, D'AGOSTINO RB. Fibrinogen and risk of cardiovascular disease. The Fragmingham Study. JAMA 258, 1183-1186, 1987.

104. KAZAMA Y, NIWA M, YAMAGISHI R, TAKAHASHI K, SAKURAGAWA N, KOIDE T. Specificity of sulfated polysaccharides to accelerate the inhibition of activated protein C by protein C inhibitor. Thromb Res 48, 179-185, 1987.

105. KRUPINSKI K, BASIC-MICIC M, LINDHOFF E, BREDDIN H. Inhibition of coagulation and platelet adhesion to extracellular matrix by unfractionated heparin and a low molecular weight heparin. Blut 61, 289, 1990.

106. LAGHI PASIMI F, PASQUI AL.

107. LAM LH, SILBERT JE, ROSENBERG RD. The separation of active and inactive forms of heparin. Biochem Biophys Res Commun 69, 570, 1976.

108. LANE B, RYAN K. Heparin and low molecular weight heparin : is anti-factor Xa activity important ? J Lab Clin Med 114, 331, 1989.

109. LANE D. Heparin binding and neutralizing proteins. In : Lane DA, Lindhal U (Eds). Heparin : Chemical and biological properties, clinical applications. Arnold E, London, 1989.

110. LANE DA, PEYLER G, FLYNN AM, THOMPSON EA, LINDAHL U. Neutralization of heparin-related saccharides by histidine-rich glycoprotein and platelet factor 4. J Biol Chem 261, 3980-3986, 1985.

111. LANE DA, FLYNN AM, PEJLER G, LINDAHL U, CHOAY J, PREISSNER KT. Structural requirements for the neutralization of heparin-like saccharides by complements protein/vitronectin. J Biol Chem 262, 16343, 1987.

112. LAURENT TC, TENGLAD A, THUNBERG L, HOOK M, LINDAHL U. The molecular weight dependence of

the anticoagulant activity of heparin. Biochem J 175, 691, 1978.

113. LEUNG L, SAIGO K, GRANT D. Heparin binds to human monocytes and modulates their procoagulant activities and secretory phenotypes. Effects of histidine-rich glycoprotein. Blood 73, 177, 1989.

114. LIJNEN HR, HOYLAERTS M, COLLEN D. Heparin binding properties of human histidine-rich-glycoprotein. Mechanisms and role in the neutralization of heparin. J Biol Chem 258, 3803-3808, 1983.

115. LINDAHL AK, ABILDGAARD U, LARSEN ML, STAALESEN R, HAMMER AK, SANDSET PM, NORDFANG O, BECK TC. Extrinsic pathway inhibitor (EPI) released to the blood by heparin is a more powerful coagulation inhibitor than is recombinant EPI. Thromb Res 62, 607-614, 1991.

116. LINDHAL U, BACKSTROM G, THUNBERG L, LEDER IG. Evidence for a 3-O-sulfated D-glucosamine residue in the antithrombin binding sequence of heparin. Proc Natl Acad Sci USA 77, 6551, 1980.

117. LINDHAL U, BACKSTROM G, THUNBERG L. The antithrombin binding sequence in heparin. Identification of an essential 6-O-sulfate group. J Biol Chem 258, 9826, 1983.

118. LJUNGBERG B, JOHNSSON H. In vivo effects of a low molecular weight heparin on platelet aggregation and platelet dependent hemostasis in dogs. Thromb Haemost 60, 232, 1988.

119. LJUNGER H., LHOLMBERG L, KJELGAARD A, NILSSON IM, ASTED B. Immunological characterization of plasminogen activators in the human vessel wall. J Clin Pathol 36, 1046, 1983.

120. LOWE GDO, FOIBES CD. Blood rheology and thrombosis. Clin Haematol 10, 343, 1981.

121. MAJACK RA, GOODMAN LV, DIXIT VM. Cell surface thrombospondin is functionally essential for vascular smooth muscle cell proliferation. J Cell Biol 106, 415, 1988.

122. MARCUM JA, ROSENGERG RD. The biochemistry, cell biology and pathophysiology of anticoagulantly active heparin-like molecules of the vessel wall. In : Lane DA, Lindahl U (Eds). Heparin chemical and biological properties,clinical applications. Edward Arnold, p 275, 1989.

123. MARCUS AJ. Thrombosis and inflammation as multicellular processes : pathophysiologie significance of transcellular metabolism. Blood 76, 1903, 1990.

124. MARDIQUIAN J. Methods of preparation of low molecular weight heparins. In : Doutremepuich C (Ed). Low molecular weight heparins in clinical practice. Marcel Dekker. New-York, p 7, 1992.

125. MARKWARDT F, KLOCKING HP. Heparin-induced release of plasminogen activator. Haemostasis 6, 370, 1977.

126. MARSH N. Does heparin stimulate fibrinolysis ? Brit J Haematol 76, 163, 1990.

127. MASTACCHI R, BARBANTI M. Inactivation of the heparin anticoagulant activity by rat kidney lysosomal enzymes. Thromb Res 47, 101-106, 1987.

128. MASTACCHI R, BARBANTI M, BIANCHINI P, OSIMA B. Interaction of a new low molecular weight heparin (OP 2123) with human platelets. Agents Actions 17, 512-514, 1986.

129. McCAFFREY TA, FALCONE DJ, BRAYTONE CF et al. Transforming growth factor ß activity is potentiated by heparin via dissociation of the transforming growth factor β/α_2 macroglobulin inactive complement. J Cell Biol 109, 441, 1989.

130. McDONALD K, HORNE MK, CHAO E. The effect of molecular weight on heparin binding to platelets. Brit J Haematol 74, 306, 1990.

131. MELANDRI G, BRANZI A, SUMPRINI F, CERVI V, GALIE N, MAGNANI B. Enhanced thrombolytic efficacy and reduction of infarct sIze by siiuh[aneius infusion of streptok!nase and heparin. Br Heart J 64, 118-120, 1990.

132. MERTON RE, THOMAS DP, HAVERCROFT SJ, BARROWCLIFFE TW. High and low affinity heparin compared with unfractionated heparin as antithrombotic drugs. Thromb Haemost 51, 254, 1984.

133. MESSMORE HL, GRIFFIN B, FAREED J, COYNE E, SEGHATCHIAN J. In vitro studies of the interaction of heparin, low molecular weight heparins and heparinoids with platelets. Ann NY Acad Sci 556, 217-232, 1989.

134. MESTRE M, CLAIREFOND P, MARDIGUIAN J, TRILLOU M, LE FUR G, UZAN J. Comparative effects of heparin and PK 10169, a low molecular weight fraction, in a canine model of arterial thrombosis. Thromb Res 38, 389-399, 1985.

135. MIKHAILIDIS DP, BARRADAS MA, MIKHAILIDIS AM, MAGNANI H, DANDONA P. Comparison of the effect of a conventional heparin and a low molecular weight heparinoids on platelet function. Br J Clin Pharm 17, 43-48, 1984.

136. MIKHAILIDIS DP, BARRADAS MA, O'DONOGHUE S, BANDONA P. Evidence for in vivo platelet activation following the injection of

conventional unfractionated heparin. Platelets 1, 189, 1990.

137. MODESTI PA, CECIONI I, COLELLA A et al. Heparin binding to and internationalization by human monocytes. Thromb Res 13, 49,1991.

138. MUSTARD JF, PACKHAM MA, KINLOUGH-RATHBONE RL. Mechanisms in thrombosis. In : Bloom A, Thomas D (Eds). Hemostasis and thrombosis. Churchill Livingstone Edinburgh, 1987.

139. NADER H, BUONASSISI V, COLBURN P, DIETRICH CP. Heparin stimulates the synthesis and modifies the sulfation pattern of heparan sulfate proteoglycan from endothelial cells. J Cell Physiol 140, 305, 1989.

140. NAGGI A, TORRI G, CASU B, PANGRAZZI J, ABBADINI M, ZAMETTA M, DONATI MB, LANZEN J, MAFFRAND JP. "Supersulfated" heparin fragments a new type of low molecular wieght heparin. Bioch Pharmacol 37, 1895-1900, 1986.

141. NORRHEIM L, ABILDGARD U, LARSEN ML, LINDAHL A. Invovement of the extrinsic pathway in the activities of low molecular weight heparins. Thromb Res (Suppl. XIV), 19, 1991.

142. NOVOTNY WF, PALMIER M, WUN TC, BROZE G, MILETICH J. Purification and properties of heparin releasable lipoprotein-associated coagulation inhibitor. Blood 78, 394, 1991.

143. O'BRIEN JR, ETHERINGTON MD, PASHLEY MA. The heparin mobilesable pool of platelet factor 4: comparison of intravenous and subcutaneous heparin and kabi heparin fragment 2165. Thromb Haemost 54, 735-738, 1985.

144. O'BRIEN JR, ETHERINGTON MD, PASHLEY M. Intra platelet factor 4 (IP PF4) and the heparin-mobilisable pool of PF4 in health and atherosclerosis. Thromb Haemost 51, 354-357, 1984.

145. OBERHOFF M, GANKE H, HANKE S et al. Reduction of smooth muscle cell proliferation by low molecular weight heparin after experimental balloon angioplasty in rabbits. Eur Heart J 12, 80, 1991.

146. OCKELFORD P. Heparin 1986 : Indications and effective use. Drugs 31, 81-92, 1986.

147. OCKELFORD PA, CARTER CJ, MITCHELL T, HIRSH J. Disordance between the anti Xa activity and antithrombotic activity of an ultra low molecular weight heparin fraction. Thromb Res 28, 401, 1982.

148. OFOSU FA, BLAJCHMAN MA, MODI GI, SMITH LM, BUCHANAN MR, HIRSH J. The importance of thrombin inhibition for the expression of the anticoagulant activities of heparin, dermatan sulfate, low molecular weight heparin and pentosane polysulfate. Br J Haematol 60, 695, 1985.

149. OKADA T, BARK DH, MAYBERG MR. Localized release of perivascular heparin inhibits intimal proliferation after endothelial injury without systemic anticoagulation. Neurosurgery 25, 892, 1989.

150. OLIVECRONA T, BENGTSSON G, MARKLUND SE, LINDAHL U, HOOK M. Heparin-Lipoprotein lipase interactions. Fed Proc 36, 60, 1977.

151. PAQUES EP, STOEHR HA, HEIMBURGER N. Study on the mechanism of action of heparin and related substances on the fibrinolytic system; relationship between plasminogen activator and heparin. Thromb Res 42, 797, 1986.

152. PARMA B, BERGONZINI GL, BIANCHINI P, OSIMA B. Antithrombotic activity of heparin and low molecular weight heparin in animals treated with anti-ATIII antibodies. Thromb Haemorrh Disorders 3, 13, 1991.

153. PERSSON E, NORDENSTROM J, NILSSON-EHLE P. Plasma Kinetics of lipoprotein lipase and hepatic lipase activities induced by heparin and a low molecular weight heparin fragment. Thromb Res 47, 151-155, 1987.

154. PESCADOR R, PORTA R, NIADA R, DIAMANTINI H, FEDELI H, MANTOVANI M. The anticoagulant, hepatic lipase-releasing activities of several natural and chemically modified heparin differ. Biochem Pharmacol 36, 253-257, 1987.

155. PREISSNER KT. Physiological role of vessel wall related antithrombotic mechanisms : contribution of endogenous and exogenous heparin-like components to the anticoagulant potential of the endothelium. Haemostasis 20(1), 30, 1990.

156. PREISSNER KT, DELVOS U, MILLER-BERGHAUS G. Binding of thrombin to thrombomodulin accelerates inhibition of the enzyme by antithrombin III. Evidence for an heparin-independent mechanism. Biochemistry 26, 2521, 1987.

157. PREISSNER KT, JENNE D. Structure of vitronectin and its biological role in haemostasis. Thromb Haemost 66, 123, 1991.

158. PREISSNER KT, MULLER-BERGHAUS G. S-protein modulates the heparin-catalyzed inhibition of thrombin bg antithrombin III. Evidence for a direct interation of S-protein with heparin. Eur J Bioch 156, 645, 1986.

159. PRINS MH, HIRSH J. Heparin as an adjunctive treatment after thrombolytic therapy for acute myocardial infarction. Am J Cardiol 67(3A), 1991.

160. RAPAPORT SI. The extrinsic pathway inhibitor : a regulator of tissue factor-dependent

blood coagulation. Thromb Haemost 66, 6, 1991.

161. REDINE F, TIXIER JM, PETITOU M, CHOAY J. Inhibition of leukocyte elastase by heparin and its derivatives. Biochem J 252, 515, 1988.

162. REILLY CF, FRITZE LMS, ROSENBERG RD. Heparin inhibition of smooth muscle cell proliferation : a cellular site of action. J Cell Physiol 129, 11, 1986.

163. REILLY CF, KINDY MS, BROWN KE, ROZENBERG RD, SONENSHEIN GE. Heparin prevents vascular smooth muscle cell progression through the G_1 phase of the cells cycle. J Biol Chem 264, 6990-6995, 1989.

164. ROGERS GM. Haemostatic properties of normal and perturbed vascular cells. FASEB J 2, 116, 1988.

165. ROSENBERG RD, DAMUS PS. The purification and mechanism of action of human antithrombin-heparin cofactor. J Biol Chem 248, 6490-6505, 1973.

166. ROSS R. The pathogenesis of atherosclerosis. On update. N Engl J Med 314, 488, 1986.

167. SABA HO, SABA SR, BLACKBURN CA, HARTMANN RC, MASON RG. Heparin neutralization of PGI2 : effects upon platelets. Science 205, 499-501, 1979.

168. SALZMAN EW, ROSENBERG RD, SMITH MH, LINDON JN, FAVREAU L. Effect of heparin and heparin fractions on platelet aggregation. J. Clin. Invest., 65, 64-73, 1980.

169. SANDSET PM., abildgaard u. Extrinsic pathway inhibitor. The key to feedback control of blood coagulation initiated by tissue thromboplastin. Haemostasis 21, 219, 1991.

170. SAWYER PM, SRINIVASSAN S. The role of electrochemical surface properties in thrombosis at vascular interfaces : cumulative experience of studies in animals and man. Bull NY Acad Med 42, 235, 1972.

171. SAWYER PM, STANCZEVSKI A., POMERANCE T. Utility of anticoagulant drugs in vascular thrombosis. Electon microscopie and biophysical studies surg 74, 263, 1973.

172. SCHARF RE, HARKER LA. Thrombosis and atherosclerosis. Regulatory role of interactions among blood components and endothelium. Blut, 55, 131, 1987.

173. SCHVED JF, GRIS FC. The mitral release of t-PA induced bu dDAVP is more important with low molecular weight heparin than with unfractionated heparin. Thromb Haemost 65, 109, 1991.

174. SIMIONESCU N, SIMIONESCU M, PALADE GE. Differentiated microdomains on the luminal surface of the capillary endothelium I-preferential distribution of aniovic sites. J Cell Biol 90, 605, 1981.

175. SINAIJ JP, JAQUINET JC, PETITOU M, DUCHAUSSOY P, LEDERMAN I, CHOAY J, TORRI G. Total synthesis of a heparin pentasaccharide fragment having high affinity for antithrombin III. Carbohydr Res 132, 5, 1984.

176. SKUTELSKY E, DANON D. Redistribution of surface anionic sites on the luminal front of blood vessel endothelium after interaction with polycationic ligand. J Cell Biol 71, 232, 1976.

177. SORIA C, SORIA J, DUNN F, THOMAIDIS A, TOBELEM G, CAEN JP. Interactions of platelets with standard heparin and low molecular weight fractions. Med J Austr 144, HS 32, 1986.

178. STASSEN JM, JUHAN-VAGUE I, ALESSI MC, De COCK F, COLLEN D. Potentiation by heparin fragments of thrombolysis induced with human tissue-type plasminogen activator or human single-chain urokinase-type plasminogen activator. Thromb Haemost 58, 947-950, 1987.

179. STERN D, BRETT J, HARRIS K, NAWROTH P. Participation of endothelial cells in the protein C. Protein S anticoagulant pathway. The synthesis and release of protien S. J Cell Biol 102, 1971-1978, 1986.

180. SUZUKI K, KUSUMOTO H, DEYASHIKI Y, NISHIOKA J, MARUYAMA I, SUSHI M, KAWAHARA S, HONDA G, YAMAMOTO S, HORIGUCHI S. Structure and expression of human thrombomodulin, a thrombin receptor on endothelium acting as a cofactor for protein C activation. EMBO J 6, 1981, 1987.

181. SZILAGYI DE, ELLIOTT JP, HAGEMAN JH, SMITH RF, DALL'OLMO CA. Biological fate of autogenous vein implants as arterial substitutes. Clinical angiographic and histologic observations in femoro-popliteal operations for atherosclerosis. Ann Surg 178, 232-244, 1973.

182. TANSEY MJB., OPIE LH. Relation between mlasma free fatty acids and aarhythmias within the first twelve hours of acute myocardial infarction. Lancet II, 419-422, 1985.

183. THOMAN DP, MERTON RE, HOCKLEY DJ. The effect of stasis on the venous endothelium : an ultrastructural study. Br J Haematol 55, 113-122, 1983.

184. THUNBERG L, LINDAHL U, TENGBLAD A, LAURENT TC, JACKSON CM. On the molecular weight dependence of the anticoagulant activity of heparin. Biochem J 181, 241-243, 1979.

185. THYBERG J, HEDIN U, SJOLUND M, PALMBERG L, BOTTGER B. Regulation of differenciated properties and proliferation of arterial smooth muscle cells. Atheriosclerosis, 10, 960, 1990.

186. TIOZZO R, REGGIANI B, CINGI MR, BIANCHINI P, CALENDRA S. Effect of heparin derived fractions on the proliferation and protein synthesis of cells in culture. Thromb Res 62, 177, 1991.

187. TOLLEFSEN DM, BLANK MK. Detection of a new heparin-dependent inhibitor of thrombin in human plasma. J Clin Invest 68, 589-596, 1981.

188. TRABUCCHI E, FOSCHI D, MARAZZI M, ABELLI P, ANDRIUOLI GILAMI F, SCAGNOL I, DEL SOLDATO P, DE SANTIS F, MONTORSI W. Heparin prevents stasis-induced thrombosisthough protection of the venous endothelial cell : an electron microscopie study in rabbits. Haemostasis 21,37-44, 1991.

189. VAIREL EG, BROUTY-BORGE H, TOULEMONDE F, DOUTREMEPUICH C, MARSH NA, GAFFNEY PJ. Heparin and low-molecular weight fraction enhance thrombolysis and by this pathway exercise a protective effect against thrombosis. Thromb Res 30, 219, 1983.

190. VAN RIFN JLML, TRILLOU M, MARDIGUIAN J, TOBELEM G, CAEN JP. Selective binding of heparins to human endothelial cells implications for pharmacokinetics. Thromb Res 45, 211-222, 1987.

191. VANNUCHI S, PASQUALI F, PORCIATTI F, CHIARUGI U, MAGNELLI L, BIANCHINI P. Binding, internalization and degradation of heparin fragments by cultured endothelial cells. Thromb Res 49, 373-383,1988.

192. VERSTRAETE H. Pharmacotherapeutic aspects of unfractionated and low molecular weight heparins. Drugs 40, 498, 1990.

193. WALSH RL, DILLON TJ, SCICCHITANO R, McLENNAN G. Heparin and heparan sulfate are inhibitors of human leukocyte elastase. Clin Sci 81, 341, 1991.

194. WALZ DA, HUNG GL. In vivo studies on the binding of heparin and its fractions with platelet factor4. Semin Thromb Haemostas 11,40-47, 1985.

195. WARKENTIN T, KELTON JG. Heparin and platelets. Hematology/oncology clinics of N America 4, 243, 1990.

196. WATAHIKI Y, SCULLY MF, ELLIS V, KAKKAR VV. Influence of heparin and various glycosaminoglycans on activation of single chain urokinase-type plasminogen activation (Scu-PA) by plasmin. Fibrinolysis 3, 31, 1989.

197. WESTWICK J, SCULLY MF, POLL C, KAKKAR VV. Comparison of the effects of low molecular weight heparin and unfractionated heparin on activation of human platelets in vitro. Thromb Res 42, 435-447, 1986.

198. WILLIAMS SP, BARROWCLIFFE TW. The effect of post-heparin plasma lipases on anti-Xa clotting activity. Thromb Res 37, 371,-377, 1985.

199. WILSON NV, SALISBURY JR, KAKKAR VV. Effect of low molecular weight heparin on intimal hyperplasia. Br J Surg 78, 1381, 1991.

200. WRIGHT TC Jr, CASTELLOT JJ. Jr, PETITOU M, LORMEAU JC, CHOAY J, KARNOVSKY MJ. Structural determinants of heparin's growth inhibitory activity : interdependence of oligosaccharide size and charge. J Biol Chem 264, 1534, 1989.

5

Native antithrombin III, an activable protein

J. Choay

It appears today that the decrease of thrombin level in various pathological situations is one of the principal means to prevent the appearance of thrombosis as well as to control its extension. For several decades this decrease has been obtained using heparin and antivitamins K. The mode of action of the latter is well documented. Heparin, the reference anticoagulant, is a glycosaminoglycan. It is highly heterogeneous in its chemical structure as well as in its molecular weight and its biological properties. Heparin acts mainly through a plasma protein; Antithrombin III (ATIII), by enhancing the rate constant of inhibition towards procoagulant serine-proteases [4]. Heparin, at low doses and by subcutaneous route, was proved to be a potent antithrombotic agent [14]. Since 1985, low molecular weight heparins, have been introduced in therapeutics [13]. These drugs are also heterogeneous; their mode of action is not yet completely understood. However, their activity, for a large part, is probably due to their capability to inhibit thrombin generation in platelet rich plasma, their weak neutralization by platelet factor 4 (PF4), their excellent bioavailability by subcutaneous route as well as to their delayed pharmacokinetics.

Despite the good therapeutical results obtained recently with low molecular weight heparins, numerous research lines are in progress with the aim to design and to develop homogeneous antithrombotic substances that are constituted of a single molecular species having a perfectly defined chemical structure and specific pharmacological targets. They concern more particularly synthetic activators of ATIII (pentasaccharide and its analogs), direct inhibitors of Factor Xa (antistasin, tick anticoagulant peptide), direct thrombin inhibitors (recombinant hirudins, hirudin synthetic fragments, synthetic derivatives, small peptides and their analogs). These chemically defined and pure substances allow to make in-depth research on their mechanism of action at the molecular level. We shall discuss here the structure and the mechanism of action of the first mentioned class of molecules, that is synthetic oligosaccharides activators of ATIII. Their mechanism of action relies on the knowledge of the structure and the activation of ATIII.

Human ATIII [2, 18] is a single chain glycoprotein having a molecular weight of 58 200 Kd. Its sequence has been determined by analysis of its constituent amino-acids and of its cDNA. It contains 432 amino-acids; its reactive bond is constituted of Arginine 393 (P1) and Serine 394 (P'1). Bovine ATIII contains 433 amino-acids; its primary structure has been established [17]. ATIII has two properties:

- It is a major serine-protease inhibitor that inhibits all the pro-coagulant serine-proteases with the exception of Factor V1la, these serine-proteases being either neutral as Factor Xa or positively charged as thrombin. ATIII is a member of the super family of the serine-protease inhibitors (serpins). This inhibition is a slow process.
- ATIII possesses also the property to be activated by a sub-family of glycosamino- glycans (heparin, heparan sulfate and their active fragments) having a high affinity for ATIII. This activation is conformational and reversible; it leads to a strong acceleration of the rate of inhibition of procoagulant serine-proteases Thus, in a purified

medium, a heparin with high affinity for ATIII and constituted of 26 osidic units leads to an acceleration of inhibition of 650 times and 4400 times towards Factor Xa and Factor IIa respectively [26]. ATIII, being an enzyme inhibitor and also being susceptible to activation is consequently a multi- functional protein. It is justified to ask whether this protein is also multi-domanial. We will consider successively:

* the enzymatic reactions of inhitibion or serine-proteases,
* ATIII slow inhibitory capability when in native form,
* the enhancement of this inhibition capability towards Factor Xa and thrombin by heparin and by one of its synthetic active fragments, a specific pentasaccharide,
* recent results on the conformation of ATIII.

We will firstly summarize some basic data on the inhibitor/serine-protease mechanism of interaction [3]. The three dimensional structure of the active site of serine-proteases is highly specific; it possesses a pocket essential for this interaction and consequently for the inhibition of proteases. Serine-protease inhibitors, belonging to the family of serpins, have also a very specific structure, that is a loop also situated into their reactive center. When the inhibitor interacts with the enzyme its loop fits well into the serine-protease pocket. This mode of interaction between an inhibitor and a serine-protease is now denominated "canonical" (Figure 2a); in contrast with other types of protease inhibitors, other modes of interaction, recently described, particularly that of hirudin with thrombin, were denominated "non canonical".

Serine-protease inhibitors act as a trap-substrate: they block the access of the substrates to the active site of the enzyme and thus prevent the subsequent specific lysis of them [16].

Let us consider the enhancement of the native ATIII inhibition towards Factor Xa by heparin. This enhancement is performed through a two steps reaction [20] mediated by heparin molecules having a high affinity for ATIII [24]. The heparin binding region to ATIII was identified as a unique pentasaccharide sequence [7, 27]. The corresponding pentasaccharide (Ps1: D-E-F-G-H) has been synthesized [8, 21] (Figure 1).

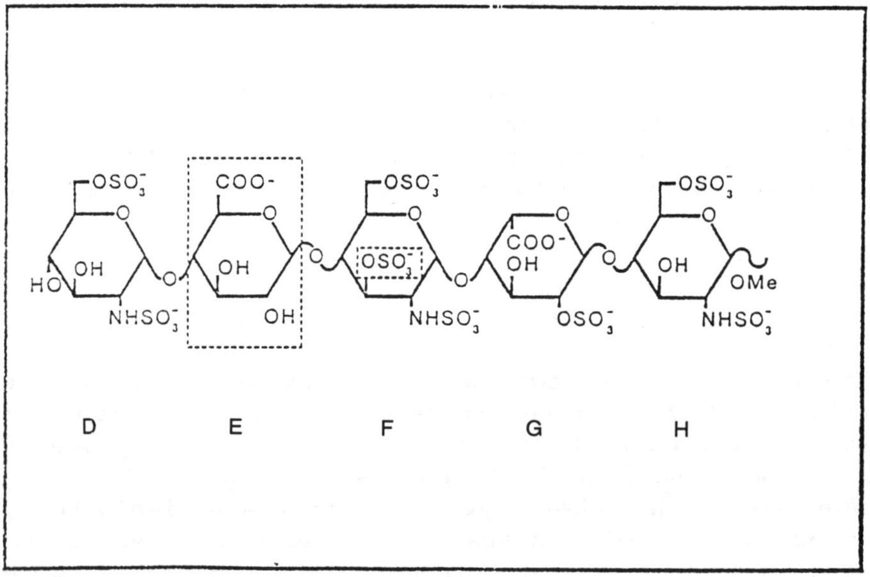

Figure 1: Pentasaccharide Ps1 and its structural irregularities.

The pentasaccharide Ps1 has the following structure: GlcNSO3-6-OSO3-(1--->4)-GlcA-(1--->4)-GlcNSO3- 3,6-di-OSO3-(1--->4)-IdoA-2-OSO3-(1--->4)-GlcN SO3-6-OSO3-1-OMe.

Ps1 possesses two irregularities compared to the major structure of heparin molecules: unit E is a non sulfated D-glucuronic acid and unit F is a trisulfated glucosamine containing in particular a sulfate group on carbon 3.
The properties of this molecule are the following:
- Ps1 binds to ATIII with a high affinity, forming with this protein a reversible complex.
- Ps1 induces in this protein a conformational change.
- Ps1 induces an acceleration of the inhibition of ATIII towards Factor Xa approximately 300-fold.

The structural and functional requirements of the synthetic pentasaccharide and consequently of the synthetic pentasaccharide sequence are well established [1, 5]. The properties of Ps1 can be explained by the formation of the binary complex Ps1-ATIII (Figure 2 c1, c2).

This latter can be considered as a ligand/receptor complex in which Ps1 is the ligand and ATIII the receptor [6]; in this complex, the protein, that is the receptor, is transconformed. In addition, the formation of the complex is independent of the ionic strength [26]. It was hypothesized that in this complex, the active site of ATIII undergoes a conformational change. This conformational change would probably lead to a reshaping of the active center of the inhibitor leading to the canonical mode of interaction and subsequently the formation of a Ps1-SP derivative [11]. It can be hypothesized that the active center of the non activated native inhibitor ATIII has not the capability to have the adequate canonical mode of interaction with Factor Xa; in the absence of heparin or pentasaccharide (Figure 2b), we propose to denominate pre-canonical "this mode of interaction".

The discovery of the conformation of the pentasaccharide Ps1 D-E-F-G-H has allowed to study the mechanism of the pentasaccharide/ ATIII interaction at the molecular level.

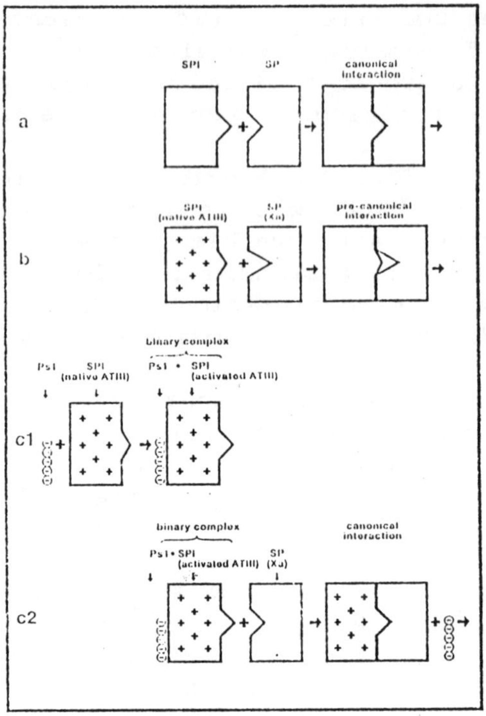

Figure 2: Simplified representation of the pentasaccharide Ps1-ATIII binary complex formation

a. Canonical serine-protease/serine-protease inhibitor interaction: the loop of the serine-protease inhibitor (SPI) is perfectly adapted to the pocket of the serine-proteases (SP).

b. "Pre-canonical" native ATIII/Factor Xa interaction: the loop is not perfectly adapted to the pocket and subsequently the rate of inhibition is slow.

c1. Activation of ATIII by pentasaccharide: the pentasaccharide (and the pentasaccharide sequence in heparin) causes a conformational change in ATIII.

c2. Pentasaccharide-ATIII complex; its interaction with Factor Xa; the loop of the transconformed ATIII is perfectly adapted to Factor Xa; its rate of inhibition by ATIII is greatly enhanced.

Thus, this conformation proves that the iduronic acid residue G exists in the form of two conformers. This characteristic generates a flexible structure for the residues G-H in opposition to the rigid structure for the residues D-E-F [23]. The structure and the function of these two sub-domains are the followings [22] (figure 3):

- the rigid D-E-F sub-domain: it is a zone of recognition of ATIII. It has an affinity for this protein, but it induces practically no biological activity.

- the flexible G-H sub-domain: when linked to the D-E-F trisaccharidic sequence. It is a zone of activation of ATIII:

* the residue G induces a liminal activity as it is shown by the activity of the tetrasaccharide D-E-F-G.

* the residues G-H, together, induce a critical biological activation as it is shown by the activity of the pentasaccharide Ps1 (D-E-F-G-H).

Structural and functional differences between these two sub-domains are in agreement with a two-step reaction for the interaction between pentasaccharide Ps1 and ATIII.

Heparin molecules larger than the pentasaccharide sequence, but containing it, have practically the three same properties as the pentasaccharide Ps1. Thus, the KD of the binding of pentasaccharide and heparin is practically the same. The variation of the fluorescence of ATIII, when bound to the pentasaccharide Ps1 and to heparin, is similar. However the acceleration of the inhibition of ATIII towards Factor Xa by heparin molecules is slightly increasing with the molecular weight of the molecules [10]; for instance, the enhancing activity of molecules containing 26 osidic units are twice that of the pentasaccharide Ps1 [26].

Let us consider the acceleration of the ATIII inhibition of thrombin by heparin and its fragments. This inhibition depends on two factors. The first is the binding of ATIII to heparin through the pentasaccharidic sequence

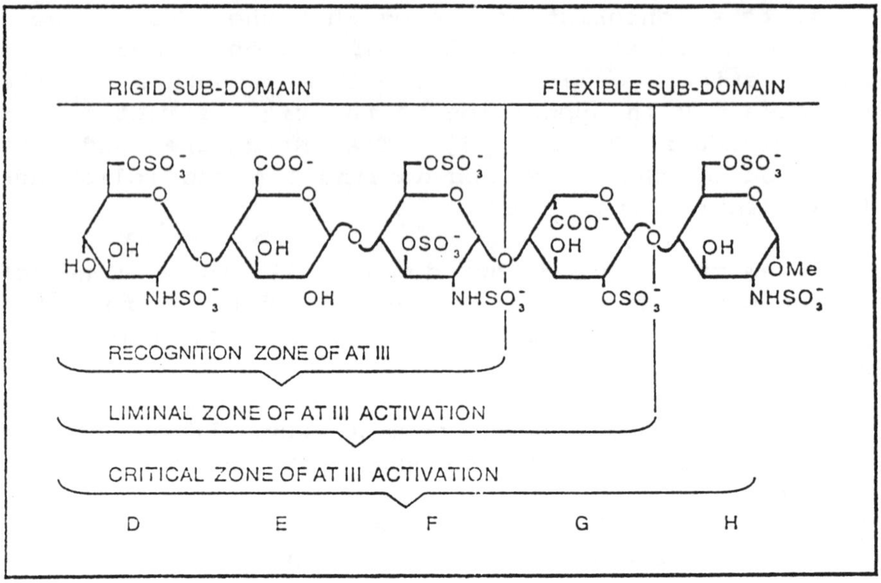

Figure 3: Structure and activity of pentasaccharide sub-domains

D-E-F-G-H. Thus, heparin molecules lacking this sequence have a weak affinity for ATIII and do not have the capability to accelerate the inhibition of thrombin by this protein.The second factor is the length of the heparin molecules [24]. Thus, in addition to the pentasaccharidic sequence, heparin molecules must possess at least 13 osidic units, that is on a whole at least 18 osidic units, to accelerate the ATIII inhibition of thrombin. It is the reason why the pentasaccharide Ps1 does not enhance the inhibition of thrombin by ATIII.

Heparin molecules, possessing the pentasaccharide sequence D-E-F-G-H plus 13 or more osidic units, have the following properties:

- they bind to ATIII, forming with this protein a reversible complex,
- they induce a conformational change in ATIII,
- they enhance the inhibitory activity of ATIII towards Factor Xa,

- they enhance the inhibitory activity of ATIII towards thrombin.

These properties can be explained by the existence of a temporary ternary complex, heparin-ATIII-Thrombin (Figure 4c). This complex would be formed following two different types of binary complexes: the binding of heparin to ATIII, due to the specific pentasaccharide sequence (Figure 4a) and the binding of heparin to thrombin [19] (Figure 4b), the requirements of which are presently poorly known with the exception of the length of the heparin molecules. The inhibitory activity of ATIII increases with the increasing length of the heparin molecule. In the ternary complex, the binding

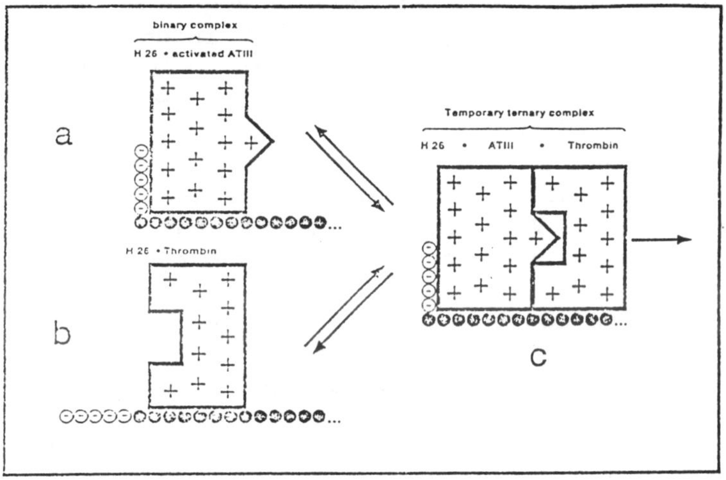

Figure 4: Schematic and partial representation of the heparin-ATIII-thrombin ternary complex formation

a. Binary complex heparin-ATIII.
b. Binary complex heparin-thrombin.
c. Ternary complex heparin-ATIII-thrombin; the formation of the binary complexes lead to the ternary temporary complex in which an approximation effect exists between positively charged ATIII and positively charged thrombin.

of heparin to thrombin would induce an approximation of thrombin and of its inhibitor ATIII, the latter acting in agreement with the canonical mode of interaction. The ternary complex leads to a covalent derivative while heparin is liberated.

Thus it is clear that the sole binding of the pentasaccharide sequence and the subsequent transconformation of ATIII are not able to induce the acceleration of thrombin inhibition. Another reaction is necessary, namely an approximation, following the heparin-thrombin binding. As a consequence, the positively charged thrombin can approximate the positively charged ATIII. The approximation effect can clearly be distinguished from the Ps1/ATIII binding. Thus, it is dependent on the ionic strength [26].

The question raised is to determine whether the binding of the pentasaccharide sequence with ATIII together with the approximation, induced by larger heparin molecules, of thrombin and ATIII are solely responsible for the acceleration of the inhibition of thrombin without the contribution of the conformational change of the active site, or whether this conformational change, essential for the inhibition of Factor Xa, contributes also to the acceleration of the inhibition of thrombin by ATIII.

Let us come now to the conformation of ATIII, of the pentasaccharide Ps1 and of the complex they form. We have in our possession four groups of data:

- The discovery of pathological variants of ATIII in patients bearing hereditary thromboembolic diseases.

A number of mutations at the molecular level were described in the ATIII structure of these patients [15]. Mutations taken here in consideration concern the ATIII binding to heparin (type IIc). They concern in particular Isoleucine 7, Proline 41, Arginine 47, located at the N-terminal end of the protein. Moreover, chemical reactions blocking the binding to heparin were described in particular for Lysines 107, 114, 125, 136 and Tryptophane 49. These localisations, at the N-terminal end, are in favour of a multi-domanial structure for ATIII.

- The discovery of the tridimensional conformation of the pentasaccharide Ps1.

This conformation was established together with force field calculation and High Field Nuclear Magnetic Resonance Spectroscopy [23].

- Modelizations realized from the tridimensional structure of the cleaved α1-antitrypsin.

From these data a modelization of the pentasaccharide/ATIII interaction has been proposed. A number of convergences between essential functional groups of the ATIII and pentasaccharide Ps1 have been shown [12].

- The cristallization of the cleaved ATIII and its analysis by X-ray diffraction.

The actual tridimensional structure of the cleaved ATIII has been described [9, 25], in particular the distribution and the orientation of alpha helix and beta sheets. This tridimensional structure is the basis to achieve a data dependent visualization of the conformation of native ATIII and of the activation of this protein by the pentasaccharide. This programme is further being carried out.

Conclusion

ATIII, in its native form, appears as a non mature protein with a limited biological activity.

ATIII comes to maturation by a conformational reversible change when engaged in a stoechiometric complex with heparin molecules having high affinity for ATIII.

Thus, this protein can be considered as a soluble activable receptor. In these molecules, the heparin binding site to ATIII is a pentasaccharide sequence. The synthetic corresponding pentasaccharide acts as a chemically pure ligand to ATIII. It is an activator of a serine-proteases inhibitor.

The conformational change is sufficient to obtain the enhancement of its inhibitory activity towards neutral enzymes as Factor Xa. It is insufficient to obtain the enhancement of its inhibitory activity towards positively charged enzymes like thrombin.

Another effect, an approximation, is necessary to obtain this enhancement of the activity. It depends on heparin molecules having the specific pentasaccharide sequence together with a minimum of 13 osidic units.

The tri-dimensional visualization of these two reactions is being elucidated. Apart from its theoretical value, this research will give a basic issue for the rational computerized design of new synthetic antithrombic drugs.

REFERENCES

1. ATHA DH, LORMEAU JC, PETITOU M, ROSENBERG RD, CHOAY J. Contribution of monosaccharide residues in heparin binding to antithrombin III. Biochemistry 24, 6723-6729, 1985.

2. BJORK I, OLSON ST, SHORE JD. Molecular mechanisms of the accelerating effect of heparin on the reactions between antithrombin and clotting proteinases. In: Lane DA & Lindahl U (Eds). Heparin: Chemical and biological properties, clinical applications. Edward Arnold, Ltd, London pp 229-255, 1989.

3. BODE W, HUBER R. Ligand binding: proteinase-protein inhibitor interactions. Curr Opin Structur Biol 45-52, 1991.

4. CASU B. Structure and biological activity of heparin. In: Advances in carbohydrate and biochemistry. Academic Press Inc., 43, 51-134, 1985.

5. CHOAY J. Chemically synthesized heparin derived oligosaccharides. Ann NY Acad Sci USA 556, 61-74, 1989.

6. CHOAY J. Structure and activity of heparin and its fragments: an overview. Semin Thromb Hemostas 15(4), 359-364, 1989.

7. CHOAY J, LORMEAU JC, PETITOU M, SINAY P, FAREED J. Structural studies on a biologically active hexasaccharide obtained from heparin. Ann NY Acad Sci USA 370, 644-649, 1981.

8. CHOAY J, PETITOU M, LORMEAU JC, SINAY P, CASU B, GATTI G. Structure-activity relationship in heparin: a synthetic pentasaccharide with high affinity for antithrombin III and eliciting high antifactor Xa activity. Biochem Biophys Res Commun 116, 492-499, 1983.

9. DELARUE M, SAMAMA JP, MOUREY L, MORAS D. Crystal structure of bovine antithrombin III. Acta Cryst B46, 550-556, 1990.

10. ELLIS V, SCULLY MF, KAKKAR VV. The relative molecular mass dependence of the anti-factor Xa properties of heparin. Biochem J 238, 329-333, 1986.

11. EVANS DLI, CARRELL RW. Heparin activation of antithrombin. International symposium on heparin and related polysaccharides. Uppsala, September 1-6, (Abstr. 24), 1991.

12. GROOTENHUIS PDJ, VAN BOECKEL CAA. Constructing a molecular model of the interaction between antithrombin III and a potent heparin analogue. J Am Chem Soc 113, 2743-2747, 1991.

13. HIRSCH J, LEVINE MN. Low molecular weight heparin. Blood 79, 1-17, 1992.

14. KAKKAR VV, SPINDLER J, FLUTE PT, CORRIGAN T, FOSSARD DP, CRELLIN RQ, WESSLER S, YIN ET. Efficacy of low doses of heparin in

prevention of deep-vein thrombosis after major surgery. Lancet 101-106, 1972.

15. LANE DA, IRELAND H, OLDS RJ, THEIN SL, PERRY DJ, AIACH M. Antithrombin III: a database of mutations. Thromb Haemost 66(6), 657-661, 1991.

16. LASKOWSKI M Jr, KATO I. Protein inhibitors of proteinases. Ann Rev Biochem 49, 593-626, 1980.

17. MEJDOUB H, LE RET M, BOULANGER Y, MAMAN M, CHOAY J, REINBOLT J. The complete amino acid sequence of bovine antithrombin (ATIII). J. Protein Chem 10(2), 205-212, 1991.

18. MOUREY L, SAMAMA JP, DELARUE M, CHOAY J, LORMEAU JC, PETITOU M, MORAS D. Antithrombin III: structural and functional aspects. Biochimie 72, 599-608, 1990.

19. OLSON ST, BJORK I. Predominant contribution of surface approximation to the mechanism of heparin acceleration of the antithrombin thrombin reaction. J Biol Chem 226(10), 6353-6364, 1991.

20. OLSON ST, SHORE JD. Demonstration of a two-step reaction mechanism for inhibition of α-thrombin by antithrombin III and identification of the step affected by heparin. J Biol Chem 257, 14891-14895, 1982.

21. PETITOU M. Chemical synthesis of heparin. In: Lane DA & Lindahl U (Eds). Heparin: chemical and biological properties, clinical applications. Edward Arnold, Ltd, London, pp 65-79, 1989.

22. PETITOU M, LORMEAU JC, CHOAY J. Interaction of heparin and antithrombin III: the role of O-sulfate groups. Eur J Biochem 176, 637-640, 1988.

23. RAGAZZI A, FERRO DR, PERLY B, TORRI G, CASU B, SINAY P, PETITOU M, CHOAY J. Conformation of the pentasaccharide corresponding to the binding site of heparin to antithrombin III. Carbohydr Res 165, C1-C5, 1987.

24. ROSENBERG RD. The heparin-antithrombin system: a natural anticoagulant mechanism. In: Lippincott JB (Ed). Hemostasis and thrombosis: basic principles and clinical practice. Colman RW et al Philadelphia, Chap. 91, pp 1373-1392, 1987.

25. SAMAMA JP, DELARUE M, MOUREY L, CHOAY J, MORAS D. Crystallization and preliminary crystallographic data for bovine antithrombin III. J Mol Biol 210, 877-879, 1989.

26. SHORE JD, OLSON ST, CRAIG PA, CHOAY J, BJORK I. Kinetics of heparin action. Ann NY Acad Sci USA 556, 75-80, 1989.

27. THUNBERG L, BACKSTROM G, LINDAHL U. Further characterization of the antithrombin-binding sequence in heparin. Carbohydr Res 100, 393-410, 1982.

6

Antithrombotic potential of the medicinal leech saliva

I.P. Baskova

The medicinal leech therapy (hirudo-therapy or leeching) is one of the oldest methods of many diseases treatment [23].

The therapeutic effect of the leeching is depended on the leech salivary gland secretion, which is injected into human organism during a leech bite through the skin and keeps going in during the period of bloodletting.

Secretion blocks the appearance of hemostatic thrombus in the damaged part of the vascular wall, putting into operation the optimum mechanisms in inhibiting platelet- vascular and plasmic hemostasis of man and vertebrate animals. These mechanisms have been elaborated during evolution as a result of adaptation to nutrition by the blood of vertebrate animals.

These mechanisms, as mirror reflexion, show the phenomena which occur as natural protective reaction of the organism to the loss of blood. Natural inhibitors of hemostasis secreted by the medicinal leech are the basis for the creation of novel efficient medicines. One of them is hirudin, thrombin enzyme inhibitor, one of the components of the leech saliva discovered by Haycraft in 1884 and studied in details by Markwardt [19]. At present recombinant hirudin and its low molecular weight fragments are used as the most effective anticoagulants with antithrombotic properties [14].

Since hirudin thus far is the only sufficiently studied component of the leech salivary gland secretion, the opinion becomes firmly rooted that the inability of blood, sucked by the medicinal leech, to form the clot is due to inhibition of thrombin. Very often the concepts "hirudin" and "leech saliva" were used as synonyms.

The possibility of obtaining the leech salivary gland secretion entirely lacking antithrombin activity of hirudin [8] made it possible to uncouple this concept and demonstrate that the inability of blood sucked by the medicinal leech, to form the clot is primarily due to the inhibition of platelet-vascular hemostasis and the early stages of plasmic hemostasis.

1. Inhibition of vascular-platelet hemostasis

Collagens of vascular-wall subendothelium play a decisive role in the initiation of vascular-platelet hemostasis [21]. The investigation of the influence of the medicinal leech saliva on platelet adhesion to collagens was conducted using the model system elaborated by Latin et al [16].

The results demonstrate that native leech saliva diluted five-fold with saline independently of its hirudin antithrombin activity is the effective inhibitor of human platelet adhesion to collagens of different genetic types (I, III et IV) and to fibrilar collagen from calf skin representing highly active substrate for platelet adhesion. The general adhesion of platelets to these substrates is 85-87 % inhibited; the initial attachment of platelets to collagen is 70-80 % blocked, while the spreading out of platelets on collagens is entirely inhibited by secretion. The degree of inhibition does not depend on the type of collagen.

This action is undoubtedly determined by the high affinity for collagen of the components of the leech secretion, since both in the case of collagen substrates pretreated with secretion and without pretreatment, the high degree of inhibition of platelet adhesion is unchanged [9].

The leech saliva does not affect the change in the form of platelets and platelet aggregation. At the same time the secretion inhibits platelet aggregation stimulated by inducers, whose action is mediated by receptors on the platelet membrane (ADP, thrombin, stable prostaglandin endoperoxide analog U-46619) and by inducers whose action is not mediated by receptors (Ca^{2+}-ionophore A23187 and arachidonic acid).

The leech saliva inhibits platelet aggregation independently of its hirudin antithrombin activity; moreover, the degree of inhibition is proportional to the volume of secretion introduced. When thrombin is used as the inducer of aggregation, the same degree of inhibition is achieved with smaller volumes of secretion possessing hirudin antithrombin activity in comparison with secretion that does not contain this activity [9]. The leech saliva activates adenylate cyclase of platelet membrane. The active ingradient is a thermostable low molecular weight trypsin-insensitive component of the leech saliva. Its activation of adenylate cyclase requires the preservation of the native membrane structure, which indirectly indicates prostaglandin receptor-mediated mechanism of its action [9].

Using radioimmuoassay method we have revealed the ability of the leech saliva and its active ingradient to interact with antibodies to 6-keto-prostaglandin $F_{1\alpha}$ (7). It is likely that secretion component activating platelet membrane adenylate cyclase is actually a substance of prostanoid nature.

2. Inhibition of plasmic hemostasis

When vascular wall integrity is broken, plasmic hemostasis is also activated.

Stimulation of the intrinsic and extrinsic mechanisms of blood coagulation is an initial stage of this activation. We failed to find out the inhibition of extrinsic of alternative pathways of blood coagulation in the presence of salivary gland secretion deprived of hirudin antithrombin activity using the test of one-stage prothrombin time. The prolongation of this time is observed only in the presence of the secretion possessing hirudin antithrombin activity. But the content of hirudin in such secretion is of course insufficient to block thrombin which was generated in rat blood after intravenous injection of sub-lethal doses of tissue thromboplastin. The leech secretion, also injected intravenously, did not protect the animals from death [2]. Actually, only high doses of hirudin preparation prevent and block disseminated intravascular blood coagulation both in experiments and in clinics that is caused by the appearance of excessive quantities of thrombin in the blood [20].

We revealed the inhibition of the contact stage of blood coagulation on intrinsic pathway by the leech saliva deprived of hirudin antithrombin activity when determining the recalcification time of blood plasma activated by dextran-sulphate [2].

Since in the activation of this mechanism an important role is played by blood plasma kallikrein; we specially studied the influence of the leech saliva on the amidolytic and kininogenase activities of purified human plasma kallikrein. It has been shown that secretion, independently of its antithrombin activity, blocks amidolytic activity of the enzyme (substrate S-2302) and reduces kininogenase activity (bradikinin substrate) of kallikrein [1]. It means that the leech secretion blocks the contact stage of blood clotting by directly inhibiting blood plasma kallikrein.

Thus, the leech Hirudo medicinalis is the source not only of hirudins, bdellins and eglins [23], but also of blood plasma kallikrein inhibitor, representing a fourth type of inhibitors of the medicinal leech proteolytic enzymes.

The experimental data demonstrate that in hemostasis induced by injury of the vascular wall comparable with that being made by a leech bite, an exclusive role belongs to the activation of the intrinsic mechanism of blood coagulation. As to hirudin, it is likely to block small amounts of thrombin, which appear as a result of the activation of the extrinsic mechanism. The low content of hirudin in the leech saliva reflects the low level of the activation of blood coagulation extrinsic mechanism during hemostasis, while small injuries of the vascular wall take place. Mathematical modelling data on kinetics of the hemostatic system also speaks in favour of these results. The threshold for the activation of the intrinsic pathway of blood coagulation is 100 times lower than that of the extrinsic one and 10 times lower than the threshold for the activation of the alternative pathway [15].

3. The protective antithrombotic effect

In the course of pathologic thrombus formation practically the same mechanisms are involved as those which occur during the formation of hemostatic thrombus. Therefore the salivary gland secretion of the medicinal leeches has been successfully used for the prophylaxis of the vein thrombosis during experiments performed on rats. Vein thrombosis was stimulated by the method of Wessler in which the activation of the intrinsic mechanism of blood coagulation and vascular stasis were combined.

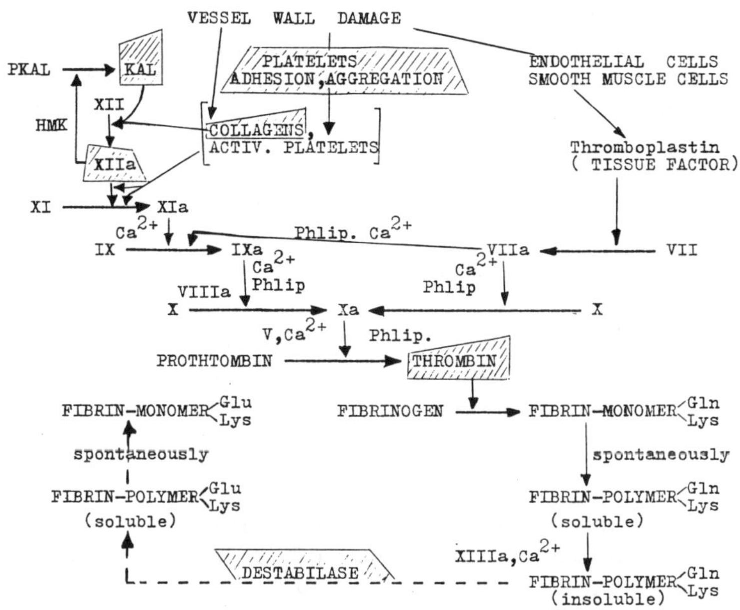

PKAL.- prekallikrein
KAL. - kallikrein
HMK - High molecular weight kininogen
Phlip. - phospholipids

Figure 1: Influence of the medicinal leech saliva on hemostasis (marked with hachures) and on stabilized cross-linked fibrin (marked with dotted lines).

The leech saliva irrespective of hirudin antithrombin activity had vividly expressed protective antithrombotic action when intravenously injected. The maximum antithrombotic effect is produced if the time period between injection of the secretion and stimulation of the thrombus formation does not exceed 4h. But even 28h later the level of thrombus formation is reduced by 40 % in comparison with the control data.

As the secretion action is directed to the inhibition of hemostasis at the stages preceding the thrombin formation (Figure 1), the secretion deprived of hirudin antithrombin activity is as active as that possessing such activity both intravenously injected and orally administered [22].

Antithrombotic action of the secretion is more profoundly pronounced in comparison with hirudin antithrombotic effect [18], which cannot be effective during oral administration.

4. Fibrinolytic action. Novel enzyme destabilase ε-(gama-Glu)-Lys-ISO- peptidase

In contrast to the known mechanisms of fibrinolysis as proteolytic degradation of fibrin by plasmin or other proteases, we have found in the medicinal leech salivary gland secretion an enzyme which we named DESTABILASE [6]. This enzyme turns insoluble stabilized fibrin into a soluble state by means of hydrolysis of ε-(gama-Glu)-Lys isopeptide bonds between selected side chains of fibrin molecules. These bonds are formed by the action of transpeptidase or factor XIIIa in the presence of Ca^{2+} from glutamine residue of one molecule of fibrin and the lysine residue of another one [17]. As a result of hydrolysis of isopeptide bonds by destabilase instead of the initial glutamine residues there are formed glutamic acid residues. This event is the key one leading to the liquifaction of fibrin caused by the spontaneous irreversible depolymerization of modified destabilized fibrin [3, 6].

Beside fibrin, D-D-dimer, a fragment of stabilized fibrin [24], isopeptide, gama-glutamyl-ε-lysine [11], as well as model analogues of isopeptide, chromogenic substrate L-gama-Glu-pNA [6, 10], are substrates of destabilase.

Semi-purified destabilase examined by SDS-PAGE showed three bands of molecular weight 12.300, 25.000 and 50.000 D, each fraction preserved amidolytic activity (substrate L-gama-Glu-pNA). After further purification it is possible to obtain a low molecular weight fraction of destabilase homogeneous on SDS-PAGE (Mr=12.3000).

Destabilase is not a simple protein. It contains a lipid component of mol. weight 390, which has cross-reactivity with antiserum to 6-keto-$PGF_{1\alpha}$. It is supposed that the lipoid component is prostanoid, which we detected in the leech saliva in the free state [7]. It is covalently bound to protein [3].

5. Thrombolytic action

Thrombolytic effect during leeching by Hirudo medicinalis is known from antiquity. Leeching of thrombophlebitis of various etiology described in many publications [23] is due to the salivary gland secretion of the leeches, but the mechanism of thrombus dissolving by secretion was unknown.

The leech saliva does not possess proteolytic activity, but is characterized by a high content of proteolytic enzyme inhibitors [8, 23]. Thrombolytic effect of the leech saliva is due to enzyme destabilase and leech prostanoids. The last ones in free state or as a component of destabilase are likely to take part in providing thrombolysis by releasing tissue plasminogen activator as prostacyclin and prostaglandin E_1 [13].

Destabilase stimulated thrombolysis in rats with induced jugular vein thrombus. 80-100 % thrombolysis was stimulated 70-100 hrs after i.v. injection or oral administration of destabilase. Prostanoid component provides protective antithrombotic effect of destabilase which was observed in experiments with rats that received i.v. injection of the enzyme [3]. Both thrombolytic and protective antithrombotic properties of the slowly acting enzyme suggest that destabilase may be favourably compared with the known thrombolytic agents.

The ability to penetrate from intestine into the blood is a particular property of destabilase. Due to the prostanoid prostetic group destabilase can partially transfer from aqueous solution into organic phase [3]. These properties permit to refer destabilase to micellar enzyme and explain its efficiency not only in intravenous, but also in oral administration to animals.

The above mentioned components of the leech saliva provide the thrombolytic properties of the extracts from the medicinal leech after intravenous injections and oral administrations to rats [5]. Proleolytic enzyme inhibitors, as components of these extracts [23] protect another biologically active substances from digestion in animal intestine.

6. Antiatherosclerotic action

In the mechanisms of initiation and development of atherosclerosis at initial stages of great importance are the composition and the level of lipoproteins of the blood plasma, the state of endothelium and proliferative activity of the vascular wall, as well as the level of activation of vascular-platelet and plasmic hemostasis. The above described properties of the leech secretion in combination with its ability to expose lipase and cholesterol-esterase activity [12] have permitted to assume that it has to show antiatherosclerotic effect too. Actually intravenous (daily, morning 7 days) injections of the leech saliva to rats reduced fibrinogen level and diminished lipid deposits in the intima of large vesicles from 20±2 % to 2.2±0.3 % in the thoracic aorta and from 4.8±5 % to 7±2 % ($p<0.01$) in the abdominal aorta. Long-term chronic oral administration of dried preparation which contained the leech salivary glands and their secretion to rats, kept on atherogenic diet, reduced the area of local edema in the intima of large vessels. The leech saliva reduced ^{3}H-thymidine incorporation into human atherosclerotic intimal cell culture [4].

7. Leech saliva as the source of potential medicines. Medicinal leech pharmacology

Obtained data destify that the leech saliva is a medicine produced by the Nature and that medicinal leech is like a syringe filled with medicine which possesses protective antithrombotic, thrombolytic, antiathero- sclerotic and other properties. Combined action of the secretion is adequate to that of a set of synthetic medicinal preparations used in the treatment of cardiovascular diseases. At the same time it is known that increasing the number of preparations simultaneously prescribed leads to an incerase of negative side effects as well. The leech secretion and the preparations containing it have neither acute nor chronic toxicity. The preparation "Piyavit" (Russian equivalent of "Leechit"), a powder for oral administration containing the salivary gland secretion has passed necessary pre-clinical tests and is admitted for clinical trials. The ability of "Payavit" to excert simultaneous protective antithrombotic, thrombolytic, antiatherosclerotic and hypotensive effects in oral administration distinguishes it positively from other well known pharmacological preparations. The leech saliva, real pharmacia, may be used for the preparation of medicines in different forms.

Biologically active isolated components of the leech saliva also have a brilliant future. The appearance of these preparations at the pharmaceutical market depends on successful solution of the problems of the medicinal leech biotechnology.

REFERENCES

1. BASKOVA IP, KHALIL S, NIKONOV GI, RABINOVICH SE, NARTIKOVA VF, PASKHINA TS. Inhibition of human blood plasma kallikrein by salivary gland secretion and an extract of the medicinal leech. Biokhimiya 53(9), 1277-1282, 1987.

2. BASKOVA IP, KHALIL S, NIKONOV GI. Influence of the salivary gland secretion of the medicinal leeches on extrinsic and intrinsic mechanisms of blood coagulation. Bul Exp Biol Med (USSR) 97, 142-143, 1984.

3. BASKOVA IP, NIKONOV GI. Destabilase, the novel ε-(gama-Glu)Lys isopeptidase with thrombolytic activity. Blood coagulation and Fibrinolysis 2, 167-172, 1991.

4. BASKOVA IP, NIKONOV GI, DOLGOV V, TERTOV VV, OREKHOV AN et al. The effect of medicinal leech preparations on atherogenesis. Cardiology (USSR) 29(5), 75-79, 1989.

5. BASKOVA IP, NIKONOV GI, KHALIL S. Thrombolytic agents of the preparation from the medicinal leeches. Folia Haematol 115(1-2), 166-170, 1988.

6. BASKOVA IP, NIKONOV GI. Destabilase - an enzyme of medicinal leech salivary gland secretion that hydrolyzes isopeptide bonds in stabilized fibrin. Biokhimiya 50 (3part1), 357-363, 1985.

7. BASKOVA IP, NIKONOV GI. Direction of prostanoids in some preparations from the medicinal leeches. Reports of Acad Sci of USSR, 292, 1492-1493, 1987.

8. BASKOVA IP, NIKONOV GI, CHERKESOVA DU. Antithrombin, antitrypsin and antichymotrypsin activities of the salivary gland secretion and intestinal chyme of medicinal leeches. Folia Haematol 111(6), 831-837, 1984.

9. BASKOVA IP, NIKONOV GI, MAZUROV AV, MISSELVITTS F, LEITIN VL, REPIN VS, AVDONIN PV, SVITINA-ULITINA IV. Mechanisms of the inhibition of vascular-platelet hemostasis by salivary gland secretion of the medicinal leech Hirudo medicinalis Biokhimia 52 (9part1), 1261-1267, 1987.

10. BASKOVA IP, NOKONOV GI, ZAVALOVA LL. Kinetics or L-gama-glu-pNA hydrolysis by destabilase form the medicinal leech Hirudo medicinalis. Biokhimiya 55, 1990.

11. BASKOVA IP, TIMOKHINA EA, NIKONOV GI, STEPANOV VM. Hydrolysis of the isopeptide ε-(gama-glutamyl)-lysine by destabilase from the medicinal leech. Biokhimiya 55 (5part2), 571-575, 1990.

12. BASKOVA IP, YUSUPOVA GI, NIKONOV GI. Lipase and cholesterolesterase activities of salivary gland secretion of the medicinal leech Hirudo medicinalis. Biokhimia 49(4), 676-678, 1984.

13. CRUTCHLEY DY, CONANON LB, MAYNARD YR. Stimulation of fibrinolytic activity of human skin fibroblasts by prostaglandins E_1, E_2, and I_2. J Pharm Exp Ther 222, 544-548, 1982.

14. FAREED Y, WALENGA YM, IYER L, HOPPENSTEADT D, PIFARRE R. Blood coagulation and fibrinolysis 2(1), 135-147, 1991.

15. KHANIN MA, BASKOVA IP, POPOV AF, SEMENOV VV. Threshold effects in blood coagulation. Thromb Res (In press).

16. LEITIN VL, LJUBIMOVA EV, SVIRIDOV DD, ZAKHAROVA OS, REPIN VS, SMIRNOV VN. Endothelial cell cultures on fibrillar collagen: partial reconstruction of the vessel wall and platelet adhesion. Thromb Res 20, 509-520, 1980.

17. LORAND L, CONRAD SM. Transglutaminases. Mol Cell Biochem 58, 9-35, 1984.

18. MARKWARDT F, HAUPTMANN Y, NOWAK G, KLESSEN C, WALSMANN P. Pharmacological studies on the antithrombotic action of hirudin in experimental animals. Thromb Haemost 47, 226-229, 1982.

19. MARKWARDT F. Pharmacology of hirudin: one hundred years after the first report of an anticoagulant agent in medicinal leeches. Biomed Biochim Acta 44, 1007-1013, 1985.

20. MARKWARDT F, NOWAK G, STURZEBECHER J, GRIESSBACH U, WALSMANN P, VOGEL G. Pharmacokinetics and anticoagulant activity of hirudin in men. Thromb Haemost 52, 160-163, 1984.

21. NIEVELSTEIN PF, DE GROOT PG. Interaction of blood platelets with the vessel wall. Haemostasis 18, 342-359, 1988.

22. NIKONOV GI, BASKOVA IP. Antithrombotic effect of the preparations from the leeches Hirudo medicinalis. Folia Haematol 115, (1-2), 47-51, 1988.

23. SAYWER RT. Leech biology and behaviour. Oxford University Press, 1986.

24. ZAVALOVA LL, NIKONOV GI, KUZINA EV, POPOVA GYu, BASKOVA IP. The stabilized fibrin fragment D-dimer a substrate for destabilase (gama-glutamyl-ε-lysyl-isopeptidase).Biokhimiya 56(1), 115-124, 1991.

7

Hirudin and hirudin fragments form the basis of new antithrombotics and anticoagulants

J. Di Maio

Heart disease remains the chief cause of morbidity and mortality in the western world accounting for almost 40 % of deaths in the US alone. Current cardiovascular drugs adequately address the usual risk factors such as hypertension and hypercholesterolemia, but plasma proteins participating in haemostasis have emerged as equally important risk considerations in vascular and cerebrovascular disorders [6, 41]. Haemostasis is controlled by an intricate web of finely tuned reactions in the blood coagulation cascade and fibrinolytic system [13, 25]. The former is brised towards negative regulation, requiring a number of zymogen to enzyme activation steps either through the intrinsic or extrinsic pathway, the latter being initiated by exposure of tissue factor to blood (Figure 1).

Accordingly, the blood coagulation cascade has evolved to respond rapidly and explosively to vascular injury. This process is manifest by highly localized reactions on membrane surfaces [25, 31], recruitment of platelets to the thrombogenic site [1] and positive feed back amplification through enzymatic activation of required cofactors [47]. However, aberrations to the normal haemostatic process leads to indications of thrombotic disorders such as coronary artery disease, cerebrovascular disease, arterial or deep vein

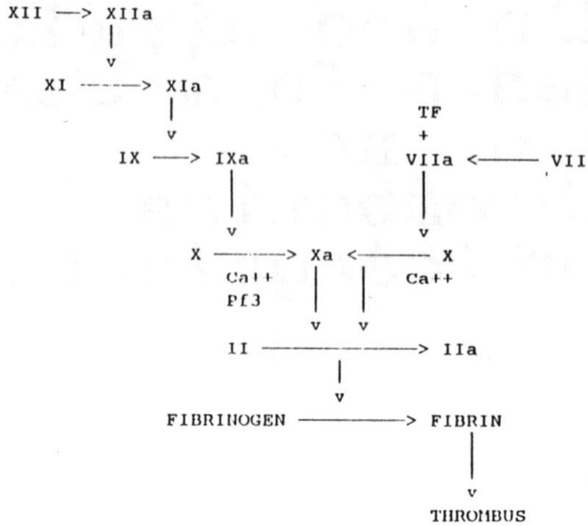

Figure 1: Enzymatic activation steps in the coagulation cascade

deep vein thrombosis and pulmonary embolism which may require therapy with a number of current antithrombotic drugs of fibrinolytic enzymes [3].

Heparin is the most widely used antithrombotic and anticoagulant drug. Mechanistically, heparin owes its therapeutic efficacy to its ability to interact with antithrombin III (ATIII) and thereby enhancing the neutralizing rate of this endogenous proteinase inhibitor by several orders of magnitude [17]. ATIII belongs to the serpin superfamily of proteinase inhibitors but does not exhibit significant selectivity toward its target proteinases [44]; its complexation with heparin potentiates the inhibition of thrombin, Factor Xa as well as other enzymes higher in the cascade.

This indiscriminant property, together with heparin's polydisperse chemical composition (Mr 6.000-40.000, Mr (av) 14.000) [23] may be viewed as contradictory to current regulatory requirements for chemically and enantiomerically homogeneous therapeutic substances that interact with a single well defined macromolecular target. This deficiency has been recognized and has stimulated efforts aimed at identifying the active pharmacophore in heparin [5]. Accordingly, size fractionation by gel filtration and controlled chemical or enzymatic depolymerization have provided low molecular weight preparations with enhanced Factor Xa/Factor IIa selectivity and improved pharmacokinetic properties [22]. There have also been major advances in the chemical synthesis of short oligosaccharide fragments that have successfully defined the core sequence responsible for binding to ATIII and catalyzing the neutralization of Factor Xa, but not thrombin [35]. However it remains to be seen whether the necessary synthetic methods become commercially viable.

Notwithstanding the potential for complications associated with anticoagulant therapy using heparin, its principal mode of action mediated by ATIII provides an efficient measure of therapeutic benefit, especially in venous thrombosis.

1. Protein anticoagulants

1.1 Hirudin and hirudin fragments

Blood sucking animals secrete a plethora of proteinaceous molecules that affect the host's haemostatic process by interfering with discrete biochemical events [38]. Notable among the proteins that have been isolated, and in some cases sequenced, is hirudin from the leech Hirudo Medicinalis (Figure 2).

Hirudin has been known for approximately 100 years, having been recognized by Alexander Haycraft as the active anticoagulant agent in leech secretions [16]. However, the pioneering work of Markwardt and his colleagues resulted in the identification of hirudin as a protein and established its property as an inhibitor of thrombin [28, 30].

This finding is fortuitous in relation to anticoagulant therapy since thrombin plays a critical role as a procoagulant enzyme and mediates feedback amplification of its action through activation of the required cofactors V and VIII, as well as the fibrin transpeptidase Factor XIII [47].

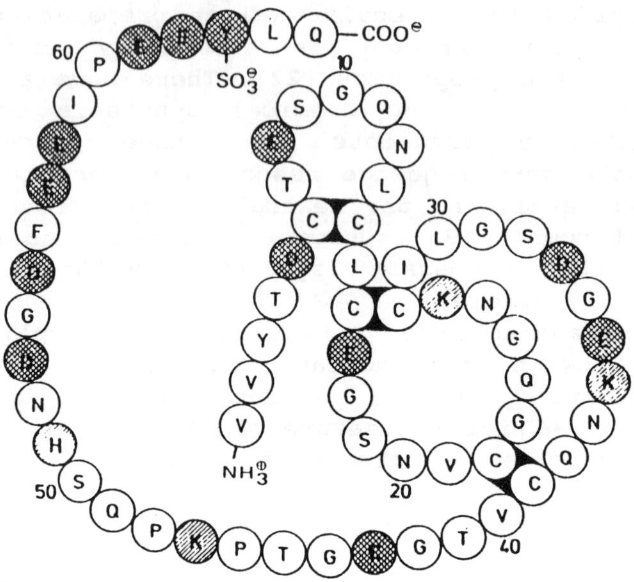

Figure 2: Primary and secondary structure of Hirudin variant HV-1.

In addition, thrombin exhibits receptor mediated platelet activation and exerts secretory activity on endothelial cells [36, 45]. These multiple functions make thrombin an attractive target for therapeutic intervention.

Hirudin is a family of isoproteins that binds to thrombin with exceedingly high affinity with reported dissociation constants in the order of 10^{-10} to 10^{-14}M [11, 42]. Using recombinant hirudin variant 2 (HV-2), association and dissociation rate constant of $1.9\pm0.2\mathrm{X}10^{8}\mathrm{M}^{-1}\mathrm{sec}^{-1}$ and $5.3\pm1.4\mathrm{X}10^{-4}\mathrm{sec}^{-1}$ respectively have been determined, having a corresponding $K_I=0.28\pm0.07$pM for human α-thrombin [10]. In agreement with previously reported isoforms, this recombinant hirudin variant lacking the typical sulfate group on the Tyr^{63} residue, belongs to the class of slow tight-binding inhibitors in accordance with the nomenclature of Morrison et al. [40]. The observed kinetics of inhibition have been previously ascribed to a propable two-step mechanism implicating an initial interaction with a high affinity site followed by a conformational change and binding to a lower affinity site.

Expectedly, one would attribute the high affinity and specificity observed for hirudin or r-hirudin toward thrombin to cumulative interactions of the inhibitor with multiple remote regions on the enzyme surface. The primary structure of hirudin indicates that it is highly acidic protein with a large content of carboxylate groups concentrated within the C-terminal tail of the protein. This observation was similar to the finding that COOH terminal fragments of hirudin comprising at least residues Asp^{55} to Leu^{64} inhibit the clotting activity of the enzyme [20] by blocking an auxiliary "anionic exosite" which is rich in basic residues and is predisposed to bind the natural thrombin substrate, fibrinogen [4]. However these same fragments, including the longer forms such as hirudin 45-65, have been reported not to inhibit the amidolytic activity of α-thrombin toward small synthetic substrates [19]. Accordingly, the functional elements of hirudin responsible for binding to the catalytic site or the putative apolar fibrinogen groove have remained conjecture until recently.

In order to use hirudin as a point of departure for the design of low molecular weight inhibitors that utilize similar primary and accessory binding loci it would be desireable to have a clear understanding of the functional domains responsible for binding, as well as the geometrical organization of the individual recognition elements when bound to the macromolecular target. Site directed mutagenesis of lysine residues were shown to have no deleterious effect on the inhibitory dissociation constant suggesting that hirudin is an atypical inhibitor of thrombin which, as a serine proteinase with trypsin specificity, would require a basic side chain within the specificy pocket. On the other hand the mutation of the N-terminal Val^1, Val^2, Tyr^3 or simple acetylation of the terminal primary amino group resulted in a significant loss in binding energy indicating a functional role for a limited number of residues located in the extreme N-terminal end of the molecule [2, 46].

The solution conformation of r-desulfato hirudin and the mutant Lys^{47}->Glu were independently solved by H^1 NMR spectroscopy [12, 15]. These findings indicated a well-defined disulfide core comprising residues 3-30 and 37-48 which forms two antiparallel ß-sheets and reverse turns. No preferred conformation could be ascribed to either exposed loop residues 31-36 or the C-terminal domain 49-65.

Seemingly contrary to the above NMR results, structure-function relationship studies of fragments corresponding to the COOH-terminal tail of hirudin have identified stringent molecular features required to maintain antithrombin activity [20, 21, 34]. From these combined studies an amphiphilic α-helix conformation was proposed with hydrophobic residues Phe^{56}, Ile^{59}, Tyr^{63} and Leu^{64} on one side and hydrophilic residues Asp^{55}, Glu^{57}, Glu^{58}, Glu^{61} and Glu^{62} on the other. Indeed an NMR study of fragments $Hirudin^{52-65}$ and $Acetyl\text{-}Hirudin^{55-65}$ in the presence of thrombin corroborated the importance of the hydrophobic side chains as evidenced by the observation of selective line broadening of the side chains of Phe^{56}, Ile^{59}, Tyr^{63}, and Leu^{64}. This effect, together with the identification of short and medium-range transferred NOEs implicated a well-defined conformation characterized by a hydrophobic (greasy) cluster involving principally the residues Phe^{56}, Ile^{59} and Leu^{64} which can insert in a complementary surface on the enzyme [48]. The positioning of the side chain of Leu^{64} adjacent to Ile^{59} results from a reverse turn centered in the last five residues.

On the other hand the hydrophilic cluster of carboxylates are exposed to solvent [33]. The assembly of this information suggests that the term "anionic exosite" may in fact be a misnomer.

In an exhaustive SAR study of COOH-terminal fragments, Krstenansky et al. [18] arrived at the same conclusion and identified MDL 28050, a modified decapeptide that binds to the putative anion exosite of human thrombin and inhibits fibrinogen clotting with an IC_{50} of 29 nM.

It is interesting to note that prothrombin time of normal human plasma is more sensitive to inhibition by hirudin peptides than plasma from other species and that this effect can be ascribed to the thrombin "anion" exosite. Using synthetic $hirudin^{53-64}$ and thrombins from various species, Maraganore et al. [27] demonstrated that the murine and human enzyme were most affected while bovine α-thrombin was least responsive. These same authors attributed this observed difference to a single mutation corresponding to Lys149E (human) which is glutamic acid in bovine α-thrombin. Investigations using acetyl-hirudin$^{55-65}$ revealed that substitution of individual residues by glycine causes a parallel potency drop for both bovine and human α-thrombin within residues Asp-Phe-Glu-Glu [32].

However, removal of the side chains of Tyr^{63}, Leu^{64}, or Gln^{65} caused a 4 to 25 fold drop in inhibitory potency against bovine thrombin but only 2 to 6 fold for human thrombin. Accordingly, the greater sensitivity of human α-thrombin to hirudin COOH terminal fragments cannot be ascribed to a single amino acid mutation, but to more salient differences within the exosite of the two enzymes.

Using this lead observation, internally deleted analogs of N-acetyl hirudin55-65 have been synthesized. These truncated analogs retained the pendant leucine residue judged to be important for formation of the hydrophobic cluster (vide supra) with Phe^{56} and Ile^{59}. The IC_{50} values for fibrinogen clotting time are shown in Table I.

Table I : Inhibition of thrombin-mediated fibrin clot formation by C-terminal deleted hirudin fragments.

Peptide		IC_{50} μM*	
		Bovine	Human
P24	Ac-D-F-E-E-I-P-E-E-Y-L-Q	4.8 ± 1.2	1.2 ± 0.2
P45	Ac-D-F-E-E-I-P-E-E-Y-L	9.0 ± 1.8	1.5 ± 0.1
P46	Ac-D-F-E-E-I-P-E-E-L	56 ± 10	25 ± 3
P47	Ac-D-F-E-E-I-P-E-L	90 ± 10	32 ± 4
P48	Ac-D-F-E-E-I-P-L	145 ± 6	50 ± 8
P49	Ac-D-F-E-E-I-L	>400	>200
P50	Ac-D-F-E-P-I-P-L	—	20 ± 3

* Mean of three determinations ± SEM

The results demonstrate that the divergent inhibitory activity observed with glycine substitutions on the native fragment (P24) was not conserved in the internally deleted series since the IC_{50} value increased 40 fold against human thrombin and 30 times for the bovine isozyme.(compare P24 & P48). However, P48 (ac-Asp-Phe-Glu-Glu-Ile-Pro-LeuOH) still has a sufficiently low IC_{50} value which could be enhanced to 20 μM upon insertion of a proline residue in position 58, analogous to the reported hirudin PA sequence [48]. It remains to be seen whether this minimal peptide segment could be manipulated into a peptidomimetic with an enhanced level of potency. But the exercise demonstrates that while both hydrophobic and ionic interactions are required for optimum binding, they are restricted to a narrow region of these inhibitors.

1.2. Bifunctional thrombin inhibitors

During the course of our laboratory's investigations on hirudin peptides, it was noted that the hirudin fragment corresponding to hirudin45-65 inhibited, albeit weakly, the thrombin-mediated proteolysis of the substrate Tos-Gly-Pro-Arg-X (where X is p-nitrophenyl or 7-amino-4-methylcoumarin). This observation is at variance with previous reports which concluded that this peptide inhibited fibrin clot formation but not the amidolytic activity toward small thrombin substrates. The explanation resided in the unexpected kinetic behaviour exemplified by the Dixon plot which showed hyperbolic reciprocal velocity with increasing inhibitor concentration. Subsequent detailed kinetic analysis suggested that the inhibition is partially competitive with respect to this substrate [9]. This conclusion has since been corroborated by other investigators [39].

Ac-Thr-Pro-Lys-Pro-Gln-Ser-His-Asn-Asp-Gly-Asp-Phe-Glu-Glu-Ile-Pro-Glu-Glu-Tyr-Leu-GlnOH

P51 $K_i=110\pm30$ nM

Ac-(D)Phe-Pro-Arg-Pro-Gln-Ser-His-Asn-Asp-Gly-Asp-Phe-Glu-Glu-Ile-Pro-Glu-Glu-Tyr-Leu-GlnOH

P53 $K_i=2.8\pm0.9$ nM

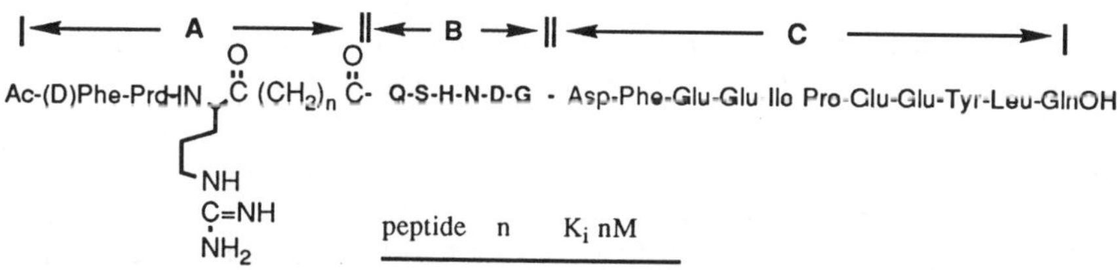

peptide	n	K_i nM
P109	1	3.8 $\pm$0.10
P79	2	0.37$\pm$0.03
P102	3	0.56$\pm$0.14
P103	4	0.14$\pm$0.02

Figure 3: Structures of bifunctional thrombin inhibitors derived from hirudin.

This observation was intrumental in the discovery of highly potent hirudin peptides that have been designated as bifunctional or bivalent thrombin inhibitors (Figure 3). The rationale for their design was that although the native hirudin 45-65 fragment had the essential recognition elements of the catalytic site, it lacked optimum primary specificity (Arg^{47}, P_1) and secondary recognition ($DPhe^{45}$, P_3) (Figure 3, compare P51 and P53). Therefore, the incorporation of thes two preferred structural elements enhanced affinity and altered the kinetic behaviour to competitive inhibition [8-10, 26].

Paradoxically, native hirudin is also a bifunctional inhibitor, but unlike the fragment hirudin45-65, mutagenesis of the analogous $lysine^{47}$ residue does not alter the affinity toward thrombin. Furthermore, in contrast to the hirudin peptide [$D-Phe^{45}$, Arg^{47}]hirudin45-65 (P53) which undergoes proteolysis between Arg^{47}-Pro^{48}, native hirudin is inert to thrombin activity. These various anomalies could be explained by the binding mode of hirudin to thrombin which has been unequivically established by X-ray crystallography [14, 37]. The complex between hirudin variant 1 or 2, shown schematically in Figure 6, revealed a number of distinctive interactions spread out across the surface of the enzyme.

As would be expected, hirudin interacts with both the "anion exosite" and the catalytic site of thrombin through its remote COOH and NH_2 terminal residues, respectively. The thrombin anion exosite is an auxiliary binding site that is unique to that enzyme. This region can bind a number of substrates or inhibitors including fibrinogen, thrombomodulin [43], hirudin [14, 37] and the extracellular domain of the thrombin platelet receptor [24]. The X-ray structure of the complex between hirudin and thrombin reveals that the amphiphilic property of the C-terminal tail of hirudin is the key feature responsible for mutual recognition. The crystal structure of this region is consistent with the bound conformation of the analogous peptide Asp^{55}-Gln^{65} determined by NMR.

Notable is that hydrophobic residues Phe^{56}, Ile^{59} and Leu^{64} form a contiguous hydrophobic surface directly in contact with the enzyme while the charged residues are exposed to solvent or make indirect electrostatic contacts with basic residues on the outer enzyme surface through intervening water molecules. Only the first three residues bind in the active site, and in a direction opposite to that of a normal substrate, with the S_1 specificity pocket unoccupied. The side chain of the putative reactive lys^{47} residue resides in the vicinity of the active site but serves only to stabilize the orientation of the NH_2 terminal backbone. Thus the deletion of the first 44 residues in the native protein (depicted by the molecular scissors in Figure 4) exposes the new recognition sequence (Thr-Pro-Lys-Pro) which is spatially aligned to fit in the active site and substitute for the native NH_2 terminal residues, albeit not as effectively.

The fibrinogenolytic activity of thrombin is confined to the N-terminal Arg^{16}-Gly^{17} bond of the A_α chain and the Arg^{14}-Gly^{15} bond of the B_β chain; in both cases the P_1' residue is glycine.

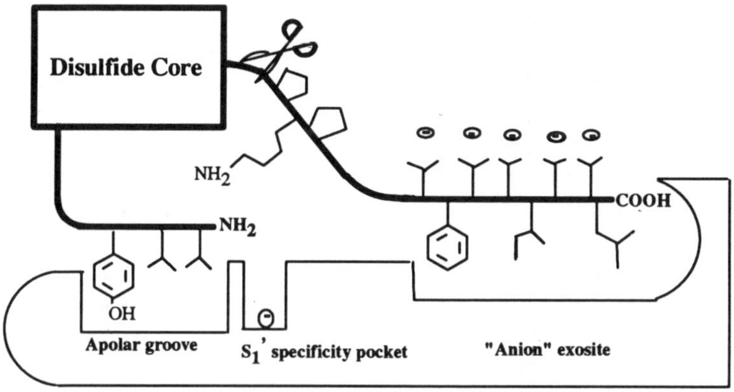

Figure 4 : Schematic diagram of the association of hirudin with thrombin in the active site and "anion exosite". Clipping the protein at residue 44 exposes lys^{47} which is complementary to the specificity pocket.

Therefore it was surprising to see the proteolysis of the scissile bond in [Ac(D)Phe^{45}, Arg^{47}, Pro^{48}] hirudin45-65 (P53) despite the presence of the amino acid proline in P_1'. This problem could be easily overcome by insertion of a ketomethylene peptidomimetic that would be structurally analogous to the situation in the native substrate, fibrinogen. The incorporation of this and related isosteres in the scissile position results in highly potent analogs with subnanomolar affinity for human α-thrombin (Figure 3, P79 and congeners). The name hirutonin has been coined to designate these bifunctional hirudin peptides. The name stems from the crucial ketomethylene function which enhances affinity and imparts complete enzymatic resistance against plasma proteases. They incorporate three essential elements:

- a component that interacts with the catalytic site of the enzyme A,
- an exosite-directed inhibitory sequence C,
- a connecting function that functions as a spacer B (Figure 3).

These novel structural prototypes prolong plasma prothrombin time, inhibit platelet aggregation mediated by thrombin and are potent antithrombotics comparable to r-hirudin in an in vivo rat arteriovenous shunt model of thrombosis [7].

Therefore through chemical manipulation of a natural thrombin inhibitory protein with molecular weight in the order of 7.5 KD, small synthetic hirudin peptides have been obtained that preserve the mechanism of interaction with the macromolecular target and exhibit high antithrombin activity. It is interesting to note that using other protein models, such as the GPIIb/IIIa antagonists decorsin, echistatin and kistrin, the essential recognition motif R-G-D could be extracted and engineered into a conformation expressing high antagonist potency. These achievements undoubtedly pave the way for a new generation of alternative antithrombotic therapy.

REFERENCES

1. ANDREWS RK, FOX JE. Platelet receptors in hemostasis. Curr Opin Cell Biol 2, 894-901, 1990.

2. BRAUN PJ, DENNIS S, HOFSTEENGE J, STONE SR. Biochemistry 27, 6517, 1988.

3. CASTAIGNE A. La Recherche 22, 425, 1991.

4. CHANG JY, NGAI PK, RINK H, DENNIS S, SCHLAEPPI JM. The structural elements of hirudin which bind to the fibrinogen recognition site of thrombin are exclusively

located within its acidic C-terminal tail. FEBS Lett 261, 287-290, 1990.

5. CHOAY J, LORMEAU JC, PETITOU M, SINAY P, FAREED J. Structural studies on a biologically active hexasaccharide obtained from heparin. Ann NY Acad Sci USA 370, 644-649, 1981.

6. COOK NS, UBBEN D. Fibrinogen as a major risk factor in cardiovascular disease. Trends Pharmacol Sci 11, 444-451, 1990.

7. DiMAIO J, GIBBS B, LEFEBVRE J, KONISHI Y, MUNN D, YUE SY, HORNBERGER W. Synthesis of a homologous serie of ketomethylene arginyl pseudodipeptides and application to low molecular weight hirudin-like thrombin inhibitors. J Med Chem 35, 3331-3341, 1992.

8. DiMAIO J, GIBBS B, MUNN D, LEFEBVRE J, NI F, KONISHI Y. In: Giralt E & Andreu D (Eds). Peptides: proceedings of the 21st European Peptide Symposium. p 774, 1990.

9. DiMAIO J, GIBBS B, MUNN D, LEFEBVRE J, NI F, KONISHI Y. Bifunctional thrombin inhibitors based on the sequence of hirudin 45-65. J Biol Chem 265, 21698-21703, 1990.

10. DiMAIO J, NI F, GIBBS B, KONISHI Y. A new class of potent thrombin inhibitors that incorporates a scissile pseudopeptide bond. FEBS Lett 282, 47-52, 1991.

11. DODT J, KOLHER S, SCHMITZ T, WILHELM B. Distinct binding sites of Ala48-hirudin 1-47 and Ala 48-hirudin 48-65 on alpha-thrombin. J Biol Chem 265, 713-718, 1990.

12. FOLKERS PJ, CLORE GM, DRISCOLL PC, DODT J, KOLHER S, GRONENBORN AM. Solution structure of recombinant hirudin and the Lys-47-Glu mutant: a nuclear magnetic resonance and hybrid distance geometry-dynamical simulated

annealing study. Biochemistry 28, 2601-2617, 1989.

13. FURIE B, FURIE BC. Cell 53, 505, 1988.

14. GRUTTER MG, PRIESTLE JP, RAHUEL J, GROSSENBACHER H, BODE W, HOFSTEENGE J, STONE SR. Crystal structure of the thrombin-hirudin complex: a novel mode of serine protease inhibition. EMBO J 9, 2361-2365, 1990.

15. HARUYAMA H, WUTHRICH K. Conformation of recombinant desulfatohirudin in aqueous solution determined by nuclear magnetic resonance. Biochemistry 28, 4301-4312, 1989.

16. HAYCRAFT JB. Proc R Soc 36, 478, 1884.

17. JORDAN RE, OOSTA GM, GARDNER WT, ROSENBERG RD. The kinetics of hemostatic enzyme anti-thrombin interactions in the presence of low molecular weight heparin. J Biol Chem 255, 10081-10090, 1980.

18. KRSTENANSKY JL, BROERSMA RJ, OWEN TJ, PAYNE MH, YATES T, MAO JT. Development of MDL 28,050, a small stable antithrombin agent based on a functional domain of the leech protein, hirudin. Thromb Haemost 63, 208-214, 1990.

19. KRSTENANSKY JL, MAO SJ. Antithrombin properties of C-terminus of hirudin using synthetic unsulfated N alpha-acetyl-hirudin 45-65. FEBS Lett 211, 10-16, 1987.

20. KRSTENANSKY JL, OWEN TJ, YATES MJ, MAO SJ. Anticoagulant peptides : nature of the interaction of the C-terminal region of hirudin with a non-catalytic binding site on thrombin. J Med Chem 30, 1688-1691, 1987.

21. KRSTENANSKY JL, OWEN TJ, YATES MT, MAO SJ. Design synthesis and antithrombin activity

for conformationally restricted analogs of peptide anticoagulants based on the C-terminal region of the leech peptide hirudin. Biochim Biophys Acta 957, 53-59, 1988.

22. LANE DA, LINDAHL U. Reviewed in heparin. (eds), Edward Arnold, London, 1989.

23. LINHARDT RJ, LOGANATHAN D, AL-HAKIM A, WANG HM, WALENGA JM, HAPPENSTEADT D, FAREED J. Oligosaccharide mapping of low molecular weight heparins: structure and activity differences. J Med Chem 33, 1639-1645, 1990.

24. LIU LW, VU TK, ESMON CT, COUGHLIN SR. The region of the thrombin receptor resembling hirudin binds to thrombin and alters enzyme specificity. J Biol Chem 266, 16977-16980, 1991.

25. MANN KG, JENNY RJ, KRISHNASWAMY S. Cofactor proteins in the assembly and expression of blood clotting enzyme complexes. Annu Rev Biochem 57, 915-956, 1988.

26. MARAGANORE JM, BOURDON P, JABLONSKY J, RAMACHANDRAN KL, FENTON JW 2d. Design and characterization of hirulogs: a novel class of bivalent peptide inhibitors of thrombin. Biochemistry 29, 7095-7101, 1990.

27. MARAGANORE JM, CHAO B, JOSEPH ML, JABLONSKI J, RAMACHANDRAN KL. Anticoagulant activity of synthetic hirudin peptide. J Biol Chem 264, 8692-8698, 1989.

28. MARKWARDT F. The comeback of hirudin- and old-established anticoagulant agent. Folia Haematol (Leip 3) 115, 10-23, 1988.

29. MARKWARDT F. Methods in enzymol. PERLMAN G.E., LORAND L. (eds), Academic Press, New York, 19, 924, 1970.

30. MARKWARDT F. Physiol Chem 308, 147, 1957.

31. NESHEIM ME, TASWELL JB, MANN KG. The contribution of bovine factor V and factor Va to the activity of prothrombinase. J Biol Chem 254, 10952-10962, 1979.

32. NI F, DiMAIO J, KONISHI Y. Unpublished observations.

33. NI F, KONISHI Y, SCHERAGA H. Thrombin-bound conformation of the C-terminal fragments of hirudin determined by transferred nuclear Overhauser effects. Biochemistry 29, 4479-4489, 1990.

34. OWEN TJ, KRSTENANSKY JL, YATES MJ, MAO SJ. N-terminal requirements of small peptide anticoagulants based on hirudin 54-65. J Med Chem 31, 1009-1011, 1988.

35. PETITOU M, LORMEAU JC, CHOAY J. Chemical synthesis of glycosaminoglycans: new approaches to antithrombotic drugs. Nature Suppl., 350, 30-33, 1991.

36. PRESCOTT SM, SEEGER AR, ZIMMERMAN GA, McINTYRE TM, MARAGANORE JM. Hirudin-based peptides block the inflammatory effects of thrombin on endothelial cells. J Biol Chem 265, 9614-9616, 1990.

37. RYDEL TJ, RAVICHANDRAN KG, TULINSKY A, BODE W, HUBER R, ROITSCH C, FENTON JW 2d. The structure of a complex of recombinant hirudin and human α-thrombin. Science 249, 277-280, 1990.

38. SAWYER RT. BIOPAPERS J 10, 11, 1990.

39. SCHMITZ T, ROTHE M, DODT J. Mechanism of the inhibition of α-thrombin by hirudin-derived fragments hirudin (1-47) and hirudin (45-65). Eur J Biochem 195, 251-256, 1991.

40. SCULLY MJ, MORRISON JF. Biochim Biophys Acta 874, 44, 1986.

41. SHEPARD LY. Tib Tech 9, 80, 1991.

42. STONE SR, BRAUN PJ, HOFSTEENGE J. Identification of regions of α-thrombin involved in its interaction with hirudin. Biochemistry 26, 4617-4624, 1987.

43. SUZUKI K, NISHIOKA J, HAYASHI T. Localization of thrombomodulin binding site within human thrombin. J Biol Chem 265, 13263-13267, 1990.

44. TRAVIS J, SALVESEN GS. Human plasma proteinase inhibitors. Ann Rev Biochem 52, 655-709, 1983.

45. VU TK, HUNG DT, WHEATON VI, COUGHLIN SR. Molecular cloning of a functional thrombin receptor reveals a novel proteolytic mechanism of receptor activation. Cell 64, 1057-1068, 1991.

46. WALLACE A, DENNIS S, HOFSTEENGE J, STONE SR. Contribution of the N-terminal region of hirudin to its interaction with thrombin. Biochemistry 28, 10079-10084, 1989.

47. WALZ DA, FENTON JW, SHUMAN MA (Eds). Bioregulatory Functions of Thrombin, vol 485, Ann NY Acad Sci USA, New York, 1986.

48. YUE SY, DiMAIO J, SZEWCZUK Z, PURISIMA EO, NI F, KONISHI Y. Characterization of the interactions of a bifunctional inhibitor with α-thrombin by molecular modelling and peptide synthesis. Protein Eng 5(1), 77-85, 1992.

8

Perspectives of the Clinical use of Hirudin

H.K. Breddin

In the pharmacological laboratory of Schmiedeberg in Strassburg John B. Haycraft in 1884 found a substance in the heads of leeches (hirudo medicinalis) which inhibited coagulation.

The name hirudin was first used by Jakoby [6]. Markwardt and coworkers isolated hirudin from leeches in the 50 ies in Erfurt [10] and characterized hirudin as a specific thrombin inhibitor with a polypeptide structure of 65 aminoacids and a molecular weight of about 7000 D. Since then hirudin has been used as an experimental anticoagulant of antithrombotic agent because it was difficult to obtain natural hirudin in larger amounts. This thrombin inhibitor has not been clinically used in a larger scale until its production by biotechnology.

1. Hirudin production

Natural hirudin is obtained from the homogenized heads or the medicinal leeches and is further purified by precipitations followed by ion exchange, chromatography and subsequent gel filtration. Hightly purified hirudin has also been obtained by affinity chromatography on matrix bound thrombin. Leeches produce a series of other proteinase inhibitors non of which has a specific effect on thrombin [18]. During a leech bite hirudin does not enter the blood circulation of its host. The leech needs hirudin to keep the blood of its victim liquid. For the prolonged bleeding from the leech bites other contents of its saliva are responsible. Some of these have been identified and are also tested as possible antithrombotic agents.

Since some years hirudin is produced by biotechnology using cultures of E. Coli and yeast. The lysed Coli or yeast cultures are purified by different chromatographic methods. The biotechnologically produced hirudins of today usually have a missing sulfate on tyr 63. Further aminoacids have been exchanged. The anticoagulant activity of recombinant hirudins is identical with that of native hirudin. Since hirudin can be produced by biotechnology larger amounts have become available and have led to its development as a possible antithrombotic drug.

2. Further developments

Starting with hirudin the development of antithrombotics of similar antithrombotic activity has proceeded. Maraganore et al. [9] analyzed the specific thrombin binding sequence of hirudin and synthetized some peptides with 17 to 18 aminoacids which they named hirulogs 1 - 5. One of these hirulogs is about as specific as hirudin and not much less active. If this preparation can be synthetized in larger amounts it may have the same effects as biotechnologically produced hirudin with possible advantages.

3. Coagulation inhibiting effects of hirudin

Hirudin is a specific thrombin inhibitor which forms equimolar complexes with thrombin, whereby the active center of the enzyme is blocked. One μg of hirudin inhibits about 15 units of human thrombin.

Markwardt and coworkers were the first to investigate the coagulation inhibiting effect of natural and biotechnologically produced hirudin in humans [10] and meanwhile some phase I-trials on the anticoagulant effects of hirudin have been published [2, 14]. Hirudin prolongs the thrombin time. For the monitoring of a treatment with hirudin the partial tromboplastin time or the measurement of the factor IIa-inhibition can be used. After a single intravenous injection the half life time is about one hour. After subcutaneous injections of 0.1 mg/kg hirudin in 8 hour intervals continuous hirudin levels between 0.05 - 2 μg/ml have been reached [10].

4. Platelet function inhibiting effects of hirudin

Hirudin inhibits platelet adhesion to glass and to subendothelial matrix [1, 4]. New results of our group which have not yet been published have shown that this effect can also be demonstrated after subcutaneous injections of hirudin in humans.

It is likely that the inhibiting effect of hirudin on platelet adhesion is caused by the inhibition of thrombin formation at the platelet surface. Platelets form thrombin if they get into contact with damaged vascular surfaces. The formation of thrombin enhances the adhesion of platelets and this process is partially inhibited by hirudin. The thrombin independent mechanisms of platelet adhesion are probably not influenced. Hirudin can also be used as a reagent to investigate different platelet functions. These reactions differ in many respects from those observed in citrate-blood or citrate-PRP because they take place at a physiological level of calcium ions. Hirudin inhibits epinephrine- induced platelet aggregation [3] and platelet spreading [1].

5. Hirudin as an antithrombotic agent

Hirudin has been used in different experimental models of thrombosis in different animals and has been identified as a potent inhibitor of thrombosis [3, 7, 8, 16-19] (table I).

The thrombosis inhibiting effect of hirudin lasts not as long as that of heparin. This had to be expected because of its shorter half life.

Table I : Effective hirudin dosage in experimental thrombosis (rats).

MODEL	ANTITHROMBOTIC EFFECTS	DOSE mg/kg	S.C. /I.V
Venous thrombosis KRUPINSKI	Increase of laser injuries	0.1-0.2	s.c.
Venous thrombosis KRUPINSKI	Increase of laser injuries	0.1-0.2	i.v.
Arterial thrombosis KRUPINSKI	Increase of laser injuries	0.1-0.2	s.c.
Vena cava JUST et al	Protein on wire coil	0.08-0.25	i.v.
Vena cava ligation DOUTREMEPUICH	Thrombus weight	0.12-0.25	i.v.
Venous thrombosis RAAKE (Jugular vein clamping)	Number of clampings	0.2-0.4	i.v.
Arterial thrombosis TALBOT et al	Incorporation of $Indium^{111}$ after mechanical surgery	3-6	s.c.

Some of the aspects for the clinical use of hirudin are listed in table I, the properties of hirudin are listed in table II.

Table II : Properties of hirudin

Hirudin :

- is a strong anticoagulant which does not need endogenous cofactors,

- has no effect on plasma proteins or enzymes,

- is a weak immunogen,

- has a high biovailability after sub- cutaneous injection,

- has a dose-dependent relatively long lasting biological half life,

- is not modulated endogenously, it is excreted to a large part in the urine,

- is not increased in different organs,

- probably does not induce bleeding complications in the doses necessary for the inhibition of thrombosis,

- can be used in patients with antithrombin III deficiency,

- can be monitored by APTT or adapted thrombin time.

The therapeutic range of hirudin, however, has to be identified in clinical trials. It is likely that overdosage will lead to increased bleeding as it is the case with heparin.

6. Methods to measure effects of hirudin (Table III)

Hirudin can be monitored using the thrombin

Table III : Possible indications for hirudin

- Prophylaxis of deep venous thrombosis in patients with a high risk of thrombosis, e.g. after hip endoprothesis or hip fractures or after knee replacements.

- Prophylaxis of arterial thrombosis, e.g. postoperatively after cardiac surgery, after PTCA or after peripheral angioplasty.

- After thrombolysis of arterial or venous thrombosis to prevent reocclusions.

- Treatment of venous thrombosis.

- Prophylaxis and treatment of consumption coagulopathy.

- In haemodialysis instead of heparin.

- For the extracorporeal circulation instead of heparin.

- In reconstructive microsurgery to improve the healing of scin flaps.

- In patients with transluminal coronary angioplasty hirudin may prevent early arterial reocclusions.

time when a human α-thrombin is used or with a chromogenic substrate test also with human α-thrombin. The APTT can also be used to monitor the effect of hirudin. Immunologic tests have been developed which detect very low concentrations of hirudin.

7. Possible clinical indications for the use of hirudin

Hirudin at present is used in clinical trials to inhibit venous thrombosis in patients with high risks, e.g. after hip endoprothesis in comparison to unfractionated heparin. The circulating levels of hirudin in clinical use have to be defined. Levels expected by interpolation from animals experiments of our group lead to those listed in table IV.

In haemodialysis hirudin is compared with heparin, in cardiac surgery it is discussed as a substiture for heparin. Hirudin may be a specific drug to treat consumption coagulopathy or disseminated intravascular coagulation.

Hirudin also may be used as an anticoagulant for the prophylaxis or reocclusions after successfull thrombolysis in patients with fresh myocardial infarction, especially since animal experiments have made it likely that hirudin enhances thrombolysis by tissue plasminogen activator [15].

Table IV: Expected circulation levels of r-Hirudin in clinical use

Indications	Levels (μg/ml)
Prophylaxis	0.1 - 0.5
Therapeutic anticoagulation	0.5 - 1.5
Extracorporeal circulation	2.0 - 5.0

8. Risks of hirudin

Table V : Hirudin and bleeding

1. Higher doses of hirudin will probably cause bleeding in postoperative situations.

2. A therapeutic "window" with sufficient antithrombotic effect without a high risk of bleeding is likely.

3. Bleeding risk lower with i.v. use of Hirudin?

The immunogenic effect of hirudin seems to be very low, as investigations in humans have shown so far. From the newly developed "hirulogs" even less immunogenic effects can be expected.

As far as animal experimental investigations allow a prediction the bleeding risk under prophylactic and therapeutic doses of hirudin will be relatively low in a therapeutic range which still has to be defined (Table V).

9. Antidot

As specific antidot against hirudin is not yet available. Such an antidot would be helpful in case of overdose. Whether an antidot is necessary in the "normal" clinical use of hirudin as an antithrombotic agent is not yet established, this seems relatively unlikely because of the short half life time.

Some investigators tried to counteract the effect of hirudin by activated prothrombin complex preparations (e.g. Feiba Immuno, Vienna) factor VIII-concentrates or desmopressinacetat (Minirin[R]). This is to some extent possible but it is not yet sufficiently clear, whether the observed changes of laboratory parameters are representative for the reduction of a bleeding tendency. It has also been suggested to reduce hirudin levels by haemoperfusion or haemoabsorption, by exchange transfusion or plasmaphoresis. In principle, it is possible to use an inactive thrombin to neutralize hirudin but it is unlikely that it will be practically used in the near future.

10. Conclusion

Hirudin which is well known for thirty years after the relevant investigations of Markwardt and his group has been revived by biotechnology which made its practical use in clinical trials possible. Whether hirudin has superior effects in comparison to its main competitor heparin or the low molecular weight heparins in some indications has yet to be validated in the near future. Hirudin itself will probably be compared with newly developed agents as hirulog and other thrombin inhibitors.

REFERENCES

1. BASIC-MICIC M, RAUSCHENBACH C, BREDDIN HK. The effects of recombinant hirudin on various platelet functions. In: Kirchmaier CM, Breddin HK, Fareed J, Markwardt F (Eds). New aspects of hirudin. Haemostasis 21 (Suppl. 1), 107, 1991.

2. BICHLER J, FICHTL B, SIEBECK M, FRITZ H. Pharmacokinetics and pharmacodynamics of hirudin in man after single subcutaneous and intravenous bolus administration. Arzneim-Forsch/Drug Es 38(1), 5, 704, 1988.

3. DOUTREMEPUICH C, LALANNE MC, DOUTREMEPUICH F, WALENGA J, FAREED J, BREDDIN HK. Comparative study of three recombinant hirudins with heparin in an experimental venous thrombosis model. In: Kirchmaier CM, Breddin HK, Fareed J, Markwardt F (Eds). New aspect of hirudin. Haemostasis 21 (Suppl. 1), 99, 1991.

4. GLUSA E. Platelet aggregation in recombinant hirudin-anticoagulated blood. In: Kirchmaier CM, Breddin HK, Fareed J, Markwardt F (Eds). New aspects of hirudin. Haemostasis 21 (Suppl. 1), 116, 1991.

5. HAYCRAFT JB. On the action of a secretion obtained from the medicinal leech on the coagulation of the blood. Proc R Soc Lond 36, 478, 1984.

6. JACOBY C. Uber hirudin. DMW 30, 1786, 1904.

7. JUST M, TRIPIER D, SEIFFGE D. Antithrombotic effects of recombinant hirudin in different animal models. In: Kirchmaier CM, Breddin HK, Fareed J, Markwardt F (Eds). New aspects of hirudin. Haemostasis 21 (Suppl. 1), 80, 1991.

8. KRUPINSKI K, BREDDIN HK. Effects of different hirudins and combinations of low doses of hirudin, heparin and acetylsalicylic acid in a rat microcirculatory thrombosis model. In: Kirchmaier CM, Breddin HK, Fareed J, Markwardt F (Eds). New aspects of hirudin. Haemostasis 21(Suppl. 1), 88, 1991.

9. MARAGANORE JM, BOURDON P, JABLONSKI J, RAMACHANDRAN KL, FENTON JW. Design and characterization of hirulogs: a novel class of bivalent peptide inhibitors of thrombin. Biochemistry 29, 7095, 1990.

10. MARKWARDT F. Die Isolierung und chemische Charakterisierung des Hirudins. Hoppe-Seylers Z Physiol Chem 308, 147, 1957.

11. MARKWARDT F. Pharmacology of hirudin: one hundred years after the first report of the anticoagulant agent of medicinal leeches. Biomed Biochim Acta 44, 1007, 1985.

12. MARKWARDT F. Past, present and futur of hirudin. In: Kirchmaier CM, Breddin HK, Fareed J, Markwardt F (Eds). New aspects of hirudin. Haemostasis 21 (Suppl. 1), 11, 1991.

13. MARKWARDT F, NOWAK G, STURZEBECHER J. Clinical pharmacology of recombinant hirudin. In: Kirchmaier CM, Breddin HK, Fareed J, Markwardt F (Eds). New aspects of hirudin. Haemostasis 21 (Suppl. 1), 133, 1991.

14. MEYER BH, LUUS HG, MULLER FO, BADENHORST PN, ROTHIG HJ. The pharmacology of recombinant hirudin, a new anticoagulant . SAMJ 78, 268, 1990.

15. MRUK JS, CHESEBRO JH, WEBSTER MWI, HERALS H, GRILL DE, FUSTER V. Hirudin markedly enhances thrombolysis with rt-PA. Circulation 82, 4 (Suppl. 3), 135, 1990.

16. RAAKE W, KLAUSER RJ, ELLING H, ZEITLER P. Antithrombotic action of recombinant hirudin in a venous thrombosis model. In: Kirchmaier CM, Breddin HK, Fareed J, Markwardt F (Eds). New aspects of hirudin. Haemostasis 21 (Suppl. 1), 127, 1991.

17. RUBSAMEN K, ESCHENFELDER V. Effect of recombinant hirudin (LU 52369) on reocclusion rates after thrombolysis in rabbits. In: Kirchmaier CM, Breddin HK, Fareed J, Markwardt F (Eds). New aspects of hirudin. Haemostasis 21(Suppl. 1), 93, 1991.

18. SAWYER RT. Leech biology and behaviour. II. Feeding biology, ecology, and systematics. Clarendon Press. Oxford 1968.

19. TALBOT MD, AMBLER J, BUTLER KD, LEES CM, MITCHELL KA, PETERS RF, TWEED MF, WALLIS RB. The effects of recombinant desulphatohirudin on arterial thrombosis in rats. In: Kirchmaier CM, Breddin HK, Fareed J, Markwardt F (Eds). New aspects of hirudin. Haemostasis 21 (Suppl. 1), 73, 1991.

9

The role of anti-myeloid series treatment in ischemic vascular disorders

M.R. Boisseau

The involvement of leukocytes in the thrombotic process has been known for many years [76], to this the more recent concept of microvascular occlusion as a result of excess adherence of these cells to the wall, under ischemic conditions, has been added [104]. At present, a number of facts have brought forth a renewed interest in these pathological deviations of white blood cells. The role of leukocytes in acute respiratory disorders pathology and during shock has been recognized [108, 117], as well as in infectious conditions [2]. These studies have led secondarily, to evaluate the effect of these cells in vascular pathology, in the domain of epidemiology and subsequently in the case of microcirculatory arrest. Concurrently with theses studies, the action mechanisms have been the subject of spectacular findings in recent years, paticularly as regards the interactions of leukocytes with endothelial cells during the cellular activation process by agonists and cytokines. The large amount of work and studies currently undertaken are rapidly allowing an evolution of the concepts (and the nomenclature...) for the development of highly interesting therapeutical applications We will consider in turn, the epidmiological contribution, the models proving the occurence of granulocyte intervention in the vascular occlusion process, the clinical structures allowing a repositionning of these various actions in the context of a direct contact with patients and finally, the therapeutical applications. Many questions still remain unanswered, but the new concept as regards the harmful effect of white blood cells in blood circulation is now accepted.

1. Epidemiological data

The epidemiological analysis allows, in a number of cases, to bring to light the prediction value of the total leukocyte concentration in the event of a thrombotic seizure in the course of vascular diseases. Thus, in the case of Japanese people exposed to atomic radiations between 1958 and 1974 the leukocyte concentration is shown to be correlated with the incidence of acute coronary seizures [87], the same applies to the true value concentration of PNNs and of monocytes, but not lymphocytes. The same study reapplied to cerebrovascular neurologic diseases gives the same results [88]. Conversely amongst the Yemenite communities who present a benign contitutional leukopenia a lower incidence of myocardial infarction is observed [107].

From 1974 onwards, an initial series of prospective studies was carried out showing the importance of total leukocyte concentration as a prediction index for the occurence of myocardial infarction [31, 37, 133, 135]. It therefore appears that the total leukocyte concentration being statistically higher in the thrombotic group is as good a prediction as the cholesterol level and blood pressure and that the risks attached are reduced after the number of white blood cells in put right [37]. In some studies, heavy smoking is held responsible for this high total leukocyte concentration [135], but in most cases, is accounted for as an independent risk, as is revealed in a recent study [19]. Secondary prospective studies, after the occurence of a first attack, yield the same results [62, 101]. In the course of a short term prognosis study (1 year), the high leukocyte concentration is predictive according to the size of the infarct, along with other haemostasis parameters [38].

These epidemilological studies can be extended further, as we will see later, to clinical tests. There are conclusive as regards the leukocyte effect which needs to be clarified at the physiopathological level. However a number of questions remain to be answered upstream of the mechanisms in play. Is there really a high leukocyte concentration absolute value? Indeed, mention can be made of a mobilization of the marginal pool, especially in the case of smokers. In fact, the readings after physical work-out tests reveal, in such patients, an increase in both circulatory and marinal pools, the mobilization of the latter being particularly enhanced by exercise [28]. Thus, the production or at least the periphal delivery of leukocytes is increased in these patients. This calls to mind the role of chronic inflammation. It is true that atherosclerosis represents a chronic inflammatory state, responsible for an haematological stress syndrome of which, the increase in the white blood cells count is one of the characteristic parmeters [94, 113]. In effect the coming into play of the inflammation, which can sometimes explain the play of inflammation, which can sometimes explain the increased production of leukocytes and independently have an harmful role, is fundamental for the triggering into action of those cells that respond to inflammatory mediators.

As a whole, the high leukocyte concentration seen in high cardiovascular risk patients, an indicator of thrombotic risk, demonstrates the activity of these cells in vascular pathology, the excess in numbers implying the excessive functional activities in the vicinity of certain vascular areas. However, leukocytes can also operate, whilst not in excess numbers in circulating blood, by exaggerating or by changing the nature of their activities.

2. The role of leukocytes in ischemia and thrombosis

Leukocytes play an active part in arterial ischemia at the level of the lower limb, brain, heart, intestine and lung [41]. They are active in the course of kidney and liver transplants which stand as models of ischemia. Besides, a number of experimental and clinical events affect principal areas: heart, liver and arteries of the lower limbs.

2.1 The two forms of ischemia

2.1.1 Ischemia per se

Ischemia per se causes an activation of the endothelium which on one hand, progressively expresses a pro-coagulant phenotype and on the other, produces free oxygenated radicals through the activation of xanthine oxydase [136]. Due to rheological conditions the polynuclear neutrophils (PNNs) swarm and adhere in "close contact" to the endothelium. Thus, were the ischemic lesion to develop further, for instance the size of the infarct, its reduction would be possible by the removal of leukocytes [26, 121]. However this phenomenon is mostly reversible and subsides following the development of a collateral supply of blood. In certain conditions, in conjunction with the amplification of reactions due to the presence of inflammatory mediators, the microvascular territories are blocked up due to the adhesion of leukocytes: phenomenon of "no-reflow" [104, 121] and this is followed by vascular seizure and thrombosis with fibrin deposits. There is doubt as to the shared responsability of leukocytes and endothelial cells towards the gravity of lesions. The presence of infectious and inflammatory lesions, as for instance at toe level in the arteriopath, must further involve the PNNs.

2.1.2. The perfusion (exchange transfusion) ischemia syndrome (I/R)

This syndrome, of which the importance is now perceived, following medical or surgical repermeabilization in the course of transplants presents a caricatural picture of the mechanisms described above. The role of the endothelial cells is primordial: transfusion leading to an input of oxygen, it leads to a considerable production of oxygenated by-products on the surface of endothelial cells as a result of xanthine oxydase activation. These by-products act strongly on the PNNS which are closely linked to endothelial cells due to rheological conditions. In such cases irreversible lesions are frequent.

A considerable amount of experimental work has recently been carried out. The setting and removal of a ligature in the rabbit has for result the causation of the I/R syndrome. The preliminary injection of anti CD10 antibodies restricts the lesions [121]. Beside the oxygenated radicals, the production of leukotriene B4 and other by-products of lipooxygenase is of importance [34, 128], these bodies being responsible at a later stage for the sub-regulation of PNN adhesion by rendering them refractory. Another well developed model is experimental ischemia in the mesenteric artery territory for the rabbit, cat and rat. The role of PNNs is shown by the use of anti CD18 antibodies [1]. The oxygenated radicals produced by xanthine oxydase play a major role as shown by the protector effect of xanthine oxydase inhibitors [36], the oxygenated metabolites establishing chemoattractant (chemotaxic) effects. The role of PAF-acether [55], of leukotriene B4 and elastase [136] have been recognized. Ischemia on the skeletal muscle of the dog has been carried out where the protector effect of anti CD18 is found again [13] and where PNNs involvement give the explanation for the occurence of a muscular contraction [124]. During the experimental infarction the size of the infarct is reduced by the anti CD11b antibodies [109]. The ischemic liver is also subject to an accumulation of PNNs [49], the shock is also enhanced by the anti CD18 [121]. Finally, the accumulation of PNNs in the skin of the rat is reduced by the inhibitors of xanthine oxydase [127].

On the whole, the experimental arguments speak for themselves and should open the way for the implementation of antiradical therapeutic methods in the human clinical domain; these to protect and regenerate PNNs and reduce leukocyte functions, however and by the same token, anti-infectious defence mechanisms should not be nullified.

Monoconal antibodies, however effective in animal models are not as yet used in man.

2.2 Main clinical perspectives

2.2.1 A chronic arteriopathy of the lower limbs (ACMI)

The active role of leukocytes in ischemic aggravation is shown in ACMI. The regidity of white blood cells in connection with their activation has been described [14, 75]. This is the case for monocytes in particular, which stay in a non exchange state for a longer period of time. The intensification of PNN functions has also been measured [75], as well as the increased formation of pseudopods. Moreover, these signs disappear after amputation of the ischmic limb [73] or following a bypass [43]. These signs become less apparent following physical exercice [110]. The physiopathology of these cell activation processes pertains to inflammatory reaction, visible at the rheological level (increased viscosity, hyperfibrinogenemia), with the predominant role played by oxygenated by-products and with the particularity of prolonged monocyte action. By and large, ACMI represents a privileged diathesis for leukocytes to take part in ischemia.

2.2.2 Cerebrovascular neurologic disease (CND)

The role of PNNs in the course of CND has for a long time been suspected since it is known that this type of cells accumulate in lesions, in particular during experimental causation of infarcts in primates [32] and as a result of histological studies, especially in poor flow areas [39].

Recently, the coming into play of PNNs has been analyzed: their accumulation in ischemic zones is linked to stasis, the activation of fragments of the complement. The white blood cells take part essentially with the creation of oxygenated radicals (encouraged by the presence of iron from haemorrhages and endothelial cells) and from lipid originated products: leukotrienes and PAF-acether [53]. They are believed to be the cause of two main types of action: the worsening of microcirculatory disorders (increase in size of the penumbra) and angiogenic oedema. These actions are to be found again, in the course of ischemic and haemorrhagic CNDs as well as cerebral traumas.

The pathogenic role at the level of the centre of infarction is, for some, associated with platelets, the consumption of which is correlated to the leukocyte influx at the early stage of CND [16]. Other have no doubt as to the predominance of the PNNs harmful effect, the animal undergoing the experiment being protected by anti-leukocyte antibodies [5]. In fact, the kinetics of intercellular actions are not known, and leukocytes certainly come into play to further aggravate the situation and perhaps, their role is also determinant. Indeed, PNNs are activated by infections known to be risk factors for CND.

The presence of activated leukocytes in the blood was made extrinsic by indirect biochemical methods [123], but mostly through the work carried out by rheologists. The deterioration of blood filtrability in the course of CNDs was already a known fact [9], and is due, as Ernst [29] described, to the leukocytal rigidity in his patients. These facts have been confirmed in transitory seizures during the chronic stages of CNDs [122] and at the onset stage of ischemic illnesses. This state of activation, characterized in this instance by poor filtrability of PNNs as well as monocytes, is correlated with age, fibrinogen and is found in subjects presenting a risk. It would appear "easier" to capture activated white blood cells in systemic blood during CNDs than in the course of other vascular diseases, however these results need confirmation with different approaches to the problem.

On the whole the deteriorating role of leukocytes in the course of CNDs seems to be a proven fact as regards microcirculatory flow and on cerebral tissue [53]. Some questions are still unsolved in particular on the exact role they play in thrombus formation. The therapeutic approach to this problem is almost non-existent in man.

2.2.3 Coronary disease (angor pectoris and myocardial infarction)

A serie of experiments in animals and human investigations have shown that leukocytes are involved in coronary disease complications. The role of these cells during experimental causation of infarct in the dog, known for about ten years [27], consists in the accumulation of microvessels close to the lesion, thus increasing the ischemic area. The collateral network allows for the inflow and involvement of the PNNs and constitutes natural reperfusion. Leukocyte depletion reduces the size of the infarction [2] and the deposit of labelled platelets on the lesion [4]. Finally, it is believed that in some cases the leukocyte count and the degree of priming are in line with the seriousness of certain complications [56]. To this former notions the reperfusion problem is added: during experimental causation of infarction in the pig and rabbit, the disorders linked to leukocytes, seen by measuring the positive myeloperoxidase areas, worsen according to the duration of reperfusion [47, 64]. Therefore, as in other vascular sectors, reperfusion whether natural or resulting from surgery, angioplasty or fibrinolysis implies leukocyte involvement. Do they have an influence in the emergence of thrombosis? This is likely, either directly via monocytal intercourse [74] or through cellular interaction.

Leukocytes, however, are only one of several pathogenetic factors involved in the intricate genesis of myocardial ischemic lesions. Therefore, in certain protocols, the depletion of the PNNs in the dog reduces the "stunning" effect; allows a better reperfusion of the collaterals but does not lead to a better myocardial functional prognosis [79]. In the rabbit, anti-CD18 antibodies limit the accumulation of PNNs that have been incubated in vitro during reperfusion but do not redress permeability. The PAF-acether inhibitors remain inactive [131]. Admittedly, the differences arise from the use of different protocols, in particular reperfusion duration.

A number of facts support the case for a step by step aggravation of PNN activation during the processes, allowing the angor pectoris to develop into an infarct. It is therefore possible to show their rigidity and the formation of pseudopods [72] with the presence of BB 40-43 fragments linked to elastase action on fibrin. Some activation tests are deleterious and are found again in patients in the event of an advanced state of ischemia. Therefore, before transluminal angioplasty, the state of priming can be seen according to the in vitro $O_2^{\cdot-}$ production capacity, but after remedial clearing of the obstruction, the level of elastase in the plasma increases [20]. Before fibrinolysis therapy the PNNs gathered in the coronary sinus become refractory on leaving the ischemic zone but recover their potentiality after treatment [46]. The fibrinolysis treatment is accompanied by a peak in plasma elastase corresponding to the activation of PNNs in the reperfusion zones that have been opened following treatment [92]. A concept can thus be established: the PNNs in circulation are in a priming state in stable angor pectoris and the stable state of coronary disease, but natural perfusion of the ischemic zones activate them in progresssive steps, the opening of previously ischemic zones speeding up their action. It would be interesting to find out if the priming stage comes first and is thus premonitory, therefore constituting a risk factor. The existence of a rheological rigidity of these cells could lead to believe that this is the case but appears to be too frequent and tied to inflammation to be a determining factor.

In these states, monocytes are also activated [72], especially as regards their procoagulant function correlated with fibrinopeptide-A genesis, whilst not knowing if this process is linked to coronary thrombosis or rather vascular thrombosis, a frequent occurence in such test cases [74].

The leukocyte action mechanisms are related to the capacity for the production of oxygenated metabolites, arachidonic acid derivatives and to the degranulation effect.

Several overview revues have recently been dedicated to the problem issued from the presence of free radicals in coronary lesions [63, 93] underlining the different origins of these products: at the endothelial cells level stemming from Xanthine Oxydase activities, the mitochondrial transports chains, the production of prostaglandins and at the level of PNNs from NADPH oxydase. The latter are not therefore the only source of active products. In any case, the relationship between PNNs, oxygenated radicals and the lesion is established: thus the lesions related to the direct activation of these cells, in the case of the coronary disease of the dog (opsonized zymozan injection), are reduced by simultaneously administrating superoxide dismutase, catalase and methionine [86]. The search, in the case of man, of oxydated and linoleic acid derivatives (phospholipidic 9-11 linoleic acid) proves positive around the 12th hour after the infarct [6]. Finally, in the rabbit, the in vitro contraction of the isolated papillary muscle is altered by PNNs and H_2O_2, enhanced by catalase [54]. Overall, activated PNNs are in the forefront of the coming into play of these products leading to the endothelial and muscle fibres lesion.

The production of arachidonic acid by- products also plays a part. The by-products of cyclo-oxygenase are incriminated [47]. However, it would appear that the most active by-products are those derived from lipooxygenase. Once produced, they first of all cause a chemoattractant effect, in particular for hydroxy-eicosatetraenoic acids (HETEs), but mostly for leukotrienes [47, 91].

The delivery of elastase by activated PNNs is obviously an essential factor and is observed in such patients, showing a peak in the plasma 40 hours after infarction of earlier in the case of thrombolytic treatment [6]. The search for BB 40-43 fibrin by-products, due to elastase activity, is equally positive [21, 69], while not knowing where the attack on fibrin has occurred.

If one is to accept the role of white blood cells in the genesis and above all in the progress of coronary ischemia lesions, several factors are still left unanswered: are they there at the origin of coronary thrombosis? Is their systematic priming important? Above all, how to combat them and what weapons to use?

2.2.4 Leukocytes and vascular thrombosis

The research bearing on the role of leukocytes in vascular thrombosis are surprisingly few when considering the clear scientific facts linking the extrinsic pathway (#tract) to the monocytal line. Monocytes have the ability to produce large quantities of tissue factor [105, 106, 130]. Besides, the clinical importance of this property is accepted [65], although few demonstrations exist.

In a study conducted in the course of surgery on the knee, the procoagulant activity of monocytes is significantly increased on the 10th day after intervention and is correlated with the presence of D-dimers on the cell surface [81]. In an other serie of studies, following hip surgery, the clotting property of monocytes is found to be significantly high on the 1st and 2nd day following intervention. Moreover, factor VII (proconvertin) decreases in the same intervals showing the parallel evolution of the extrinsic pathway along with monocytal activation [78]. In both these series of studies no correlation was found with the occurence of thrombosis.

Several interpretation hypotheses have been put forward following these studies. The coming into play of a new line of macrophagic monocytes bears little probability. The role of the C5a and C3b complement fragments which are known to activate monocytes [84] seems to be elective. The C-reactive protein is also particularly active on these cells and a correlation is established between such patients and monocyte activation [130]. The parallel between these factors kinetics at the post-operative stage and the activation of the coagulant capacity of the cells, is still to be formally established.

One important point, is the relationship between monocytes and factor VII: the liaison between this factor activated cells, in particular by endotoxin has been shown, [83] leading to clotting properties. At this point, the question is to find out at which stage the pathway is influenced by the macrophagic contingent under the conditions of operative risk.

By and large, the exact placing and behaviour of monocytes in the genesis of vascular thrombosis still remain to be determined. Questions that arise are the following: what are the right kinetics in the post-operative period and the connection with the acute phase of the inflammatory reaction? Does a preliminary priming occur and how important is it? How can an explanation be found for the important individual variations observed in the monocyte clotting capacity between different patients? Finally, what could the therapeutic repercussions be since little data is available concerning the effects of modern anithrombotics on monocytes, either at the direct or indirect level through the moderating influence on cytokinins, TNFα in particular of which the action is primordial in this lineage.

No approach concerning the activation of PNNs need be retained in the case of vascular thrombosis.

3. Physiopathogenesis and therapeutic targets

Outside the role of monocytes in the course of vascular thrombosis (not dealt with in this review), the stages at which leukocytes come into play during ischemia are principally located in the microcirculatory framework engaging considerable surface areas, especially in the muscles. However, in stasis conditions, leukocytes are prone to attach to the walls of large vessels, more so at the level of atherosclerosed plates of valvular folds. Nevertheless, the level at which most of the phenomena, under scrutiny here, take place are on the vascular side of microcirculation, the seat of particularly reactive endothelial cells [58].

The following stages can be recognized:

3.1 Rheological conditions

Leukocytes usually establish contact with the vascular wall because of the appropriate rheological conditions, in accordance with the slowing down of the flow (weak shear) and the high hematocrit values in the area. The presence of red blood cells aggregates induces the projection of white blood cells towards the wall and a number of them make contact, thus forming the leukocytal flux or "rolling". These phenomena gather momentum during stasis and ischemia. "Rolling" is followed by unstable adhesion, bringing the leukocytes to a standstill and then by stable adhesion or "sticking" before trans-parietal migration.

On the whole, two therapeutic targets can be identified here: " rolling" and unstable adhesion which are reversible phenomena and "sticking" which is irreversible.

3.2 Immunobiochemistry

Unstable adhesion is linked to the expression of a heavy molecular weight selectin by endothelial cells, GMP-140 which is capable of trapping leukocytes ("catching"). The up-regulation of this ligand is rapid but transient (table I) under the influence of agonists such as, thrombin, histamine and bradykinin. Due to lectin-like properties, it recognises sugar patterns and creates reversible links.

Table I: Stages in granulocyte adhesion to the endothelium

Consequences of the adhesion Stages	1-Margination 2-Trans-modulation of the Mac-1 receptor	1-Granulocytes accumulation 2-Setting up of [PAF et Rx Oxy.] activations	Migration Trans-endothelial of leukocytes as a whole
Endothelium adhesion repression factors	unknown	**1-Cytokines** Interleukin-6 Interleukin 2&4 GM-CSF TGF-ß INF-Γ TNF-α **2-Prostaglandins** PGE_2 **3-Endothelial inhibitor**	ditto
Stages of adhesion (*)	leukocyte flow ("rolling")	2-unstable adhesion ("catching", "tethering")	3-stable adhesion ("sticking") then migration
Agonists	unknown (Gran.? Endoth.?)	thrombin histamine leukotriene B4 P.A.F.	Interleukin-1 TNF-α primers: INF-Γ (IL-1 synergy) Interleukin-8

Leukocytal and endothelial ligands	Leukocytes : Selectins : LAM-1	Endothelium : Selectins : 1-GMP-140 2-ELAM-1	Endothelium : Immunogl. superfamily 1-ICAM-1 2-ICAM-2
Duration of regulation positive	LAM-1 5 mn (max: 5mn)	GMP-140 10 mn (max: 30 mn) ELAM-1 60 mn (max: 4 hours)	ICAM-1 4 hours (max: 24 hours)
negative	LAM-1 10 mn (after gran. activation)	GMP-140 60 mn ELAM-1 12 hours	ICAM-1 > 72 hours
Endothelial and leukocytal receptors	**Endothelium** Clustered Oligo-saccharides	**Granulocytes** GMP-140 tetra-saccharides Sialyl-Le^x or CD15) ELAM-1 Sulfate rich protein SOD (and sialyl-Le^x)	**Granulocytes** ß2-integrins CD11a/CD18 [LPA-1] CD11b/CD18 [Mac-1]

(*) : on the venous side of microcirculation, in precise rheological conditions (see text)

Abbreviations : LAM-1 : leukocyte adhesion mol., GMP-140 : glycoprotein of mol. weight 140, ELAM-1 : endothelial leukocyte adhesion mol., ICAM-1 : intercellular adhesion mol., LFA-1 : lymphocyte function activated antigen, Mac-1 : macrophage antigen (as well as, CR3 : complement receptor n°3), GM-CSF : granulocyte colonies proliferation factor, TGF-ß : tumor growth factor, TNF-α : tissue necrosis factor or cachectin, INF-Γ : gamma interferon.

3.2.1 Stable adhesion is associated with the following stages:

- Endothelial cell activation: the activation takes place because of the presence of extracellular products (like liposaccharides or formyl-peptides) or intracellular products originating from monocytes but more so from granulocytes (leukotriene B4, PAF-acether, TNF-α and H_2O_2) At the endothelial cells level, activation triggers the synthesis of interleukine 1 and of PAF-acether, close to the membrane surface. Intricate up and down regulation phenomena follow one another at the endothelial cells level depending on the intensity and duration of activation, with in particular the expression of the tissue factor that, by generating cytokines (especially interleukine 8), ties up with the formation of thrombin and with regulations.
- Activation of the PNNs: granulocytes are activated on the surface of endothelial cells [136] principally by PAF-acether but also by leukotrienes and free radicals, thus allowing the expression of ß2 integrins.
- Irreversible adhesion: linked to the ELAM1 and ICAM1 systems, followed by leukocyte migration.

On the whole, the therapeutic targets at this level are mainly to do with the endothelium because of its role as PNN activator. The proof of the matter appears to lie in the important role played by the xanthine oxydase inhibitors and due to the fact that in ischemic reperfusion, the reactions are mostly to do with the incoming PNNs in the blood flow, which are probably not strongly activated. However, especially in the course of intense paroxysmal phenomena such as prolonged ischemia, it is easy to believe that PNNs activation plays an important part.

3.2.2 Phenomena associated with ischemia:

- PNN activation: in the ischemic zones, the activation conditions for granulocytes increase, either due to the presence of inflammatory products or because of cellular interaction (monocytes and platelets). They generate thrombotic phospholipids (PAF- acether), products of lipooxygenase (leukotrienes) and oxygenated radicals of the H_2O_2 type. The latter appear to be important as they can associate with the radical activity of the endothelium, which would also be facilitated by a converting factor for xanthine dehydrogenase of leukocyte origine [61]. The presence of d and e type agonists (fMLP), induces also the "spreading" of PNNs, putting them in "close contact" with the endothelial surface, leading to the formation of a pseudo-phagosome favouring the development of proteolytic activities protected from blood inhibitors.

- Endothelial cell activation: the endothelium down-regulates a number of anticoagulant properties in step with the intensity of activation (thrombomodulin t-PA) and up-regulates coagulant activities tissue factor PAI1. The activities of the prostacyclin type (PGI_2) and of the relaxant factor ($NO^{\cdot}$) are increased. The up-regulation of xanthine oxydase is one of the characteristics of endothelial activity in the course of ischemia. This enzyme is unevenly distributed in the endotheliums and tissues and is particularly low in the heart and in the ombilical endothelium. Nevertheless, it would appear that it can be synthesized during ischemia but this is still a matter of discussion [23].

Two phenomena come into play in the course of ischemia and the distress that it brings: the rupture of phosphate bonds from ATP leading to an excess of hypoxanthin and the presence of proteases which, at the level of the endothelium, transform xanthine dehydrogenase into xanthine oxydase. The proteases may stem from PNNs, either as elastase or an undertermined converting factor. Antiproteases are rendered inactive due to the PNNs-endothelium close contact.

Besides, PNNs when activated supply H_2O_2 to endothelial cells by activation of NADPH oxydase, bound to the membrane according to the following reactions:

$NADPH + 2O_2 \Longrightarrow 2O_2^{\cdot-} + NADP + H^+$

Followed dismutation of $O_2^{\cdot-}$

$2O_2^{\cdot-} + 2H^+ \Longrightarrow H_2O_2 + O_2$

At the time of reperfusion, an excess of oxygen allows the following reactions to take place [23, 126]

- formation of a superoxyde ion $O_2^{\cdot-}$, due to the action of xanthine oxydase on hypoxanthin
- formation of the hydroxyl radical, according to the Fenton reaction:

$O_2^{\cdot-} + Fe^{3+} \Longrightarrow Fe^{2+} + O_2$

$Fe^{2+} + H_2O_2 \Longrightarrow Fe^{3+} + HO + HO^{\cdot}$ (hydroxyl radical)

$HO^{\cdot}$, the ultimate product of this pathway, is the most toxic of all oxygenated radicals when iron is present and is held responsible for cellular lysis. Furthemore, the myeloperoxidase formed during the secretion of PNN cells can lead to the formation, from H_2O_2, of chloride or bromide, of hypochloric acids (HOCl, HOBr), which have powerful oxidation poperties.

The general picture is therefore one where the activation of endothelial and circulatory cells in the course of ischemia allows to define all therapeutic targets (table II).

Table II

Increase in micro-circulatory blood fow
- Effect on vasomotion
  - Buflomedil
- Effect on endothelial permeability
  - Calcium antogonists, dextrane sulfate

Reduction of adhesion to the endothelium
- Unstable adhesion
  - Fucoidin, protamine
  - Sulfate rich polysaccharides, Heparin
- Stable adhesion
  - Buflomedil

Action on the activation of endothelial cells

- Effect on xanthine oxidase
  - Allopurinol, Oxypurinol
  - AINS
  - Pterin-aldehyde
  - Flavonoids
  - Calcic inhibitors
  - Deferoxamine
  - Anthraquinones, Iodoxamide
  - Methylene blue
- Action on other systems
  - supply of glutamine (ATP)
  - Effect on PGI_2: Vit E
  - Effect of prostanoids of the Iloproste type

Action on the activation of neutrophils

- Decrease in the production of $O_2^{\cdot -}$ ions
  - Glucocorticoids, Lipocortin 1
  - Vit E
  - SOD
  - Gingkolides
  - Prostanoids
  - AINS
  - Antiallergic drugs
- Anti-myeloperoxidase effect
  - Dimethylurea
  - Naphtalenes
  - Flavonoids
  - Propylthiouracil
- Anti-HOCl effect
  - AINS
- Antiproteases
  - Aprotinin, Trasylol
  - Eglin Ce (antielastase)
  - α-2-macroglobulin
- Various actions
  - Antichemoattractants: Gingkolides
  - Pentoxifylline: restores cAMP, reduces F-actin and α-monocyte TNF

Flux recovery is of course necessary but in some cases it would be preferable to perform it in the absence of leukocytes and with hypo-oxygenated blood. Adhesion limiting should mostly be restricted to the unstable adhesion stage, the first stage of the phenomenon. Activation prevention or reduction remains the most sought after strategy: first and foremost at the endothelial cells level and above all, in connection with the genesis of toxic oxygen radicals. However, various means are on offer, especially as regards anti-protease actions.

4. Current picture of anti-myeloid series treatments

Despite the advanced knowledge of ischemic conditions at the experimental and clinical levels, no current therapeutic protocol is in place. There is too much disagreement as to the beneficial effects of the proposed treatment due to the variations of experimental conditions, the duration of ischemia, the treatment application methods, before or after. Nonetheless, there is no doubt that positive effects are on the whole always present.

There are wide ranging strategies, currently on offer, aiming at the targets that we have defined: flux, PNNs, endothelial cells, cellular functions and products that are released.

4.1 Medications for the microcirculatory flow

A number of medications are suggested in order to increase vasomotion and therefore the flow in microvessels, amongst these, Buflomedil appears to be of primary importance [15]. In the course of stasis and ischemia the permeability disorders of the endothelium are constant, due to contact with PNNs: some calcium inhibitors abate this phenomenon [59]. The presence of dextran sulfate limits fluid escape [60].

4.2 Restriction of PNN adhesion

The restriction of unstable adhesion, in other words the coming into play of selectins homing on sugars found on the endothelial cell can be obtained in the presence of fucoidin [10], protamine and sulfate rich polysaccharides [48]. Dextran sulfate appears to act in this fashion. It is possible to assume, within reason, that this preventive role is played by heparins and synthetic heparin substitutes bonding with the cellular coat.

The interference with stable adhesion involving ß2 integrins of PNNs and the ICAM1 ligand can be obtained with buflomedil, in particular [134]. A moderate response has to be sought due to the fundamental nature of this adhesion in immunological defence.

4.3 Restriction of endothelial cell activation

4.3.1 Inhibition of xanthine oxydase

The drug studied most is allopurinol and its derivative oxypurinol, its use in human clinical terms being widespread. In the rat, allopurinol reduces the cerebral oedema linked to ischemia [60], likewise in the kidney [129], but in this case the effect of the drug is not restricted to the inhibition of xanthine oxydase. This is found in models involving the rabbit heart [82], of which the myocardium seems to be lacking the enzyme. The positive effect of allopurinol is hence attributed to an action on PNNs, on the $HO^{\cdot}$ radical stemming from inside the muscular fibres and by a restorative effect on the mitochondrial ATP pool. Other inhibitors, outside allopurinol itself, have no effect in this case [125]. But in the model of an isolated rabbit leg without transfusion, the effect of allopurinol is seen again, hence in the absence of PNNs [125]. In this case, the effect is attributed to the inhibition of skeletal muscular endothelial xanthine oxydase where this enzyme is plentiful, which shows the importance of these phenomena in skeletal muscles [18, 89]. In man, the necessary concentrations to achieve the inhibition of this enzyme are easily obtained as can be verified by measuring the dosage of 1-methyl uric acid [50]. Therefore, allopurinol is active in situations with or without the presence of PNNs or xanthine oxydase in the target organ, which shows the wider restorative power of nucleotide adenins [36]. In addition, its low molecular weight allows it to diffuse inside sarcolemmas when in contact with cells [82].

The non steroid anti-inflammatory products, such as azapropazone and tinoridin inhibit xanthine oxydase [42] in a microsomal peroxidation model in the rat (scavenger effect on $OH^{\cdot}$).

The pterin-aldhyde present in folic acid preparations, with a long life span in the blood system, inhibits xanthine oxydase [52].

A number of flavonoids exert an anti-xanthine oxydase action [51]. Among the drugs used in cardiology, propanolol [71] and calcic inhibitors [95] have an effect. Such products seem interesting in as much as they easily diffuse at cellular level and since they build up in membrane lipids. Finally, some cafein extracts have an anti-xanthine oxydase action [77].

Iron being essential for the formation of the hydroxyl $OH^{\cdot}$ (Fenton reaction): a suggestion for using iron chelating agents to inhibit xanthine oxydase has been put forward. Analyses of endothelial cell cultures show the important effect of deferoxamine [66].

Were also tested: anthraquinones [100], lodoxamide [44] and methylene blue that could effectively be injected in patients [33].

4.3.2 Other systems acting on endothelial cells

The supplementing of glutamine to endothelial cells makes them less susceptible to the action of H_2O_2, in protecting the mitochondrial GAPDH activity tied to ATP synthesis [80]. Polystyrene catalase complexes bind to the surface of endothelial cells and act as protection against H_2O_2 [96].

The increase in production of PGI_2 by endothelial cells is almost constant when the cells experience distress, in such a way that it is above all important to identify the cases when drugs inhibit its secretion. However, a number of facts have been reported: Vitamin E increases the production of PGI_2 [67] and the stable analogue lioprost, reduces the PMN adhesion to the endothelium (isolated rat lung) increasing AMPc and has no action on $O_2^{\div}$ [138].

4.4 Restriction of PNN activation

4.4.1 Slowing down of the superoxide $O_2^{\div}$ ion production

Glucocorticoids and Lipocortin 1 inhibitit NADPH-oxydase when it is activated by phopholipase A_2 [68].

The use of superoxydismutase (SOD) has mostly taken place in the course of experimental models, as in the ischemic heart [116], liver grafts with rh-SOD [25]. The bond with polyethylene glycol prolongs the SOD effect [12].

Vitamin E reduces the production of $O_2^{\div}$ by PNNs [137] but not per os [67].

certain anti-allergic or anti-inflammatory drugs act upon white blood cells: aselastin [102], H2-antagonists, cimetidine and ranitidin [7], ibuprofen in a septic shock model [85], piroxicam [111].

Ginkgo biloba is a scavenger or $O_2^{\dot{-}}$ but also develops a SOD activity, that other flavonoids may also have [3].

Prostacyclin analogues, such as taprosten, slow down the production of $O_2^{\dot{-}}$ [99].

Pentoxifylline reduces NBT spontaneous activation, partly linked to O_2 formation [24].

4.4.2 Action on myeloperoxydase (MPO)

Dimethylurea blocks the MPO pathway, protecting α1-antitrypsin [120]. Naphtalenes bind to the enzyme and act as inhibitors [115].

Anti-inflammatory compounds, such as indometacine, piroxicam and ibuprofen, block the formation of HOCl by acting on the oxydation of Cl in the same way as clofazimine and dapsone [57].

Flavonoids inhibit MPO [35], as well as propylthiouracil, an anti-thyroid drug which binds to the enzyme [40].

4.4.3 Action of protease inhibitors

The use of antiproteases is an indirect way of reducing the effect of oxygen toxic radicals, this being made easy by the presence of such products in the human pharmacopeia [17]. Thus, aprotinin is active during reperfusion [114], as well as trasylol in the occlusion of the mesenteric artery [22].

Eglin C as an inhibitor of elastase and cathepsin G, reduce the PNN functions [90].

α_2-macroglobulin, acting on PNN proteases, has an antiradical action and could be used in therapeutics [119]. Some authors, however, get negative results using these products, in particular on vascular permeability breakdown [60].

4.4.4 Action on various PNN functions

The chemotaxy associated to PAF acether is inhibited by gingkolides [11].

Numerous studies are devoted to pentoxifylline which is unquestionably of interest in situations where activated PMN play an harmful role. Moreover, its use over the years in vascular pathology indicates good tolerance. The clinical studies have dealt mainly with degenerative and thrombotic vascular pathology of the brain and lower limbs. However, its action in the course of respiratory distress syndromes is convincing. The basic action of this methyl xanthin consists in the inhibition of phospho-diesterase thus increasing the level of $_c$AMP [30]. The adhesion of PNNs treated in this fashion seems to decrease [24, 112]. In other respects, pentoxifylline reduces the polymerisation of F-actin, following activation by fMLP [70]. In addition this drug reduces the synthesis of α-TNF by monocytes.

5. Conclusion

In the last ten years, especially in animal models, numerous trials have shown the efficacy of an action on targets involving the role of PNNs and of monocytes in the course of microvascular occlusion, either in the case of respiratory phenomena of the lungs or in the course of vascular ischemia of the bowel, myocardiac and also at the skeletal muscles level.

In fact, the drugs used often go beyong the endothelium, the leukocytes and their liaisons: some involve muscular fibres directly, in particular for the myocardium deprived of xanthine oxydase.

Even with such encouraging results, no universal strategy has, to this day, been put forward. The absence of a consensus stems partly from the difficulty in identifying PNN activation in patients, the PNN generally being trapped in the ischemic zones, which in turn does not allow to establish correlations with the evolution of ischemia.

The best priming analysis of circulating PNNs, in order to quantify their activation, the use of always improved therapeutic protocols for white blood cells, should open the door to the applications of anti-granulocyte therapy in human pathology, especially in preventive and per-operatory medecine.

REFERENCES

1. ARGENBRIGHT LW, LETTS LG, ROTHLEIN R. Monoclonal antibodies to the leukocyte menbrane CD18 glycoprotein complex and to intercellular adhesion molecule-1 inhibit leukocyte-endothelial adhesion in rabbits. J Leuk Biol, 49, 253-257, 1991.

2. BAGGE U, AMUNDSON B, LAUITZEN C. White blood cells deformability and plugging of skelatal muscle capillairies in hemorrhagic shock. Acta Physiol Scand 108, 159-163, 1980.

3. BARROSO-ARANDA J, SCHMID-SCHONBEIN GW. Pentoxifylline pretreatment decreases neutrophil activation during endotoxic shock and improves survival. In: Hakim J & Mandell GL (Eds). Pentoxifylline and analogues: effects on leukocyte function. Vol 1, pp 97-103, 1990.

4. BEDNAR M, SMITH B, PINTO A, MULLANE KM. Neutrophil deplation suppresses ^{111}I-labeled platelet accumulation in infarcted myocardium. J Cardiovas Pharmacol 7, 906-912, 1985.

5. BEDNAR MM, RAYMOND S, Mc AUTILLE T, LODGE A, CROSS CE. The role of neutrophils and platelets in rabbit model of thromboemboic stroke. Stroke 22, 44-50, 1991.

6. BELL D, FACKSON M, NICOLL JJ, DAWES J, MUIR AL. Inflammatory response, neutrophil ativation and free radical production after acute myocardial infarction: effect of thrombolytic treatment. Br Heart J 63, 82-87, 1990.

7. BIEMOND PE, SWAAD AJG, PINDERS JMA, BIENDORFF CM, KOSTER JF. Superoxide production by polymorphonuclear leukocyte in rheumatoid arthritis and ostioarthritis: in vivo inhibition by the antirheumatic drug piroxicam due to interference with the activation of the NADPH-oxidase. Ann Rheum Dis 45, 249-255, 1986.

8. BLEBEA J, KERR JC, HOBSON RW, PADBERG FT. The effects of oxygen free radical scanvengers on skeletal muscle ischemia and reperfusion injury. Curr Surg Sept-Oct, 396-398, 1987.

9. BOISSEAU MR. Hemorheological disorders in cerebrovascular accident: relationship to inflammatory processes and thrombogenesis. In: Hartmann A & Kuschinsky W (Eds). Cerebral ischemia and hemorheology. Berlin: Springler-Verlag, pp 69-75, 1987.

10. BOISSEAU MR, FREYBURGER G, BELLOC F, SEIGNEUR M. Hemorheological effects of buflomedil: action on shape and functions of the human neutrophils. Blood Vessels 28, 15-20, 1991.

11. BOOGAERTS MA, MALBRAIN S, MEEUS P, VAN HOVE L, VERHOEF GEG. In vitro moduation of normal and diseased human neutrophil function by pentoxijylline. Blut 61, 60-64, 1990.

12. BUSSE W , RANDLEV B, SEDGWICK L. The effect of azelastin in neutrophil and eosinophil generation of superoxide. J Allergy Clin Immunol 83, 400-405, 1989.

13. CARDEN DL, SMITH JK, KORTHUIS RJ. Neutrophil-mediated microvadcular dysfunction in postichemic canine skeletal muscle. Role of granulocyte adherence. Circul Res 66, 1436-1444, 1990.

14. CIUFFETTI G, MANNARINO E, PASQUALINI L, MERCURI M, LENNIE SE, LOWE GDO. The hemorheological role of cellular factors in peripheral vascular disease. VASA 17, 168-170, 1988.

15. CLISSOLD SP, LYNCH S, SORKIN EM. Buflomedeil, a review of its pharmacodynamic and pahrmacokinetic properties. Drugs 33, 430-460, 1987.

16. D'ERASMO E, SAVERIO-CELI F, ACCA M, MAZZUOLI G. Relationship between platelet and white blood cell count during the early phase of cerebral infarction. Stroke 22, 283, 1991.

17. DADOUKIS I, ANGAIRIDAKIS K, ALETRAS H. The action of the basic trypsin inhibitor Trasylol on shock resulting from occlusion of the superior mesenteric artery: an experimental study. Int Med Res 9, 31-39, 1981.

18. DAY RO, MINERS J, BIRKETT DJ, GRAHAM GG, WHITEHEAD A. Relationship between plasma oxipurinol concentrations and xanthine-oxidase activity in volunteers dosed with allopurinol. Br J Clin Pharmac 26, 429-434, 1988.

19. DE LABRY LO, CAMPION EW, GLYNN RJ, VOKONAS PS. White blood cell count as predictor of mortality: results over 18 years from the normative aging study. J Clin Epidemiol 43, 153-157, 1990.

20. DE SERVI S, MAZZONE A, RICEVUTI G, FIORAVANTI A, BRAMUCCI E, ANGOLI S, STEFANO G, SPECCHIA G. Granulocyte activation after coronary angioplasty in humans. Circulation 82, 140-146, 1990.

21. DINERMAN JL, MEHTA JL, SADEEN TG, EMERSON S, WALLIN R, DAVDA R, DAVIDSON A. Increased neutrophil elastase release in unstable angina pectoris and acute myocardial infarction. J Am Coll Cardiol 15: 1559-1563, 1990.

22. DONNELYY PK, BOOTH H, WHITE M, SHENTON BK. α-2-macroglobulin and generation of oxygen radicals by granulocytes: potential role in prevention and treatment of reperfusion injury. Clin Chim Acta 302, 55-64, 1991.

23. DOWNEY JM. Free radicals and their involvement during longterm myocardial ischemia and reperfusion. Annu Rev Physiol 52, 487-504, 1990.

24. EGAN RW, HAGMANN WK, GALE PH. Naphtalenes as inhibitores of myeloperoxidase: direct and indirect mechanisms of inhibition. Agents and Actions 29, 266-276, 1990.

25. ENGLE WA, YODER MC, BAURLEY JL, PAO-LO Y. Vatamin E decreases superoxide anion production by polymorphonuclear leukocytes. Ped Res 23, 245-248, 1988.

26. ENGLER RL, DAHLGREN MD, MORRIS D, PETERSON M, SCHMID6SCHONBEIN GW. Role of leukocytes in response to acute myocardial ischemia and reflow in dogs. Am J Physiol 252, 314-322, 1986.

27. ENGLER RL, SCHMID-SCHONBEIN GW, PAVELEE RS. Leukocyte capillary plugging in myocardial ischemia and reperfusion in the dog. Am J Pathol 111, 98, 1983.

28. ERNEST E, HAMMERSCHMIDT DE, BAGGE U, MATRAI A., DORMANDY JA. Leukocytes and the risk of ischemic diseases. JAMA 257, 2318-2324, 1987.

29. ERNST E, MATRAI A, PAULSEN F. Leukocyte rheology in recent stoke. Stroke 18, 59-62, 1987.

30. FREYBURGER G, BELLOC F, BOISSEAU MR. Pentoxfylline inhibits actin polymerization in human neutrophils after stimulation by chemoattractant factor. Agents Actions 31, 72-78, 1990.

31. FRIEDMAN GD, KLATSKY AL, SIEGELAUB MS. The leukocyte count as a predictor of myocardial infarction. N Engl J Med 290, 1275-1278, 1974.

32. GARCIA JH, KAMIJYO Y. Evolution of histological change after occlusion of a middle cerebral artery in primates. J Neuropathol 33, 408-421, 1978.

33. GIBBS D, VARANI J, GINSBURG I. Formation and use of poly-L-histidine catalase complexes: protedtion of cells from hydrogen peroxid-mediated injury. Inflammation 13, 465-474, 1989.

34. GOLDMAN G, WELBOURN R, PATERSON IS, KLAUSNER JM, KOBRIK L, VALERI CR, SHEPRO D, HECHTMAN HB. Ischemia-induced neutrophil activation and diapedisis is lipoxygenase dependent. Surgery 107, 428-433, 1990.

35. GOLDSTEIN BD, WITZ G, TROLL W. Protease inhibitors antagonise the activation of polymorphonuclear leukocyte oxygen

consumption. Biochem Biophys Res Commun 88, 854-860, 1979.

36. GRANGER DN, Mc CORD JM, PARKS DA, HOLLYWARTH ME. Xanthine oxidase inhibitors attenuate ischemia-induced vascular permeability changes in the cat intestine. Gastroent 90, 80-84, 1986.

37. GRIMM RH, NEATON JD, LUDWIG W. Prognostic importance of the white blood cell count for coronary, cancer and all-cause mortality. JAMA 254, 1932-1937, 1985.

38. HAINES AP, HOWARTH D, NORTH WRS, GOLDENBERG E, STIRLING Y, MEADE TW, RAFTERY EB, MILLAR CRAIG MW. Haemostatic variables and the outcome of myocardial infarction. Thromb Haemost 50, 800-803, 1983.

39. HALLENBECK J, DUTKA A, TANISHIMA T et al. Polymorphonuclear leukocyte accumulation in brain regions with low blood flow during the early posischemic period. Stroke 17, 246, 1986.

40. HALLET MB, SHANDALL A, YOUND HL. Mechanism of protection against reperfusion injury by aprotinin. Roles of polymorphonuclear leukocytes and oxygen radicals. Biochem Pharmacol 34, 1757-1761, 1985.

41. HARLAN JM. Neutrophil-mediated Vascular Injury Acta Med Scand (Suppl.), 715, 123-129, 1987.

42. HATANO T, YASUHARA T, YOSHIHARA R, IKEGAMI Y, MATSUDA M, YAZAKI K, AGATA I,. NISHIBE S, NORO T, YOSHIZAKI M et al . Inhibitory effects of galloylated flavonoids on xanthine oxidase. Planta Med 57, 83-84, 1991.

43. HICKEY NC, GOSTLING P, BAAR S, SHEARMAN CP, SIMMS MH. Effect of surgery on the systemic inflammatory response to intermittent

claudicatuin. Br J Surgery 77, 1121-1124, 1990.

44. HINSHAW DB, BURGER JM, DELIUS RE. Mechanism of protection of oxidant-injured endothelial cells by glutamine. Surgery 108, 298-305, 1990.

45. HOGG N. Human monocytes are associated with the formation of fibrin. J Exp Med 157, 473-485, 1983.

46. HOSHIDA S, KUZUYA T, NISHIDA M, KIM Y, FUJI H, MINAMINO T, KITABATAKE A, TADA M, KAMADA T. Transcardiac alteration of neutrophil function before and after coronary thrombolysis in human myocardial infarction. Int J Cardiol 30, 49-54, 1991.

47. ITO T, ASAI F, USHIYAMA S, MATSUDA K, OSHIMA T. Reduction of infarct size and infiltration of polymorphonuclear leukocytes by a thromboxane synthetase inhibitor. Arzneim-Forsch/Drug Res 40, 23-24, 1990.

48. ITOH T, KAWAKAMI M, YAMAUCHI Y, SHIMIZU S, NAKAMURA M. Effect of allopurinol on ischemia and reperfusion-induced cerebral injury in spontaneously hypertensive rats. Stroke 17, 1284-1287, 1986.

49. JAESCHKE H, FARHOOD A, SMITH W. Neutrophils contribute to ischemia/reperfusion injury in rat liver in vivo. FASEB J 4, 3355-3359, 1990.??

50. JAHN U, THIELE K. In vitro inhibition of xanthine-oxidase by azapropazone and 8-hydroxy-azapopazone. Arzneim-Forsch/Drug Res 38, 507-508, 1988.

51. JANERO DR, BURGHARDT B. Antiperoxidant effects of dihydropyridine calcium antagonists. Bioch Pharma 38, 4344-4348, 1989.

52. JANERO DR, LOPEZ R, PITTMAN J, BURGHARDT B. Propanolol as xanthine oxidase inhibitor: implications for antioxidant activity. Life Sc 44, 1579-1588, 1988.

53. KOCHANEK PM, NEMOTO EM, EVANS RW, SCHOETTLE RJ. Polymorphonuclear leukocyte, platelets and lipid mediators in the pathogenesis of ischemic and traumatic central nervous system injury. In: Bazan NG (Ed). Lipid mediators in ischemic brain damage and experimental epilepsy. Basel: Karger, pp 220-240, 1990.

54. KREAMER R, SELIGMANN B, MULLANE KM. Polymorphonuclear leukocytes reduce cardiac function in vitro by release of H_2O_2. Am J Physiol 258, 1847-1855, 1990.

55. KUBES P, SUZUKI M, GRANGER DN. Platelet activating factor induced microvascular dysfunction: role of adherent leukocytes. Am J Physiol 258, 158-163, 1990.

56. KUZUYA T, HOSHIDA S, SUZUKI K, SASAKI T, KITABATAKE A, KAMADA T, MINAMINO T, TADA M. Polymorphonuclear leukocyte activity and ventricular arrhytmia in acute myocardial infarction. Am J Cardiol 62, 868-872, 1988.

57. LEE E, MIKI Y, KATSURA H, KARIYA K. Mechanism of inactivation of myeloperoxidase by propylthiouracil. Biochem Pharmacol 39, 1467-1471, 1990.

58. LEY K, GAETHGENS P. Endothelial, not hemodynamic differences are responsible for preferencial leukocyte rolling in rat mesenteric venules. Circ Res 69, 1034-1041, 1991.

59. LEY K, GAETHGENS P. Inhibition of leukocyte rolling by sialic acid. Int J Microcirc Clin Exp, 1 (Suppl.), 135 (Abst.), 1990.

60. LEY K, LUNDGREN E, BERGER E, ARFORS KE. Shear-dependent inhibition of granulocyte adhesion to cultured endothelium by dextran sulfate. Blood 73, 1324-1330, 1989.

61. LO BALSAMO L, BERGSLAND J, LAJOS P, FELDMAN MJ. Prevention of reperfusion injury in ischemic-reperfused hearts by oxipurinol and allopurinol. Transplant Int 2, 218-22, 1989.

62. LOWE GDO, MACHADO SG, KROL WF, BARTON BA, FORBES CD. White blood cell count and hematocrit as predictor of caronary recurrence after myocardial infarction. Thromb Haemost 54, 700-703, 1985.

63. LUCCHESI BR. Modulation of leukocyte-mediated myocardial reperfusion injury. Ann Rev Physiol 52, 561-576, 1990.

64. LUO WS, GUO ZG, TANG XL. Neutrophil infiltration in eschemic porcine myocardium and protective effect of verapamil. Acta Pharmacol Sinica 11, 435-438, 1990.

65. LYBERG T. Clinical significance of increased thromboplastin activity on the monocyte surface, a brief review. Haemostasis 14, 430-439, 1984.

66. LYNCH MJ, GRUM CM, GALLAGHER KP, BOLLING SF, DEEB M, MARGANROTH ML. Xanthine oxidase inhibition attenuates ischemic reperfusion lung injury. J Surg Res 44, 538-544, 1988.

67. MARIDONNEAU-PARINI I, ERRASTA M, ROUSSEAU-MARIE F. Inhibition of $O_2^{\cdot-}$ generation by dexamethasone is minicked by lipocortin 1 in alveolar macrophages. J Clin. Invest 83, 1936-1940, 1989.

68. MARZI I, KNEE J, BUHREN V, MENGER M, TRENTZ O. Reduction by superoxide dismutase of leukocyte-endothelial adherence after liver transplantation. Surgery 111, 90-97, 1992.

69. MEHTA J, DINERMAN J, MEHTA P, SALDEEN TGP, LAWSON D, DONNELLY WH, WALLIN R. Neutrophil function in ischemic heart disease. Circulation 79, 549-556, 1989.

70. MENASCHE P, GROUSSET C, GAUDUEL Y, MOUAS C, PIWNICA A. Enhancement of cardioplegic protection with the free-radical scavenger peroxidase. Circulation (suppl. III), 74, 111-138, 1986.

71. NAKANISHI T, NISHI M, INADA A, OBATA H, TANABE N, ABE S, WAKASHIRO M. Two new potent inhibitors of xanthine oxidase from leaves of Perilla frutescens Britton var. acuta Kudo. Chem Pharm Bull (Tokyo) 38, 1772-1774, 1990.

72. NASH GB, CHRISTOPHER B, MORRIS AJR, DORMANDY JA. Changes in the flow properties of white blood cells after acute myocardial infarction. Br Heart J 62, 329-334, 1989.

73. NASH GB, THOMAS PRS, DORMANDY JA. Abnormal flow properties of white blood cells in patients with severe ischaemia of the leg. Brit Med J 296, 1669-1702, 1988.

74. NERI SERNERI GG, ABBATE R, GENSINI GF, GORI AM, ATTANASIO M, MARTINI F. Monocyte activation and increased procoagulant activity in unstable angina. Lancet 336, 1444-1445, 1990.

75. NEUMANN FJ, WAAS W, DIEHM C, WEISS T, HAUPT HM, ZIMMERMANN R, TILLMANNS H, KUBLER W. Activation and decreased deformability of neutrophils after intermittent claudication. Circulation 82, 922-929, 1990.

76. NIEMETZ J. Coagulant activity of leukocytes: tissue factor activity. J Clin Invest 51, 307-313, 1972.

77. NORO T, NORO K, MIYASE T, KUROYANAGI M, UMEHARA K, UENO A, FUKUSHIMA S. Inhibition of

xanthine oxidase by anthraquinones. Chem Pharm Bull 35, 4314-4316, 1987.

78. NYGAARD OP, UNNEBERG K, REIKERAS B, OSTERUD B. Thromboplastic activity of blood monocytes after total hip replacement. Scand J Clin Invest 50, 183-186, 1990.

79. O'NEILL PG, CHARLAT ML, MICHAEL LH, ROBERTS R, BOLLI F. Influence of neutrophil depletion on myocardial function and flow after reversible ischemia. Am J Physiol 256, 341-351, 1989.

80. OKANO T, TAMAI H, MINO M. Superoxide generation in leukocytes and vitamin E. Internat. J Vit Nutr Res 61, 20-26, 1990.

81. OLLIVIER V, SHEIBANI A, CHOLLET-MARTIN S, VIE P, BENACERRAF R, DUPARC J, DE PROST D. Monocyte procoagulant activity and membrane associated D-Dimer after knee replacement surgery. Thromb Res 55, 179-185, 1989.

82. OREDSON S, PLATE G, QVARFORDT P. Allopurinol - a free radical scavenger - reduces reperfusion injury in skeletal muscle. Eur J Vasc Surg 5, 47-52, 1991.

83. OSTERUD B, BJORKLID E. Human factor VII associated with endotoxin-stimulated monocytes in whole blood. Biochem Biophys Commun 108, 620-626, 1982.

84. OSTERUD B, OLSEN JO, BENJAMINSEN AW. The role of complement in the induction of thromboplastin synthesis. Haemostasis 14, 386-392, 1984.

85. PINCEMAIL J, DUPUIS M, NASR C, HANS P, HAAG-BERRURIER M, ANTON R, DEBY C. Superoxide anion scavenging effect and superoxide dismutase activity of Ginkgo biloba extract. Experientia 45, 708-712, 1989.

86. PRASAD K, KALRA J, CHAUDHARY AK, DEBNATH D. Effect of polymorphonuclear leukocyte-derived oxygen free radicals and hypochlorous acid on cardiac function and some biochemical parameters. Am Heart J 119, 538-545, 1990.

87. PRENTICE RL, SHIMIZU Y, LIN CH, PETERSON AV, KATO H, MASON MW, SZATROWSKI TP. Leukocyte counts and coronary heart disease in a Japanese cohort. Am J Epidemiol 116, 496-506, 1982.

88. PRENTICE RL, SZATROWSKI TP, KATO H. Leukocyte counts and cerebrovascular disease. J Chronic Dis 35, 703-714, 1982.

89. PUIG JG, MATEOS FA, DIAZ VD. Inhibition of xanthine oxidase by allopurinol: a therapeutic option for ischemia induced pathological processes? Ann Rheum Dis 48, 883-888, 1989.

90. RABIER M, DAMON M, CHANEZ P, MENCIA-HUETA JM, BOUSQUET J, MICEL FB, GODARD P. Platelet-activating factor neutrophil chemotaxis and ginkgolides. In: Braquet P (Ed). Ginkgolides, chemistry, biology, pharmacology and clinical perspectives. J.R. Prous Science Publishers, vol 1, p 105, 1989.

91. RADOMSKI M, HERBACZYNSKA-CEDRO K, CEREMUZYNSKI L. Increased activity of circulating polymorphonuclear leukocytes in acute myodardial infarction. Int J Cardiol 27, 392-393, 1990.

92. RANJADAYALAN K, UMACHANDRAN V, TIMMIS A, GUTTERIDGE CN. Neutrophil activation and reperfusion during fibrinolytic therapy of myocardial infarction. Br J Haematol 77, 13, 1991.

93. REIMER KA, MURRY CE, RICHARD VJ. The role of neutrophils and free radicals in the ishemic-reperfused heart: why the confusion

and contreversy. J Mol Cell Cardiol 21, 1225-1239, 1989.

94. REIZENSTEIN P. The haematological stress syndrome. Br J Haematol 4, 329-334, 1979.

95. RINALDO JE, GORRY M. Protection by deferoxamine from endothelial injury: a possible link with inhibition of intracellular xanthine oxidase. Am J Respir Cell Mol Biol 3, 533-535, 1990.

96. RIVA CM, MORGANROTH ML, LJUNGMAN AG, SCHOENEICH SO, MARKS RM, TODD III RF, WARD PA, BOXER LA. Iloprost inhibits neutrophil induced lung injury and neutrophil adherence to endothelial monolayers. Am J Resp Cell Med Biol 3, 301-309, 1990.

97. ROMSON JL, HOOK BG, KUNKEL SL, ABRAMS GD, SCHORK MA, LUCCHESI BR. Reduction of the extent of ischemic myocardial injury by neutrophil depletion in the dog. Circulation 67, 1016-1023, 1983.

98. ROSENGREEN S, ARFORS KE. Neutrophil-mediated vascular leakage is not suppressed by leukocyte elastase inhibitors. Am J Physiol 259, 1288-1294, 1990.

99. SAGONE AL, HUSNEY RM, WEWERS MK, HERZYK DJ, DAVIS WB. Effects of dimethylthiourea on the neutophil myeloperoxidase pathway. J Appl Physiol 67, 1056-1062, 1989.

100. SALARIS SC, BABBS CF, VOORHEES III WD. Methylene blue as an inhibitor of superoxide generation by xanthine oxidase. Biochem Pharm 42, 499-506, 1991.

101. SCHLANT RC, FORMAN S, STAMLER J, CANNER PL. The natural history of coronary heaty disease: prognostic factors after recovery from myocardial infarction in 2789 men. Circulation 66, 401-414, 1982.

102. SCHMELING DJ, DRONGOWSKI RA, CORAN AG. The beneficial effects of ibuprofen on a lathal live E. Coli septic shock model and the relationship of these effects to superoxide radical production. Prog Clin Biol Res 299, 53-61, 1989.

103. SCHMID-SCHONBEIN G, ENGLER RL. Perspectives of leukocyte activation in the microcirculation. Biorheology 27, 859-869, 1990.

104. SCHMID-SCHONBEIN GS. Granulocyte activation in capillary obstruction. In: Liepsch DW (Ed). Blood flow in large arteries: applications to atherogenesis and clinical medecine. Basel: Karger, pp 150-159, 1990.

105. SEMERARO N, LATTANOIO A, MONTEMURRO P, PAPANICE M, DE LUCIA O, DE BELLIS G, GIORDANO D. Mechanisms of blood clotting activation in inflamation: the role of mononuclear phagocytes. Int J Tissue React 7, 313-320, 1985.

106. SHELLEY WB, JUHLIN L. Induction of fibrin in thrombi by monocytes. Nature 270, 343-344, 1977.

107. SHOENFELD PJ. Leucopenia and low incidence of myocardial infarction. Lancet 1, 1606, 1981.

108. SIBILLE Y, REYNOLDS HY. Macrophages and ploymorphonuclear neutrophils in lung defense and injury. Rev Resp Dis 141, 471-501, 1990.

109. SIMPSON PJ, TODD III RF, FANTONE JC et al. Reduction of experimntal canine myocardial reperfusion injury by a monoclonal antibody (anti-mo1, anti-CD11B) that inhibits leukocyte adhesion. J Clin Invest 81, 624-629, 1988.

110. SMITH JA, TELFORD RD, MASON IB, WEIDEMAN MJ. Exercice, training and neutrophil

microbicidal activity. Int J Sports Med 11, 179-187, 1990.

111. STAHLBERG HJ, LOSCHEN G, FLOHE L. Inhibition by prostacyclin analogs of O_2^{-} production in human plymorphnuclear leukocytes. Basic Life Sc 49, 991-995, 1988.

112. STRIETER RM, REMICK DG, WARD PA, SPENGLER RN, LYNCH JP, LARRICK J, KUNKEL SL. Cellular and molecular regulation of tumor necrosis factor-α production by pentoxifylline. Biochem Biophys Res Commun 155, 1230-1236, 1988.

113. STUART J, GEORGE AJ, DAVIES AJ, AUKLAND A, HURLOW RA. Hematological stress syndrome in atherosclerosis. J Clin Pathol 34, 464-467, 1981.

114. SUTTER S, CHEVALLIER S. The effect of Eglin-C on the function of human neutrophils in vitro Biol Chem Hoppe-Seyler 369, 573-578, 1988.

115. T HART BA, IP VAI CHING TRAM, VAN DIJK H, LABADIE RP. How flavinoids inhibit the generation of luminol-dependent chemo-luminescence by activated human neutrophils. Chem. Biol. Interactions 73, 323-335, 1990.

116. TAMURA Y, CHI LG, DRISCOLL EM Jr, HOFF PT, FREEMAN BA, GALLAGHER KP, LUCCHESI BR. Superoxide dismutase conjugated to polyethylene glycol provedes sustained protection against myocardial ischemia/ reperfusion injury in canine heart. Circ Res 63, 944-959, 1988.

117. TANAKA H, SUGIMOTO H, YOSHIOKA T, SUGIMOTO T. Role of granulocyte elastase in tissue injury in patients with septic shock complicated by multiple-organ failure. Ann Surg 213, 81-85, 1991.

118. TANGELDER GJ, ARFORS KE. Inhibition of leukocyte rolling in venules by protamine and sulfated polysaccharides. Blood 77, 1565-1571, 1991.

119. THIEL M, BARDENHEUER M, POCH G, MADEL C, PETER K. Pentoxifylline does not act via adenosine receptors in the inhibition of the superoxide action production of human polymorphonuclear leukocytes. Biochem Biophys Res Commun 108, 53-58, 1991.

120. VAN ZYL JM, BASSON K, KRIEGLER A, VAN DER WALT BJ. Mechanism by which clofazine and dapsone inhibit the myeloperoxidase pathway. Biochem Pharmacol 42, 599-608, 1991.

121. VEDDER NB, WINN RK, RICE CL, CHI EY, ARFORS KE, HARLAN FM. A monoclonal antibody to the adherence-promoting leukocyte glycoprotein, CD18, reduces organ injury and improves survival from haemorrhagic shock and resuscitation in rabbits. J Clin Invest 81, 939-944, 1988.

122. VERMES I, STRIK F. Altered leukocyte rheology in patients with chronic cerebrovascular disease. Stroke 19, 631-633, 1988.

123. VIOLI F, RASURA M, ALESSANDRI C? INTISO D, GERMANI M, SERVI M, FIESCHI C, BALSANO F. Leukocyte response in patients suffering from acute stroke. Stoke 19, 1283-1284, 1988.

124. WALDEN DL, Mc CUTCHAN HJ, ENQUIST EG, SCHWAPPACH JR, SHANLEY PF, REISS OK, TERADA LS, LEFF JA, REPINE JE. Neutrophils accumulate and contribute to skeletal muscledysfunction after ischemia-reperfusion. Am J Physiol 259, 1809-1812, 1990.

125. WALKER PM, LINDSAY TF, LABBE R, MICKLE DA, ROMASHIN AD. Salvage of skeletal muscle with free radical scavengers. J Vasc Surg 5, 68-75, 1987.

126. WARD PA. Mechanisms of endothelial cell injury. J Lab Clin Med 118, 421-426, 1991.

127. WARREN JS, YABROFF KR, MANDEL DMM, JOHNSON KJ, WARD PA. Role of O_2^{-} in neutrophil recrutment into sites of dermal and pulmonary vasculitis. Free Rad Biol & Med 8, 163-172, 1990.

128. WELBOURN R, GOLDMAN G, KOBZIK L, PATERSON I, VALERI CR, SHEPRO D, HECHTMAN HB. Neutrophil adherence receptors (CD18) in eschemia. Dissociation between quantitative cell surface expression and diapedesis mediated by leukotriene B_4. Immunol 145, 1906-1911, 1990.

129. WERNS SW, GRUM CM, VENTURA A, HAHN RA. Ho PPK, TOWNER RD, FANTONE JC, SCHORK MA, LUCCHESI BR. Xanthine oxidase inhibition does not limit canine infarct size. Circulation 83, 995-1005, 1991.

130. WHISLER RL, PROCTOR VK, DOWNS EC, MORTENSEN RF. Modulation of human monocyte chemotaxis and procoagulant activity by human C-reactive protein (VRP). Lymphokine Research 5, 223-228, 1986.

131. WILLIAMS FM, COLLINS PD, TANNIERE-ZELLER M, WILLIAMS TJ. The relationship between neutrophils and increased microvascular permeability in a model of myocardial ischaemia and reperfusion in the rabbit. Br J Pharmacol 100, 729-734, 1990.

132. YAMADA Y, YOKODA M, FURUMICHI T, FURUI H, YAMAUCHI K, SAITO H. Protective effects of calcium channel blokers on hydrogen peroxide incuced increases in endothelial permeability. Cardiov Res 24, 993-997, 1990.

133. YARNELL JWG, SWEETNAM PM, ELWOOD PC, EASTHAM R, GILMOUR RA, O'BRIEN JR. Haemostatic factors and ischaemic heart disease: the

Caerphilly study. Br Heart J 53, 483-487, 1985.

134. ZAGER RA, GMUR DJ. Effects of xanthine-oxidase inhibition on ischemic acute renal failure in the rat. Am J Physiol 257, 953-958, 1989.

135. ZALOKAR JB, RICHARD JL, CLAUDE JR. Leukocyte counts, smoking and myocardial infarction. N Engl J Med 304, 465-468, 1981.

136. ZIMMERMAN BJ, GRISHAM MB, GRANGER DN. Role of oxidants in ischemia/ reperfusion-induced granulocyte infiltration. Am J Physiol 258, 185-190, 1990.

137. ZIMMERMAN J, MILLARD J. H_2-antagonist inhibition of human neutrophil superoxide anion synthesis. Clin Pharmacol Ther 45, 487-494, 1989.

138. ZWEIER JL, RAYBURN BK, FLAHERTY JT, WEISHFELDT ML. Recombinant superoxide dismutase reduces oxygen free radical concentrations in reperfused myocardium. J Clin Invest 80, 1728-1734.

10

Thrombomodulin - a novel anticoagulant

J. Morser

Thrombomodulin is a membrane associated endothelial cell glycoprotein that binds thrombin. The binding of thrombin to thrombomodulin changes thrombin's substrate specificity from a procoagulant to an anticoagulant. In the figure below (Figure 1), the procoagulant activities of thrombin (fibrinogen to fibrin conversion, platelet activation and clotting cascade activation) are shown with thin lines, while the anticoagulant activity (via the protein C pathway and antithrombin III (ATIII) inactivation of thrombin) are shown with thick lines. After thrombin binding to thrombomodulin, the rate of activation of protein C is enhanced by at least 100 fold, the procoagulant activities are inhibited and the rate of inhibition of thrombin by ATIII is enhanced.

We show here that a recombinant thrombomodulin that is soluble is a safe and efficacious anticoagulant because of its mechanism of action. This discussion of thrombomodulin is divided into two parts, a section on structure/function relationships and a section on the potential therapeutic uses of thrombomodulin.

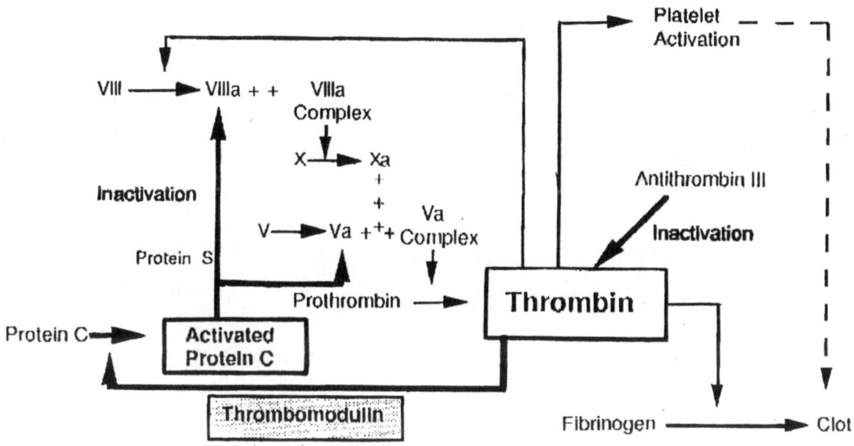

Figure 1: The role of thrombomodulin

1. Thrombomodulin structure

The protein structure of thrombomodulin can be subdivided into five domains of which three are extracellular: a lectin domain, 6 copies of the EGF-like domain, an O-linked glycosylation domain, and then a transmembrane domain and a cytoplasmic domain (Figure 2). We have produced numerous deletion mutants of human thrombomodulin which have been rendered soluble by removal of the transmembrane and cytoplasmic domains. These mutants have been tested in "in vitro" assay systems and the regions of the thrombomodulin molecule required for thrombin binding and protein C conversion cofactor activity have been identified.

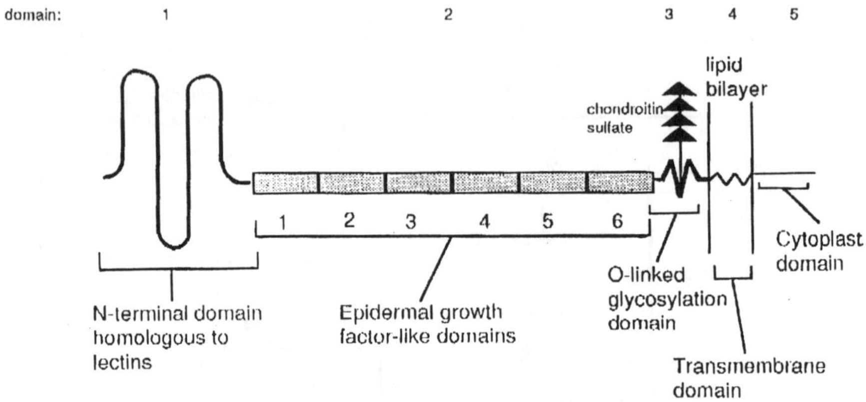

Figure 2: Domain structure of thrombomodulin

Two different structures appear to be important for the protein C activation cofactor activity of thrombomodulin. The first is a region of the protein structure encompassing EGF-like domains 4, 5 and 6. This region was identified by constructing a serie of deletion mutants from the N-terminus and C-terminus of thrombomodulin. This fragment will bind to thrombin and activate protein C. The binding site for thrombin is located within the C loop of EGF5 while EGF4 is required for protein C activation.

The second region important for cofactor activity is the chondroitin sulfate moiety that is post-translationally added to the O-linked glycosylation domain. The addition of the chondroitin sulfate moiety increases the binding affinity between thrombin and thrombomodulin eight fold and hence increases cofactor activity. The interaction of the chondroitin sulfate and thrombin occur at a second site on thrombin, different from the one that EGF5 binds to. Although the chondroitin sulfate increases the affinity between thrombomodulin and thrombin, it does not enhance the rate at which protein C is activated. We have shown that the amount and type of chondroitin sulfate added, as well as the site of addition, is dependent on the cell line.

Recombinant thrombomodulin and its truncated analogs are susceptible to oxidation. Their sensitivity to oxidation is similar to that of α1-antiprotease, suggesting that the inactivation of thrombomodulin may have a physiological role. We identified the sites of oxidation as the methionine residues within the 6 EGF-like domains. Site specific mutants of the 2 methionines in this fragment by either glutamine or leucine did not lose activity after oxidation when the substitution was at methionine 388. Thus oxidation of methionine 388 was responsible for the loss of activity.

Mutants with all possible amino acids substituted for methionine 388 were tested. It was shown that the leucine substitution had an increased specific activity two fold higher than the wild type. This was mainly due to an effect on the Km of the thrombomodulin/thrombin complex for protein C.

In addition we have substituted alanine for all amino acids except glycine, alanine, proline and cysteine in the minimal active fragment of EGFs 4, 5 and 6. Of the 77 substitutions tested, 22 were shown to lead to a protein that was significantly less active in activation of protein C. This analysis allowed identification of critical residues for binding to thrombin and activation of protein C.

2. Therapeutic potential of throbomodulin

In order to demonstrate the therapeutic potential of recombinant soluble thrombomodulin we have been characterizing the mode of action and "in vivo" activity of a fragment of thrombomodulin consisting of the 6 EGF-like domains that had been produced in insect cells.

Soluble thrombomodulin has been tested in standard coagulation assays and shown to prolong the thrombin time, PT and APTT. In addition it has been tested in a thrombin generation assay in platelet rich plasma. In this assay coagulation is triggered with addition of a high dilution of thromboplastin and aliquots are removed for determination of thrombin concentration. The results were compared with those of heparin and hirudin. All agents tested strongly influenced the thrombin generation curve. While hirudin, in a dose dependent manner, postponed the thrombin burst, supporting the irreversible thrombin inhibition as its major mode of action, heparin showed both an inhibition of maximal thrombin generation as well as a delay of the thrombin burst. These results underline the catalytic mode of action of heparin in not only inhibiting thrombin directly but also its formation.

In contrast, thrombomodulin, in a dose dependent manner, decreased maximal thrombin generation without a significant effect on the time to the thrombin burst. The effect of thrombomodulin was demonstrated to be protein C dependent by use of protein C deficient platelet rich plasma, in which thrombomodulin was much less active. Thus thrombomodulin is highly effective in inhibiting the generation of thrombin in thromboplastin activated platelet rich plasma by a mechanism that is clearly distinct from that of heparin or hirudin. This mechanism is protein C dependent and can be explained by the anticoagulant activity of activated protein C.

We investigated the pharmacokinetics of several of the soluble thrombomodulin fragments that we had produced in different cell lines. The determinants responsible for clearance were identified as the presence of chondroitin sulfate, the other carbohydrate and the length of the molecule. On this basis a molecule was selected for further testing.

We compared the effects of randomized and blinded doses of thrombomodulin, hirudin, heparin to a saline control on thrombus formation in a rat vena cava model of thrombosis. In addition APTT, thrombin time and platelet function were tested "ex vivo". All three agents prevented vena cava thrombosis. At therapeutically equivalent doses, thrombomodulin did not prolong the APTT or thrombin time, as did heparin and hirudin. Neither platelet aggregation nor platelet secretion in response to thrombin was affected by thrombomodulin, but it was inhibited by both heparin and hirudin at therapeutically equivalent doses. When bleeding time was tested in a model consisting of venipuncture of a mesenteric vein thrombomodulin caused significantly less bleeding than haparin or hirudin at equivalent therapeutic doses.

Soluble recombinant human thrombomodulin has been shown to have a novel mode of action, inhibiting thrombin generation by causing the activation of protein C. When tested in a rat model of venous thrombosis it inhibits thrombus formation with less effect on hemostatic parameters than either heparin or hirudin, suggesting that it will possess a more attractive safety profile.

11

Anticoagulation for neonates, infants and children

N. Schlegel, M.F. Hurtaud-Roux, F. Beaufils

Although rare in pediatric patients, thrombotic complications are observed since birth, with a first peak of frequency in the neonatal period and a second peak near the adolescence period.

Due to the great heterogeneity of the thrombi localization and the corresponding symptoms but also due to the impossibility of obtaining large homogeneous series of cases, the antithrombotic strategy is not codified in the pediatric age group. In most of the cases, this strategy is extrapolated from guidelines for adults. Interesting informations are also supplied by in vitro and ex vivo studies comparing the effects of one anticoagulant in neonatal and adult plasma [7, 23], and by pharmacokinetic studies in animal models [7]. However, due to immediate or potential severity of thrombosis, the preventive or curative treatment of such a disorder has to be considered with the highest attention. Anticoagulation always carries the danger of haemorrhage. Therefore, the indications of such a treatment must be carefully assessed in the clinical context. In some cases, it should be better to forego doing this treatment, where the risk of haemorrhage, for example the risk of intracranial haemorrhage in very premature babies, and the resulting consequences are not justified by the potential benefit.

Two categories of anticoagulant agents, both synthetic, are currently available for the treatment of thrombosis: heparins are antivitamins K. An other category of anticoagulants, coagulation inhibitors concentrates, from human origin, are also available for special cases.

The aim of this article is to summarize the guidelines which can be proposed today for using these agents in the pediatric age group patients.

1. Heparins

1.1 Indications

The use of heparins is indicated for preventing the constitution of a thrombus or, if the thrombus is already constituted, for preventing its extension and its recurrence.

1.1.1 Prevention of a thrombus formation

Preventive indications can be proposed in two different situations: catheterization or thrombogenic pathological situations.

Catheters are now widely used for pediatric patients and catheter related thrombotic complications, either venous or arterial, have been reported. Venous thrombosis are observed during long-term parenteral nutrition, or long-term catheterization in children with leukemia or cancer. These complications seem to decrease with time, due to the progress in biomaterials and the improvement of the catheter placement techniques. But, the true frequency of asymptomatic catheter thrombosis is not known. In the largest recent series [8, 15, 17, 26, 33], symptomatic catheter related thrombotic complications have been reported to occur in 13 to 31 per cent of cases, or 0.03 to 0.09 per 100 days of catheter use. Short-term jugular venous catheterization is also at risk of thrombosis [27]. Femoral artery thrombosis is the most frequent thrombotic complication of arterial catheters in children and has been reported to occur in 3.6 per cent to 8.6 per cent of cases in the two largest recent publications [18, 40].

Various thrombogenic pathological situations are observed in children, and represent indications for preventive treatment with heparin. The risk of deep vein thrombosis and pulmonary embolism or arterial thrombotic complications is associated with a wide variety of disorders [30]. Among them, nephrotic syndrome is a very peculiar situation where the risk of thrombosis is as much due to an acquired antithrombin III (ATIII) deficiency as to an excessive synthesis of coagulation factors [20]. The optimal doses and regimen of heparin treatment cannot be standardized and are variable with time and with the response to the specific treatment of the nephrotic syndrome itself. The details of the heparin treatment should thus be adapted to the ATIII concentration which can be lower than 20 per cent, and the coagulation factors concentration which can be over 200 per cent. For these reasons, heparin is not the best candidate for preventing thrombosis in these patients.

1.1.2 Treatment of a thrombosis

Heparin is the anticoagulant of choice for the initial treatment of the majority of acute thrombotic episodes whatever the age. In pediatric patients, heparin is used for the treatment of catheter related arterial or venous thrombosis, deep vein thrombosis, renal vein thrombosis, coronary arteries thrombosis occuring during the Kawasaki syndrome. Intracranial venous thrombosis is an exception as heparin therapy carries a significant risk of haemorrhage, and the possible benefit is debatable. Acquired or congenital ATIII deficiency related thrombosis is of particularly difficult management due to the fact that the action of heparin is precisely related with the ATIII concentration. In these cases, an ATIII concentrate infusion can be usefully associated with heparin.

The benefit of heparin comparatively with other anticoagulant treatment, with other antithrombotic strategy, with antiplatelet drugs administration or with supportive care alone has not been evaluated in the different thrombotic complications observed in children patients.

In some cases, an association of several of these treatments might be more efficient but the associated haemorrhagic risk has to be evaluated very carefully.

1.2 Dosage and regimen

The modalities of heparin treatment in children are adapted from the knowledge coming from adult patients treatment [13, 38].

1.2.1 Unfractionated heparin (UFH)

Prevention

The usual dose of UFH for children at low risk of thrombosis is similar to the one injected to adult patients: 100 IU/Kg/day subcutaneously. This dose does not induce detectable modifications of the usual tests, which are therefore considered to be unnecessary. For children at "high risk" of thrombosis, the goal of the heparin treatment is to obtain a patient's plasma Activated Partial Thromboplastin Time (APTT) 1.2 to 1.3 time the control's plasma APTT.

Despite controversy, it had appeared that the addition of heparin to a concentration of 1 IU/ml to the infusion was reducing significantly the risk of thrombosis during catheterization [9, 28]. Theoretically, this dose carries no haemorrhagic risk in patients with normal levels of coagulation factors and normal platelet count, as the total dose of heparin does not exceed 200 to 250 IU/Kg/day. However, recently, a randomized trial did not show a significant difference between two regimens, either once a week saline or heparin prophylaxis, to maintain catheter patency in children with central venous catheters [34].

Treatment

Basically, the heparin treatment of a thrombosis starts with a loading dose injected as a bolus. The bolus is followed by a maintenance dose intravenously, according to the results of the biological tests. The usual bolus dose is 50 IU/Kg, and the initial maintenance dose is 500 IU/Kg/day. In several cases, this maintenance dose has to be increased further, during the neonatal period (see below) or during peculiar diseases like nephrotic syndrome. The goal of the treatment is to maintain the patient's plasma APTT 1.5 to 3 times the control's plasma one, and an heparinemia of 0.3 to 0.6 IU/ml.

The heparin dose has to be selected according to the type of thrombosis, arterial or venous, and to the haemorrhagic risk, specific for each patient.

The indications related to the optimal duration of the heparin treatment are not definitively defined yet for pediatric patients, as well as for adult patients. The usual duration for heparin therapy during limbs venous thrombosis is as short as possible, ie between 7 to 10 days. The optimal heparin treatment duration is more difficult to determine for arterial thrombosis, peripheric or deep, and for deep thrombosis venous or arterial. In most of the cases, it appears that the treatment duration should not exceed 2 weeks, and is often limited by technical difficulties of UFH infusion in children patients.

1.2.2 Low molecular weight heparins (LMWH)

Owing to their subcutaneous administration, LMWH might be considered to be theoretically more suitable than UFH in pediatric patients. Unfortunately, specific pharmacological studies concerning LMWH in a pediatric population are rare, and there is no scientific data indicating that the plasmatic anti-Xa activity should be different from the one recommended for adult patients, ie 0.15 to 0.30 IU/ml for prevention of thrombosis, and 0.50 to 1 IU/ml for treatment of a thrombosis. In our experience the "prevention" concentration is generally obtained by one subcutaneous injection of 30 to 50 IU anti-Xa/Kg/day. But, in some of the cases where haemorrhagic risks are associated to thrombotic complications, like haemorrhagic colitis, Crohn disease, we prefer to start with lower doses (20 to 40 IU anti-Xa/Kg/day) and, subsequently, to adapt the dose taking in account both the plasmatic anti-Xa activity and the absence, apparition or increase of digestive haemorrhage.

If there is a high risk of thrombosis, for instance in case of important inflammatory syndrome with high concentrations of coagulation factors (Factors II, VII+X, V higher than 120 per cent, fibrinogen higher than 600 mg/dl and Factor VIII higher than 150 per cent), it is recommendable to start with a preventive dose of 50 IU anti-Xa/Kg/day and, if necessary, to increase the dose till 0.65 IU or more in order to obtain a plasmatic anti-Xa activity not lower than 0.30 IU/ml, and preferably between 0.30 and 0.50 IU/ml.

1.3 Biological monitoring

Blood samples for biological controls must be drawed by a line different from the one used for heparin infusion. In several cases of difficult drawing or prolonged heparin treatment, it is useful to position a special line, arterial or venous, for blood drawing.

A full study of the coagulation system is absolutely necessary before starting the heparin therapy, in order to detect a putative contra-indication. This initial study includes platelet numeration, hemoglobin concentration determination, APTT, Prothrombin Time (PT) and fibrinogen concentration evaluation. ATIII concentration is also to be measured if a decreased concentration of this molecule is suspected.

In pediatric as well as in adult patients, three tests are available for monitoring heparin therapy: APTT, anti-Xa activity, heparinemia. The APTT of the patient's plasma is expressed in seconds comparatively to the APTT of a control plasma. Anti-Xa activity is expressed in international units per ml of plasma. Heparinemia, which corresponds to the coagulation time of the patient's plasma in presence of thrombin, is expressed in units per ml of plasma. The three tests are generally used for evaluating the effect of UFH. By contrast, anti-Xa assay is usually thought to be sufficient for evaluating the effect of LMWH, but APTT is useful for the detection of an overdosage. In case of LMWH therapy, anti-Xa activity is determined in a blood sample obtained exactly 4 hours after the subcutaneous injection.

A biological monitoring does not seem to be absolutely necessary during the prophylactic treatment of adult patients with LMWH [13, 38]. By contrast, we think that, due to the absence of specifically pediatric conditioning of LMWH and the rare pharmacological data related to the use of LMWH for neonates and children, it seems better to propose a specific biological monitoring for pediatric patients, at least at day 2, and day 4 after starting the treatment. Further controls will be necessary in different circumstances: modification of the dose, suspicion of overdosage, new pathological event, introduction of drugs able to interfere with LMWH.

1.4 Undesirable effects

The practical difficulties of infusion and blood sampling for biological control in a pediatric population increase the risk of undesirable effects as compared to the adult patients.

1.4.1 Haemorrhage

Whatever the heparin injected, UFH or LMWH, the risk of haemorrhage is always present.

Haemorrhage are generally the consequence of an overdosage which can be detected by abnormally prolonged APTT and thrombin time. Heparins can be neutralized by protamine sulphate [38]. In adults, the dose of protamine sulphate is depending of the half life of the drugs: about 1 hour for intravenous UFH and 2 hours for subcutaneous LMWH. The dose of protamine sulphate is also depending on the neutralization reaction between protamine sulphate and heparin :

- 100 IU of UFH are neutralized by 1 mg of protamine sulphate
- the neutralization of LMWH by protamine sulphate is not completely determined today; it might be acceptable to say that 100 IU anti-Xa of LMWH are

approximately neutralized by 1 mg of protamine sulphate. In absence of specifically pediatric studies, these recommendations might be used also for children.

1.4.2 Heparin-induced thrombocytopenia [38]

Heparin-induced thrombocytopenia, as a consequence of an immunological decrease of platelet number, is a severe unforseeable event which can be observed during the first treatment with heparin, as early as the fifth day of the treatment and whatever the dosage and the mode of administration. If the frequency seems to be higher during UFH treatment, heparin-induced thrombocytopenia can also be observed during LMWH therapy. The diagnosis is based on an acute or progressive decrease of the number of platelets, or the worsening of the thrombosis although a theoretically efficient treatment. This severe accident would be prevented by shortening the heparin therapy duration. In case of UFH induced thrombocytopenia, LMWH must be checked in vitro before being injected to the patient.

The frequency of heparin-induced thrombocytopenia in a pediatric group is not known yet and cautious measures similar to measures applied to the adult group must be taken.

1.4.3 Osteoporosis [38]

Although the true risk of developing a heparin induced osteoporosis is unknown, the clinical and radiological symptoms of this uncommon but real complication must be regularly researched in the rare cases of long term heparin therapy in children, whatever the type of heparin [22].

1.5 Are there specific recommendations about the use of heparins for neonates?

The recommendations for the use of heparins for adults cannot be simply extrapolated to newborns [2, 7]. The neonatal hemostatic system is characterized by low levels of vitamine K dependent factors and contact factors, which are approximately half of the adult values [4, 6]. Consequently, the neonatal APTT is spontaneously and moderately prolonged by an average 1.3 times the APTT of the adult. This physiological immaturity could explain an increased "sensitivity" to heparin in neonates. However, the levels of physiological inhibitors of coagulation, specially ATIII, are also lower than adult levels. Furthermore, the volume of distribution of heparin is increased in newborns as compared with adults [7]. From these data, one can expect an increased "resistance" to heparin in neonates. Schmidt et al [32] speculate that newborns should be more resistant when heparin treated for a thrombosis but more sensitive during a heparin preventive therapy. Recently, Andrew et al [2] have proposed the following guidelines for initiating heparin therapy in newborns: initial bolus of 50 to 100 IU/Kg, and then infusion of 20 to 30 IU/Kg/hour. After this initial period, the treatment will be adjusted according to the biological tests.

As to LMWH, in vitro systems and pharmacokinetic studies have shown important differences between newborns and adults in humans [39] as well as in the piglet model [3].

With the lack of official recommendations based on clinical trials, which are particularly difficult to perform in the pediatric population, the general rules for the use of heparins for adults should apply to the very young children and newborns. Besides, the biological monitoring of the treatment should include the APTT and the heparinemia in order to weigh the respective importance of heparin therapy and hepatic immaturity in the prolongation of the APTT. The anti-Xa activity assay and the thrombin clotting time measurement are dependent of the ATIII concentration. Due to the low AT III concentration in the newborn plasma, the results of the very usual assays underestimate the heparin concentration in neonatal plasma [31]. The biological monitoring should be more watchful due to the high risk of intracranial haemorrhage in the newborn and the high risk of overdosage.

2. Antivitamins K

2.1 Indications

In a pediatric age group, the use of antivitamins K is characterized by two main difficulties: 1) treatment equilibration, 2) high haemorrhagic risk. For these reasons, the indications are limited to pathological conditions associated with a lasting risk of thrombotic complications, mainly: nephrotic syndrome, mechanical heart valves, inherited prethrombotic states such as heterozygous ATIII, Protein C or Protein S deficiencies, decreased fibrinolytic activity, recurrent thrombotic episodes, long time immobilization.

2.2 Pharmacological agents, dosage and regimen

Different antivitamins K are available for adults and can be theoretically used for children. The pharmacokinetic characteristics should be carefully examined when selecting an antivitamin K for a children treatment. This treatment is based on two principles: safety and efficiency. What is the ideal antivitamin K for children patients? In order to have the best control of the competitive inhibition of the vitamine K, the two most important criteria might be: 1) an initiation of action not too fast, and 2) a stability of action as reliable as possible. For these reasons, warfarin sodium (Coumarin) could be the agent of choice. But different characteristics of warfarin might be considered as disadvantages: long half-life of 35 hours, alteration of the warfarin requirement by many drugs in relation with different mechanisms. Children who are fed with milk formulae that contain high concentrations of vitamin K need theroretically higher dosage of warfarin. More questionable is the high risk of frequent and important variations of the warfarin requirements due to possible sudden variations of their milk formulas intake. Furthermore, there is no pediatric conditioning, thus the usual initial dosage of 0.03 to 0.16 mg/Kg/day corresponds to approximately 1 to sixth to three quaters of a 2 mg tablet for a 10 Kg body weight baby!

Two other antivitamins K, acenocoumarol and ethyl biscoumacetate, are also prescribed. The initial time nessecary to obtain an efficient action is between 24 to 36 hours, and between 24 to 48 hours respectively. Both have an action duration of 24 hours. The half life is 8.7 hours for acenocoumarol and 2.5 hours for ethyl biscoumacetate.

An antivitamin K treatment induces the decrease of all the vitamin K dependent proteins, including coagulation factors (II, VII, X, IX) but also coagulation inhibitors like Protein C and Protein S. When starting the treatment, the decreasing rate of the concentration of these proteins is related to their half-life: Fact V = 5 hours, Fact IX = 14 hours, Fact X = 40 hours and Fact II = 60 hours. The anticoagulation is obtained after a variable period from 24 hours to 120 hours and is stabilized after one week of treatment. Therefore, the dosage must be adapted during all the treatment as strictly as possible. Due to the evolutive and therefore variable concentrations of the coagulation factors and their inhibitors during the growth of the child, the variations of the dosages considered as efficient are more frequent in a pediatric than in an adult patients group. It has been reported that the dosage requirements may be higher in infants and adolescents than in adults [10, 41]. Different regimens of long term anticoagulant therapy isolated or associated with antiplatelet therapy are used for patients with prosthetic heart valves [41]. The safety and efficiency of these pharmacological agents remain controversial as to their use is concerned in the pediatric group. The minimum amount of oral anticoagulant necessary to remain symptom free and the targeted therapeutic range which might be selected according to the nature and to the anatomic localization of the heart valves are not defined yet [29]. The main problem remains the bleeding risk [19].

2.3 Biological monitoring

The biological monitoring is based on the International Normalized Ratio (INR) [37], which is based itself on the different sensitivities of the reagents used to measure the PT. The INR is calculated as follows: $[\text{patient PT/control PT}]^{ISI}$ where ISI represents the International Sensitivity Index, and is indicated by the manufacturer of each reagent used for the PT determination.

No specific recommendations have been established for INR in a pediatric age patients group. Therefore, the INR values recommended for adults are the only data available today to monitor an antivitamin K treatment, whatever the age [14, 16, 35]. The INR value is from 2.0 to 3.0 for the prevention of venous thrombosis and systemic embolism, as well as for the treatment of venous thrombosis and pulmonary embolism. A higher value of INR, from 3 to 4.5 is deemed necessary for the treatment of recurrent embolism and thrombosis of patients with mechanical heart valves.

The frequency of biological control during antivitamin K therapy should be more frequent for children than for adults, due to the possibly more frequent variations in the equilibrium of their coagulation system. During the initial period of the treatment, the PT has to be controlled every two days, and, after one week, once or twice a week. If any possibility of a coagulation variation is suspected, for instance due to an unexpected new illness or to the administration of other drugs, the PT must be immediately controlled.

In case of a shift from heparin to antivitamin K therapy, the biological monitoring will include APTT, PT and heparinemia as long as both anticoagulant agents are simultaneously administered. Heparin can be stopped when INR is at least at 2.5 during 48 hours.

Heparin is substituted to antivitamins K before surgery. During the surgical operation, heparin itself is generally suspended as shortly as possible taking in account both the haemorrhagic risk of the surgical procedure and the thrombotic risk in the patient. In case of emergency surgery, the injection of 5 to 10 mg of vitamine K or Solvent-Detergent treated PPSB can balance the pharmacological inhibition of vitamin K.

As already mentioned for the biological monitoring of heparins, there are practical difficulties for the monitoring of antivitamins K treatement in children. Blood sampling is often difficult, and always traumatic for young people, and the repetition of the venipunctures may represent a problem. For these reasons, the benefit/risk ratio must be carefully discussed. Recently, Adams et al [1] have evaluated a whole blood PT monitor (512 Coagulation Monitor, Biotrack, LA, USA). They concluded from their studies that this monitor was well received by children and parents and was an accurate method for monitoring coumadin treated children.

2.4 Side effects

The rare studies which have attempted to evidence putative effects of coumarin derivatives in different animal or human tissues have not found out significant anomalies. More precisely, non-carboxylated proteins were not found in these tissues, including liver, kidney, lung, spleen, testes, muscles and heart [11]. No specific data in relation with pediatric patients are available.

Haemorrhagic risk of long term oral anticoagulation has been reported to be comparable to that in adults [36].

2.5 Are there specific recommendations about the use of antivitamins K for neonates?

During the neonatal period, the antivitamin K treatment is very hazardous and therefore exceptionnally administered. If it is decided to make this choice, it is necessary to consider the low physiological concentration of the vitamin K dependent coagulation factors and inhibitors and the very unstable equilibrium between procoagulants and anticoagulants. Consequently, the effects of antivitamin K therapy cannot be predicted in a precised way.

As for heparins, Andrew et al [2] have proposed the following guidelines for initiating Coumadin therapy in newborns: loading dose of 0.2 mg/kg for 2 days and maintenance dose adjusted to INR value desired. There is no reference for the INR value in the neonatal period.

3. Purified ATIII and Protein C concentrates

Concentrates of purified coagulation inhibitors represent new interesting approaches for the prevention and treatment of thrombotic episodes due to congenital or acquired ATIII or Protein C deficiencies.

In patients with congenital ATIII deficiency, the first thrombotic episode usually occurs in the second decade. Nevertheless, the use of ATIII concentrate has already been reported in rare cases of children

thrombosis associated with hereditary ATIII deficiency [24, 25]. Short-term ATIII concentrate treatment can also be helpful in cases of thrombosis due to acquired ATIII deficiencies. Heparin treatment can be associated with ATIII concentrate infusions.

Homozygous and double heterozygous forms of congenital Protein C deficiency are responsible of massive venous thrombosis and purpura fulminans in neonates [12, 21]. Recently, purified Protein C concentrates became available. Such a concentrate has been used for the successful treatment of a newborn with severe Protein C deficiency and purpura fulminans [12]. Moreover, a long-term therapy with this highly purified concentrate was well tolerated.

4. Conclusion

In brief, the anticoagulation mechanisms are interesting to prevent and to treat the thrombotic complications occuring in pediatric patients. Even though the basic mechanisms are similar for all human beings at any age, specific guidelines are needed for young children, mainly in the neonatal period and in the two or three first years of life, until the coagulation system is completely mature. Due to the limited knowledge on pharmacological characteristics of anticoagulants in neonates, infants and children, and due to the practical difficulty of the biological monitoring, and due to the impossibility to get large series, only multicentric studies will be able to define these specific guidelines.

REFERENCES

1. ADAMS M, VEGH P, MARZINOTTO V, ANDREW M. Monitoring coumadin therapy in children (personal communication).

2. ANDREW M. An approach to the management of infants with impaired haemostasis. Baillière's Clinical Haematology, 4, 251-289, 1991.

3. ANDREW M, OFOSU FA, BROOKER L, BUCHANAN M. The comparison of the pharmacokinetics of a low molecular weight heparin in the newborn and adult pig. Thromb Res 56, 529-540, 1990.

4. ANDREW M, PAES B, JOHNSTON M. Development of the hemostatic system in the neonate and young infant. Am J Pediatr Hematol Oncol 12, 95-104, 1990.

5. ANDREW M, PAES B, MILNER R, JOHNSTON M, MITCHELL L, TOLLEFSEN DM, CASTLE V, POWERS P. Development of the human coagulation system in the healthy premature infant. Blood 72, 1651-1657, 1988.

6. ANDREW M, PAES B, MILNER R, JOHNSTON M, MITCHELL L, TOLLEFSEN DM, POWERS P. The development of the human coagulation system in the fullterm infant. Blood 70, 165-172, 1987.

7. ANDREW M, SCHMIDT B. Use of heparin in newborn infants. Semin Thromb Haemostas 14, 28-32, 1988.

8. BAGNALL HA, GOMPERTS E, ATKINSON JB. Continuous infusion of low-dose urokinase in the treatment of central venous catheter

thrombosis, in infants and children. Pediatrics 83, 1963-1966, 1989.

9. BOSQUE E, WEAVER L. Continuous versus intermittent heparin infusion of umbilical artery catheters in the newborn infant. J Pediatr 108, 141-143, 1986.

10. BRADLEY LM, MIDGLEY FM, WATSON DC, GETSON PR, SCOTT LP 3d. Anticoagulant therapy in children with mechanical prosthetic cardiac valves. Am J Cardiol 56, 533-535, 1985.

11. DE BOER-VAN DEN BERG M. Thèse, Maastricht March 13, 1987. (Professor H.C. HEMKER).

12. DREYFUS M, MAGNY JF, BRIDEY F, SCHWARZ HP, PLANCHE C, DEHAN M, TCHERNIA G. Treatment of homozygous protein C deficiency and neonatal purpura fulminans with a purified protein C concentrate. N Engl J Med 325, 1565-1568, 1991.

13. GROUPE D'ETUDES SUR L'HEMOSTASE ET LA THROMBOSE. Utilisation des héparines en pratique médicale courante. STV 3, n° 5(suppl), 4-10, 1991.

14. Guidelines on oral anticoagulation: second edition. British society for haematology. British committee for standards in haematology. Haemostasis and thrombosis task force. J Clin Pathol 43, 177-183, 1990.

15. HARVEY WH, PICK TE, REED K, SOLENBERGER RI. A prospective evaluation of the Port-a-Cath implantable venous access system in chronically ill adults and children. Surg Gynecol Obstet 169, 495-500, 1989.

16. HIRSCH J, POLLER L, DEYKIN D, LEVINE M, DALEN JE. Optimal therapeutic range for oral anticoagulants. Chest 95 n°2 (suppl), 5S-11S, 1989.

17. HOCKENBERRY MJ, SCHULTZ WH, BENNETT B, BRYANT R, FALLETTA JM. Experience with minimal complications in implanted catheters in children. Am J Pediatr Hematol Oncol 11, 295-299, 1989.

18. INO T, BENSON LN, FREEDOM RM, BARKER GA, ZIPURSKY A, ROWE RD. Thrombolytic therapy for femoral artery thrombosis after pediatric cardiac catheterization. Am Heart J 115, 633-639, 1988.

19. LEVINE MN, RASKOB G, HIRSH J. Hemorrhagic complications of long-term anticoagulant therapy. Chest 95 n°2 (suppl), 26S-36S, 1989.

20. LOIRAT C, PILLION G, SCHLEGEL N, DOUENIAS R, MATHIEU H. Etude des protéines de la coagulation et de la fibrinolyse au cours des syndromes néphrotiques de l'enfant. Arch Fr Pediatr 36(suppl), LVI-LXIII, 1979.

21. MARLAR RA, BROEKMANS AW, and the Working Party. Diagnosis and treatment of homozygous protein C deficiency. Report of the working party on homozygous protein C deficiency. The Subcommittee on protein C and protein S, International Committee on Thrombosis and Haemostasis. J Pediatr 114, 528-534, 1989.

22. MATZCH T, BERQVIST D, HEDNER U, NILSSON B, OSTERGAARD P. Effects of low molecular weight heparin on induction of osteopororis in rats. Thromb Haemost 63, 505-509, 1990.

23. Mc DONALD MM, HATHAWAY WE. Anticoagulant therapy by continuous heparinization in newborn and older infants. J Pediatr 101, 451-457, 1982.

24. MENACHE D. Replacement therapy in patients with hereditary antithrombin III Deficiency. Semin Haematol 28, 31-38, 1991.

25. MENACHE D, O'MALLEY JP, SCHORR JB, WAGNER B, WILLIAMS C, et al. Evaluation of the safety, recovery, half-life and clinical efficacy of Antithrombin III (Human) in patients with hereditary antithrombin III deficiency. Blood 75, 33-39, 1990.

26. MIRRO J Jr, RAO BN, STROKES DC, AUSTIN BA, KUMAR M, DAHL GV, COLTEN M, BALA SL, RAFFERTY M, HANCOCK M et al. A prospective study of Hickman/Broviac catheters and implantable ports in pediatric oncology patients. J Clin Oncol 7, 214-222, 1989.

27. MOORE RA, Mc NICHOLAS KW, NAIDECH H, FLICKER S, GALLAGHER JD. Clinically silent venous thrombosis following internal and external jugular central venous cannulation in pediatric cardiac patients. Anesthesiology 62, 640-643, 1985.

28. RAJANI K, GOETZMAN BW, WENNBERG RP, TURNER E, ABILGAARD C. Effect of heparinization of fluids infused through an umbilical artery catheter on catheter patency and frequency of complications. Pediatrics 63, 552-556, 1979.

29. RAO PS, SOLYMAR L, MARDINI MK, FAWZY ME, GUINN G. Anticoagulant therapy in children with prosthetic valves. Ann Thorac Surg 47, 589-592, 1989.

30. ROBIN M, BOYER C. Causes des thromboses veineuses de l'enfant et de l'adolescent en dehors de la période néonatale. Arch Fr Pediatr 44, 467-472, 1987.

31. SCHMIDT B, MITCHELL L, OFOSU FA, ANDREW M. Standard assays underestimate the concentration of heparin in neonatal plasma. J Lab Clin Med 112, 641-643, 1988.

32. SCHMIDT B, OFOSU FA, MITCHELL L, BROOKER LA, ANDREW M. Anticoagulant effects of heparin in

neonatal plasma. Pediatr Res 25, 405-408, 1989.

33. SHULMAN RJ, RAHMAN S, MAHONEY D, POKORNY WJ, BLOSS R. A totally implanted venous access system used in pediatric patients with cancer. J Clin Oncol 5, 137-140, 1987.

34. SMITH S, DAWSON S, HENNESSEY R, ANDREW M. Maintenance of the patency of indwelling central venous catheters: is heparin necessary ? Am J Pediatr Hematol Oncol 13, 141-143, 1991.

35. STEIN PD, KANTROWITZ A. Antithrombotic therapy in mechanical and biological prosthetic heart valves and saphenous vein bypass grafts. Chest 95 n°2 (suppl), 107S-117S, 1989.

36. STEWART S, CIANCIOTTA D, ALEXSON C, MANNING J. The long-term risk of warfarin sodium therapy and the incidence of thromboembolism in children after prothetic cardiac valve replacement. J Thorac Cardiovasc Surg 93, 5S1-4, 1987.

37. VAN DEN BESSELAAR AMPH. Scientific and standardization committee communication: recommended method for reporting therapeutic control of oral anticoagulant therapy. Thromb Haemost 63, 316-317, 1990.

38. VERSTRAETE M. Pharmacotherapeutic aspects of unfractionated and low molecular weight heparins. Drugs 498-530, 1990.

39. VIEIRA A, OFOSU FA, ANDREW M. Heparin sensitivity and resistance in the newborn: an explanation. Pediatr Res 25, 274-275, 1989.

40. WESSEL DL, KEANE JF, FELLOWS KE, ROBICHAUD H, LOCK JE. Fibrinolytic therapy for femoral arterial thrombosis after cardiac

catheterization in infants and children. Am J Cardiol 58, 347-351, 1986.

41. WOODS A, VARGAS J, BERRI G, KREUTZER G, MESCHENGIESER S, LAZZARI MA. Antithrombotic therapy in children and adolescents. Thromb Res 42, 289-301, 1986.

12

Anticoagulation in the elderly : indications and limitations

G. Pinganaud, PJ. Louvet, JP. Emeriau

Anticoagulants are not often prescribed in elderly people because of the risk of haemorrhage. But during the last few years, the results of many large controlled double blind trials have been published, which have specified indications. Chronological age by itself is not a contra-indication, the limitations being the diseases associated with ageing.

1. Myocardial infarction (MI) and ischaemic cardiopathy

The elderly coronary artery disease (CAD) is one of the major causes of death and disability. For patients aged 75 years or more, the MI mortality rate exceeds 50 % (for the overall population itself, not those being treated). The interest of anticoagulation treatment is based on three points:

- first: a substantial reduction of mortality after acute MI with intravenous thrombolytic therapy,

- second: to avoid thromboembolic complications and MI extent with heparin and antiplatelet agents,
- third: to decrease the reinfarction rate and the risk of death after MI with oral anticoagulants.

1.1 Acute myocardial infarction

1.1.1 Thrombolytic therapy

In most procedures for MI treatment, beyond the age of 70 is considered a contra-indication to thrombolytic therapy. However, mortality after MI is higher in elderly patients (Table I) [6].

Before MI, elderly have a more extensive CAD, which may impair non-infarct-zone contractility, and relatively more left ventricular (LV) dysfunction due to impaired healing. Thrombolytic therapy preserves the LV function, which is directly correlated with MI artery patency. In White et al study thrombolytic therapy significantly improved LV ejection fraction, by 4.3 % in younger patients and 7.5 % in older patients [38]. In this study, streptokinase (SK) and recombinant tissue plasminogen activator (rtPA) significantly reduced end-systolic volume and end-systolic volume is more important prognostic factor than ejection

Table I : Worcester heart Attack Study [6]

OVERALL HOSPITAL MORTALITY	
< 55 years	5 %
55 - 64	7.9 %
65 - 74	16.1 %
> 75 years	32.1 %

fraction after MI. Thrombolytic therapy did not affect end-diastolic volume. Thrombolysis after acute MI may confer greater benefits in older patients.

However most thrombolytic trials in patients with MI have restricted randomization on the basis of age because of concern about the possibility of an increased risk of hemorrhage. This restriction was not confirmed by two large trials GISSI [12] and ISIS [7]. In GISSI I study, the two most feared events, with SK. major bleeding (defined as need for transfusion of at least 2 units of blood) and anaphylactic shock (documentation of which was required in ad-hoc forms) proved to have a low incidence: 0.3 % major bleed and 0.7 % for anaphylactic shock: no specific adverse reactions of bleeding or negative clinical events were recorded in older age group (35 % of patients were aged > 65) than in the younger group. In ISIS II study, there was a not unusual excess of bleeding among the 401 patients who were aged 80 or over, with SK. Other informations concerning hemorrhagic complications with intravenous rTPA in the elderly are available from the Thrombolysis and Angioplasty in Myocardial Infarction (TAMI) [35] and from the Thrombolysis in Myocardial Infarction (TIMI) [27] trials, although both restricted entry to patients aged < 76 years. In the TAMI trial (in which 150 mg of rtPA was administered) factors associated with increased bleeding risk were invasive procedures femelle gender smaller size and older age. In the TIMI trial, factors associated with increased bleeding risk were the dose of rTPA per kilogram of body weight, age and elevated diastolic blood pressure. These results suggest that complications might be reduced especially by adjusting rtPA dose for body weight.

These results confirm that advanced age alone should not be considered a contra-indication to thrombolytic therapy.

1.1.2 Heparin

Generally, intravenous therapy with heparin for acute MI is started few hours after the onset of symptoms. The second indication is unstable CAD (unstable angina and non Q wave MI). But, in most studies, age more than 70-75 years represents a cause for exclusion.

The Risk Group have published a study concerning the risk of MI and death during treatment with low dose aspirin and intravenous heparin in men with unstable CAD [25]. 796 men aged under 70 years with unstable CAD (unstable angina or non Q wave MI) were randomized to double-blind placebo-controlled treatment with oral aspirin 75 mg/day and/or 5 days of intermittent intravenous heparin. The group treated with aspirin and heparin had the lowest number of events during the initial 5 days. In this group there was a 75 % risk reduction compared with placebo or heparin alone (Table II) [25].

In the Risk Group, heparin alone has no significant influence on event rate (MI or death) compared with placebo.

In earlier studies in unstable CAD, a seven day treatment with heparin IV reduced the risk of Q wave infarction by 80 %, but treatment was started earlier and by continuous infusion [10, 19, 30].

Subcutaneous heparin treatment showed little clinical benefit in unstable angina [10] and acute MI (the SCATI group) [26]. In the SCATI study, 711 patients of either sex, up to age 80 were considered for inclusion if acute MI was suspected on clinical and electrographic grounds. These patients were randomized to a group receiving calcium-heparin 12500 U, subcutaneous every 12 hours (360 with 192 patients age 61 to 89 years), or to a group receiving no heparin (351 with 182 patients aged 61 to 81 years), beginning within 24 hours of the onset of symptoms. 433 of those patients, admitted within 6 hours, were given intravenous SK.

Table II: MI and death with aspirin (A) 75 mg/days or placebo (P) and heparin (H) or placebo Risk Group [25]

TREATMENT		FOLLOW UP		
		5 days	30 days	90 days
PP (n=199)		12	28	35
PH (n=198)		11	25	33
AP (n=189)		7	9	14
AH (n=210)		3	8	12
PP/PH	P	NS	NS	NS
PP/AP	P	NS	0.0037	0.0042
PP/AH	P	0.027	0.005	0.0003
PH/AP	P	NS	0.012	0.009
PH/AH	P	0.045	0.002	0.0007
AP/AH	P	NS	NS	NS

Electrocardiographically confirmed transient ischaemic episodes occured in 60 (16.6 %) of the heparin group and 67 (19 %) of the controls, not a significant difference. In the subset of 433 patients who received SK, myocardial ischaemia recured in 14.2 % and 19.6 % respectively, a difference just short of significance (p=0.08). Mortality was significantly lower in the calcium-heparin treated patients, both in the overall groups (21/360 VS 35/351, p=0.03) and in the SK subgroups (10/218 VS 19/215, p=0.05). On predischarge two-dimensional echography, the prevalence of thrombus was significantly lower in the heparin group than in the

Table III summaries the frequency distribution of endpoint events.

	SK GROUP (433)			NON SK GROUP (278)		
EVENTS	HEPARIN (218)	CONTROL (215)	P	HEPARIN (142)	CONTROL (136)	P
RECURRENT ISCHAEMIA	31 (14.2%)	42 (19.6%)	0.08	29 (40.4%)	25 (18.3%)	0.88
NON FATAL REINFARCTION	18 (8.2%)	21 (9.7%)	0.47	2 (1.4%)	3 (2.2%)	0.59
MORTALITY	10 (4.5%)	19 (58.8%)	0.05	11 (7.7%)	16 (11.7%)	0.10
SCATI GROUP [11]						

control group (19/107 VS 3/93, p<0.01). These findings indicate that mortality, post MI recurrent ischaemic events and mural thrombus formation after acute MI, may be reduced by heparin in patients given fibrinolytic treatment [26].

The critical issue in treating elderly patient with an anticoagulant is whether the benefit outweighs the risk of therapy.

To determine the nature, incidence and predictors of in-hospital bleeding, Landefeld [14, 15] have examined 617 hospitalised patients, who started long-term anticoagulant therapy. The mean age was 62±14 years (range, 18 to 92 years). Therapy was initiated with heparin in 177 (29 %) patients and with warfarin in 440 (71 %). At some point during their in-hospital courses, 570 patients (92 %) were treated with warfarin alone, 156 patients (25 %) with heparin alone, and 155 patients (25 %) with warfarin and heparin simultaneously. Five patients (1 %) received streptokinase. Bleeding is a serious iatrogenic problem in patients starting anticoagulant therapy: 25 patients among 411 have minor bleeding (6 %) and 19 patients among 411 have major bleeding (5 %). Four independant risk factors for major inhospital bleeding were identified and weighed using univariate and multivariate discriminant analysis in a randomly chosen group of 411 patients:

* Co-morbid conditions other than the indication for anticoagulant therapy

* The use of heparin to begin therapy in patients aged 60 years or older: compared with younger patients, such patients had major bleeding 4.7 times as frequently if 60 to 79 years old and 8.5 times as frequently if more than 80 years old.

The risk of heparin-related bleeding was greater in patients aged 60 years or older who started therapy with intravenous heparin, but age was not associated with bleeding during the hospital course of patients treated with warfarin alone. Age has previously been related to bleeding more often in patients treated with heparin [36] than in those treated with oral anticoagulants [3].

* The intensity of therapy: compared with patients whose maximal prothrombin and partial thromboplastin times were less than twice the control-value, major bleeding was 3.2 times as frequent in patients with a 2.0 to 2.9 prolonged times control and 7.9 times as frequent in patients with a 3.0 or more prolonged times control.

* Liver dysfunction that worsened during treatment.

Identified specific risk factors may lead to rational risk reduction strategies and may be useful in weighing the risk against the benefits of anticoagulant therapy in individual patients especially in elderly patient, elderly being itself a risk factor.

1.1.3 Antiplatelet agents

The pathogenesis of unstable angina and myocardial ischaemia is the same, with a fissure in an atherosclerotic plaque which becomes covered with thrombotic material and decreases coronary blood flow [4]. Treatment with antiplatelet agents is effective in a prevention of complications.

In a review [1] thirty one randomized trials of antiplatelet treatment for patients with an history of transient ischaemic attack, occlusive stroke, unstable angina, or MI including a total of some 29000 patients, antiplatelets treatment had no apparent effect on non-vascular mortality but reduced vascular mortality by 15% (SD 4 %) and no fatal vascular events (stroke or MI) by 30 % (SD 4 %). The risk reduction in the new vascular events rate were 23 % (SD 4 %) for 900-1500 mg aspirin, 24 % (SD 8 %) for 300-325 mg aspirin, 17 % (SD 8 %) for sulphinpyrazone and 31 % (SD 5 %) for aspirin plus dipyridamol. The most convenient and least expensive type of antiplatelet agent is low dose aspirin. But, we have direct evidence about the antithrombotic effects of very low doses (for exemple, less than 100 mg/day).

But the Risk Group observed 57 to 69 % reduction of Q wave and non Q wave MI with 75 mg aspirin/day [25].

The discussion is therefore centered on 2 points:

* What is the optimum dosage for aspirin to obtain a full inhibition of platelets aggregation with the lowest frequency of side effects? Is a low dose (75 or 80 mg aspirin) sufficient? Several studies have found a protective effect of high doses of aspirin after MI [40] unstable angina [33] and in the prevention of MI [13], but in a comparative study of heparin and low dose aspirin (80 mg) added to rtPA heparin achieved higher rates of sustained patency of the infarct-related artery than did aspirin during the first 24 hours after MI [9]. The dose of aspirin may have been insufficient to halt reocclusion of the infarct-related artery after successful thrombolysis. At the present time, the optimum dose of aspirin is not clearly defined.

* What is the efficacy of aspirin in the primary prevention of angina? In the United States, the

Physicians Health Study conclusion was that low dose aspirin does not alter the incidence or delay the onset of confirmed angina pectoris [18]. In this study, aspirin dosage was 325 mg on alternative day. The results of an essay in a californian retirement community were comparable [21]. However, low doses aspirin seems an interesting treatment especially in unstable angina and during the acute period after MI onset. The higher doses are less convenient and more gastrotoxic than 300 mg/day.

Pharmacological studies, however, suggest that cyclo-oxygenase dependant platelet aggregation is inhibited just as effectively by 300 mg of aspirin as by higher doses: indeed some pharmacologist have suggested that doses substantially lower than 300 mg/day might actually be preferable, and doses of only 100 mg/day have a substantial antithrombotic effect in man. If to reduce gastrotoxicity still further an enteric coated preparation was used than the dose should probably not be reduced much below 80 mg/day [1].

1.2 After acute myocardial infarction

Beneficial effect of oral anticoagulants after MI has been highly controversial, although a number of clinical trials are conclusive.

The Warfarin Reinfarction Study [28] was initiated to assess the effect of long term treatment with oral anticoagulant after MI. A clear advantage emerged for the group that received warfarin (Table IV).

Table IV: Distribution of events according to treatment group

	WARFARIN	PLACEBO	RISK REDUCTION	p VALUE
TYPE OF ANALYSIS AND EVENTS	n = 607	n = 607	95%	
INTENTION OF TREAT				
DEATH	94	123	24 (40-44)	0.0267
REINFARCTION	82	124	34 (19-54)	0.0007
CEREBROVASCULAR ACCIDENT				
"ON TREATMENT"	20	40	55 (30-77)	0.0015
DEATH	60	92	35 (17-57)	0.005
REINFARCTION	70	122	43 (29-61)	0.0001
CEREBROVASCULAR ACCIDENT	16	41	61 (38-81)	0.0003

The warfarin reinfarction [24]

In the Risk Group, heparin alone has no significant influence on event rate (MI or death) compared with placebo.

In earlier studies in unstable CAD, a seven day treatment with heparin IV reduced the risk of Q wave infarction by 80 %, but treatment was started earlier and by continuous infusion [10, 19, 30].

In this study 1241 patients, who were 75 years of age or younger, were randomized 27 days after the onset of a MI, in 2 groups warfarin versus placebo for an average of 37 months. At the end of the treatment period there had been 133 deaths in the placebo group and 94 in the warfarin group with 24 % risk reduction. 124 patients in the placebo group had reinfarctions as compared with 82 in the warfarin group (-34 %). Furthermore, a reduction of 55 % in the number of total cerebrovascular accidents in the warfarin group was observed.

Venous bleeding was noted in 0.6 % on the warfarin treated patients for year. The target range for anticoagulation was an international normalized ratio of 2.8 to 4.8.

The influence of anticoagulants on the cerebrovascular accident rate is a difficult problem to appreciate, particularly in older patients. The Sixty Plus Reinfarction Study reported a statistically non-signifiant reduction of cerebrovascular accidents in old patients who received warfarin for 6 years or more after a first MI [32]. The aim of this trial was to compare the results of oral anticoagulant during a 2 years period: 878 patients over 60 years of age was randomized in 2 groups anticoagulant versus placebo. The 2 years total mortality was 13.4 % in the placebo group and 7.6 % in the group treated with anticoagulant (p=0.017). The other results are particularly interesting: the 2 years incidence of recurrent myocardial infarction was 15.9 % in placebo group and 5.7 % in the anticoagulant treated group (p=0.0001). The incidence of intracranial events was 5.6 % in placebo group and 3.1 % in the group of anticoagulants (p=0.28) with an important reduction for non haemorrhagic events: 13 in placebo and 2 in anticoagulant group. In this selected group of elderly patients, an intensive and stable oral anticoagulant therapy have substantically reduced the risk of cardiac death and recurrent MI.

In conclusion, for this 2 trials and for the first time, long term oral anticoagulation was associated with a reduction of morbidity and mortality a long time after MI. Moreover, there is a significant diminution of cerebral embolism.

One limit is represented by the intensity of treatment which is related to the incidence of bleeding [39]. In the Sixty Plus Reinfarction Study, when supervision of treatments was particularly attentive, accident were relatively rare and related to the age of the patients: one death due to bleeding per 206 patients-years at risk and one major bleeding episode per 55 patients-years at risk [32]. In the Warfarin Reinfarction Study, the rate was lower [28]. The difference may be explained by the higher proportion of patients with an international normalized ratio (INR) exceeding 4.8 in the Sixty Plus Group.

In the future, managment of oral anticoagulation will be carried out with a certain security. Four factors are identified with heparin. The risk of bleeding may be appreciated by a risk index: the number of specific co-morbid indications, intravenous heparin use in patients over age 60, a maximum prothrombin time or partial thromboplastin time ratio >2 and worsening liver function during therapy [14]. An other interesting approach is the reduction of the level of the anticoagulation. In the prevention of stroke due to atrial fibrillation, low levels of INR (1.5 <INR<2.5) are associated with a significant reduction of cerebrovascular accident [29, 31].

2. Atrial fibrillation

Atrial fibrillation (AF) is probably the most common cause of cardiac embolism to the brain.

In 1988, LODDER published a paper concerning the value of long term anticoagulation in patients with a first stroke due to a non rheumatic AF. 50 patients from the Oxfordshire Community Stroke Project who did not receive anticoagulations were compared that of 70 patients from Maastricht who were treated with anticoagulants. After a mean follow up of 27 months no significant difference was observed [16].

In the Copenhagen Study [22], 1007 patients were divided into 3 equal groups: warfarin with an international normalized ratio between 2.8 and 4.2, aspirin 75 mg daily and placebo. The mean age was 74.2 years. The incidence of thromboembolic complications was significantly reduced: 5 with warfarin, 20 with aspirin and 21 with placebo. 71 patients died during this study with a 3 vascular death in the warfarin group, 12 in the aspirin group and 15 in the placebo group. The difference was significantly different.

In the Boston Study [31], the principal difference in the protocol was about the level of anticoagulation: the target range was an International Normalized Ratio of 1.5 to 2.7. 420 patients entered the study and were randomized in anticoagulant group and placebo group: the mean age was 68 years. There were 2 strokes in the warfarin group compared with 13 strokes in the placebo group. The stroke risk reduction was 86 % for the Warfarin Group. The death ratio was markely lower in the warfarin group: 2.25 as compared with 5.57 % per year in the placebo group.

These 2 geriatric series are of particular interest: warfarin is able to reduce stroke incidence and cardiovascular death incidence. The second trial demonstrates that low level of anticoagulation give the same results with a significative reduction of hemorrhagic risk which is the principal problem for elderly patients.

The third and last point about the coagulation problem concerns aspirin: in the Copenhagen trial, aspirin is not able to prevent thromboembolism due to AF.

3. Cardiopathies with an increased embolism risk

The embolic risk is increased with:

- rheumatic mitral valve diseases
- prosthetic heart valves
- idiopathic dilated cardiomyopathy

and anticoagulation prophylaxis is easily justified [37].

4. Venous thromboembolism

4.1 Acute treatment of venous thromboembolism

In elderly patients as in younger ones, the need of anticoagulant treatment at the begining of venous thrombosis (VT) or pulmonary embolism (PE) is indiscutable but there is no universally accepted approach to the initial anticoagulant treatment. Possible variations include the duration of initial heparin treatment before oral anticoagulant therapy is started, the method of giving heparin (intravenous infusion or injection, or subcutaneous injection), the length of overlap between heparin and the oral anticoagulant and details of laboratory control.

In two studies [5, 11] a shorter course (3 to 5 days) compared with conventional treatment (8 to 10 days), the short course of heparin is as effective as a conventional course. In treating VT or PE in shorter course, warfarin was begun on the first day of heparin treatment. Furthermore, using the shorter course would permit earlier discharge from the hospital and thus after substantial most savings.

Heparin continues to be the prefered drug for the initial treatment of thromboembolic disease. But a low molecular weight fraction may be used with the same levels of tolerance to therapy and similar therapeutic efficacy in the extent of improvement of PE obstruction or deep VT. In order to determine the efficacy and safety of low molecular weight (LMW) heparins, several randomized trials in which the LMW heparin was compared to a fractionated heparin, have been published [17, 20, 24, 34]. All the results confirm interest of LMW heparins. A later study [23] compare 170 symptomatic patients randomized in two groups: 85 received an adjusted dose intravenous standard heparin and 85 received fixed-dose subcutaneous LMW heparin. The frequency of recurrent

VT did not differ significantly between the two groups (12-14 % Vs 6-7 %).

4.2 Prevention of venous thromboembolism in elderly patients

Thromboembolic disorders such a DVT and PE are a frequent cause of mortality in elderly patients. Additional risk factors like surgery or prolonged bed rest are followed more often by venous thromboembolism. Blood stasis, damaged vessel walls and hypercoagulability contribute to thrombophilia, which increases the risk of thromboembolic events.

In a previous study [8], the effect of prophylactic low-dose heparin on mortality was tested in 1358 consecutive patients

Table V: Distribution of age and results in the two groups [40].

	PLACEBO GROUP (n = 685)	TREATED GROUP (n = 669)	
	% OF TOTAL PATIENTS		
YEAR OF BIRTH			
1930 - 1939	8.0	8.4	
1920 - 1929	19.7	16.7	
1910 - 1919	29.0	31.4	
1900 - 1909	32.1	32.9	
BEFORE 1899	11.2	10.6	
MORTALITY	7.8	10.9	p = 0.025

admitted to the medical wards on an acute cure hospital. The treatment was started no later than 12 hours from admission and was randomized: a group treated with 5000 U of sodium heparin injected substaneously at 12 hours interval and a second group receiving placebo (Table V).

Mortality was significantly lower in the treated group: 7.8 % (52 of 669 patients) versus 10.9 % (75 of 689 patients) in the placebo group. The estimated mortality reduction attribuable to heparin was 31.1 %.

Low doses of heparin significantly reduce the incidence of deep VT after MI, stroke heart failure, chest infection and acute stroke.

Heparin therapy is currently used in geriatric internal medicine as a preventive measure of thromboembolic disorders. The development of low molecular weight heparins (LMWH) provided not only an improvement in tolerance to therapy but also in its simplified administration. This fact has been translated into by the improved acceptibility of treatment by the patient.

In a recent prospective study [2] comparing a LMWH (Nadroparine) to unfractionated heparin (calcium heparin), 99 patients (49 for Nadroparine and 50 for calcium heparin) were included. Age was 83.5±6.1 years an average for the first group and an average 84.8±6.7 years for the second group. Two major hemorrhages were observed with calcium heparin (4 %), zero with Nadroparine. Only one deep venous thrombosis was diagnosed by doppler ultrasound in the group of patients on unfractionated heparin and one in the Fraxiparine group.

5. Conclusion

Anticoagulant drugs reduce the morbidity and mortality from venous and arterial thrombotic disease especially in older patients who have the highest risk. Also age alone is not a contra-indication to full dose anticoagulation. But elderly people are more susceptible to the side effects of drugs and anticoagulant drugs are no exception. Good reasons especially the risk of bleeding exist for being extremely cautious before prescribing anticoagulant drugs to elderly patients. Finally the decision to use anticoagulants in elderly patients depends on the individual opinion of the doctor and the efficacy of supervision.

REFERENCES

1. Antiplatelets trialists collaboration. Secondary prevention of vascular disease by prolonged antiplatelet treatment. Brit Med J, 296, 320-331, 1988.

2. AQUINO JP, GAMBIER A, DUCROS JJ. Prevention of thromboembolic accidents in elderly subjects with Fraxiparine[R]. Second international symposium. Recent pharmacological and clinical data. Bounamoux H, Samama M, Ten Cate JW (Eds). Schattauer, Stuttgart, New York, 189, pp 51-54, 1990.

3. COON WW, WILLIS PW. Hemorrhagic complications of anticoagulant therapy. Arch Inter Med 133, 386-392, 1974.

4. FUSTER V, BADINON L, BADINON JJ, CHESEBRO JH. The pathogenesis of coronary artery disease and the acute coronary syndromes. N Engl J Med 23, 242-250, 1992.

5. GALLUS A, TILLET J, JASKAMAN J, MILLS W, WYCHERLEY A. Safety and efficacity of warfarin started early after submassive venous thrombosis or pulmonary embolism. Lancet 2, 1293, 1986.

6. GOLDBERG RJ, GORE JM, GURWITZ JH, ALPERT JS, BRADY P, STROHSNITTER W, CHEN ZY, DALEN JE. The impact of age on the incidence and prognosis of initial acute myocardial infarction: the Worcester Heart Attack Study. Am Heart J 117, 543-549, 1989.

7. Gruppo Italiano Per Lo Studio Della Streptochinasi Nell' Infarcto Miocardico (GISSI). Effectiveness of intravenous thrombolytic treatment in acute myocardial infarction. Lancet 1, 397-402, 1986.

8. HALKIN H, GOLDBERG J, MODAN M, MODAN B. Reduction of mortality in general radical in-patients by low dose heparin prophylaxis. Ann Int Med 96, 561-565, 1982.

9. HSIA J, HAMILTON WP, KLEIMAN N. Heparin aspirin reperfusion trial. A comparison between heparin and low dose aspirin as adjunctive therapy with tissue plasminogen activator for acute myocardial infarction. N Engl J Med 323, 1433-1437, 1990.

10. HUBER K, RESCH T, ROSC D, PROBST R, DAINDL F, BINDER BR. Heparin induced increase of t-PA antigens plasma levels in patients with unstable angina: no evidence for clinical benefits of heparinization during the initial phase of treatment. Thrombos Res 55, 779-784, 1989.

11. HULL RD, RASKOB GE, ROSENBLOOM D, PANJU AA, BRILL-EDWARDS P, GINSBERG JS, HIRSH J, MARTIN GJ, GREEN D. Heparin for 5 days as compared with 10 days in the initial treatment of proximal venous thrombosis. N Engl J Med 18, 322, 1990.

12. ISIS 2. Collaborative group randomized trial of intravenous streptokinase, oral aspirin, both or neither among 17187 cases of suspected acute myocardial infarction. Lancet 1, 349-360, 1988.

13. KLINT CR, KNATTERUD GL, STAMLER H. Persantin-aspirin reinfarction study. Part II. Secondary prevention with persantin and aspirin. JACC 7, 251-269, 1986.

14. LANDEFELD CS, MAC GUIRE EI, ROSENBLATT MW. A bleeding risk index for estimating the possibility of major bleeding in hospitalized patients starting anticoagulant therapy. Am J Med 89, 569-578, 1990.

15. LANDEFELD CS, COOK EF, FLATLEY M, WEIGBERG M, GOLDMAN L. Identification and preliminary validation of predictors of major bleeding in hospitalized patients starting anticoagulant therapy. Am J Med 82, 703-713, 1987.

16. LODDER J, DENNIS NS, VAN RAAK L, JONES LN, WARLOW CP. Cooperative study on the value of long term anticoagulation in patients with stroke and non-rheumatic atrial fibrillation. Brit Med J 296, 1435-1438, 1988.

17. MANCIET G, VERGNES C, VAISSIE J, BOISSEAU MR. A study on the efficacy and tolerance of Fraxiparine[R] during long-term therapy on the elderly. A randomized double blind clinical trial. An european multicenter randomized clinical trial. Second international symposium. Recent pharmacological and clinical data. Bounamoux H, Samama M, Ten Cate JW (Eds). Schattauer, Stuttgart, New York, pp 55-59, 1990.

18. MASON JE, GROBEE DE, STAMPFER MJ et al. Aspirin in the primary prevention of angina pectoris in a randomized trial of United States Physicians. Am J Med 89, 772-776, 1990.

19. NERI SERNERI GG, GENSINI GF, POGGESI L, TROTTA F, MODESTI PA, BODDI M, IERI A, MARGHERI M, CASOLO GC, BINI M et al. Effects of heparin, aspirin or alteplase in reduction of myocardial ischaemia in refractory unstable angina. Lancet 335, 615-618, 1990.

20. NINET J, DUROUX P. Treatment of proximal deep venous thrombosis with the low molecular weight subcutaneous heparin (Fraxiparine[R]) or unfractionated intravenous heparin. An european multicenter randomized clinical trial. Second international symposium. Recent pharmacological and clinical data. Bounamoux H, Samama M, Ten Cate JW (Eds). Schattauer, Stuttgart, New York, 65-75, 1990.

21. PAGANINI HILL A, CHAO A, ROSS RK, ANDERSON BE. Aspirin use and chronic diseases: a cohort study of the elderly. Brit Med J 299, 1247-1250, 1989.

22. PETERSON P, BOYSEN G, GODFREDSEN J, ANDERSEN ED, ANDERSEN B. Placebo-controlled, randomized trial of warfarin and aspirin for prevention of thromboembolic complications in chronic atrial fibrillation. The Copenhagen AFALSAK Study. Lancet 28, 175-179, 1989.

23. PRANDONI P et al. Comparison of subcutaneous low molecular weight heparin with intravenous standard heparin in proximal deep vein thrombosis. Lancet 339, 441-445, 1992.

24. PRANDONI P, VIGO M, CATTELAN AM, RUOL A. The treatment of deep venous thrombosis by fixed doses of a low molecular weight fraction (CY 216). Second international symposium. Recent pharmacological and clinical data. Bounamoux H, Samama M, Ten Cate JW (Eds). Schattauer, Stuttgart, New York, pp 77-80, 1990.

25. RISK GROUP. Risk of myocardial infarction and death during treatment with low dose aspirin and intravenous heparin in men with unstable coronary artery disease. Lancet 336, 827-830, 1990.

26. SCATI GROUP. Randomized controlled trial of subcutaneous calcium heparin in acute myocardial infarction. Lancet 11, 182-186, 1989.

27. SHEEHAN F, BRAUNWALD E, CANNER P, DODGE HT, GORE J, VAN NATTA P, PASSAMANI ER, WILLIAMS DO, ZARET B et al. The effect of intravenous thrombolytic therapy on left ventricular function: a report on tissue-type plasminogen activator and streptokinase from thrombolysis in myocarcial infarction (TIMI phase 1) trial. Circulation 75, 817-829, 1987.

28. SMITH P, ARNESEN H, HOLMIE I. The effect of warfarin on mortality and reinfarction after myocardial infarction. N Engl J Med 323, 147-152, 1990.

29. Stroke prevention in atrial fibrillation study group investigators. Preliminary report of the stroke prevention in atrial fibrillation study. N Engl J Med 322, 863-868, 1990.

30. TELFORD AM, WILSON C. Trial of heparin versus Atenolol in prevention of myocardial infarction in intermediate coronary syndrome. Lancet, 1225-1228, 1991.

31. The Boston area anticoagulation trial for atrial fibrillation investigators. The effects of low-dose warfarin on the risk of stroke in patients with non-rheumatic atrial fibrillation. N Engl J Med 323, 1501-1511, 1990.

32. The Sixty Plus Reinfarction Study Research Group. A double blind trial to assess long

term oral anticoagulant therapy in elderly patients after myocardial infarction. Lancet 2, 989-993, 1980.

33. THEROUX P, OUIMET H, MAC CANS J. Aspirin, heparin or both in unstable angina. N Engl J Med 319, 1105-1111, 1988.

34. THERY C. Treatment of pulmonary embolism with CY 216 dose finding study. French study group on Fraxiparine[R] therapy. Second international symposium. Recent pharmacological and clinical data. Bounamoux H, Samama M, Ten Cate JW (Eds). Schattauer, Stuttgart, New York, pp 81-85, 1990.

35. TOPOL EJ, CALIFF RM, KEREIAKES DJ, GEORGE BS. Thrombolysis and angioplasty in myocardial infarction (TAMI) trial. J Am Coll Cardiol 10, 65B-74B, 1987.

36. WALKER AM, JICK H. Prediction of bleeding during heparin therapy. JAMA 244, 1209-1212, 1980.

37. WESSLER S. Anticoagulants in the prevention of embolic stroke. Part I. Geriatrics 42(2), 29-35, 1987.

38. WHITE H, CROSS D, SCOTT M, NORRIS R. Comparison of effects of thrombolytic therapy on left ventricular function in patients over with those under 60 years of age. Am J Cardiol 67, 913-918, 1991.

39. WITZEN AR, TIJSSEN JG, DEVRIES WA, LOELIGER EA, ROOS J. Risk of long term oral anticoagulant therapy in elderly patients after myocardial infarction. Lancet 1, 64-68, 1982.

40. YUSUF S, WITTES J, FRIEDMAN L. Overview of results of randomized clinical trials in heart disease. Treatment following myocardial infarction. JAMA 260, 2088-2093, 1988.

13

Pregnancy and anticoagulation

F.X. Roques, S.A.M. Nashef, E.M. Baudet, C. Doutremepuich

Anticoagulation during the course of pregnancy, whether by heparin or vitamin K antagonists, exposes both mother and fetus to the risk of serious adverse effects. Nevertheless, there are situations with definite indications for anticoagulant treatment during pregnancy and the treatment modalities available differ little from those used in the non-pregnant state. A therapeutic strategy designed to minimise the risk of anticoagulation in pregnancy must take into consideration the indication for which anticoagulation is required, the relative risks of individual anticoagulants to mother and fetus and the stage of pregnancy during which anticoagulants are administered.

1. Indications for anticoagulation during pregnancy

These fall whithin two broad categories :

established, long-term indications or de novo indications arising or expected to arise during the course of the pregnancy.

1.1 Established indications

There are situations in which long-term anticoagulation has been justifiably established before pregnancy occurs, such as mitral valve disease with atrial fibrillation, the presence of a mechanical prosthetic heart valve or a history of life-threatening venous thromboembolic disease. In such cases, there is no alternative to maintaining anticoagulation throughout pregnancy. Other situations may arise where long-term anticoagulation may have been established for less clearcut indications: in such cases the need for anticoagulation should be carefully reassessed in the context of pregnancy, evaluating every case individually.

1.2 De novo indications

It is known that women with a previous history of thromboembolic disease have a 5-10 % risk of recurrence during pregnancy. Prophylactic anticoagulation should be considered in relation to every patient's individual history: in women with a recent thromboembolic episode, it would be reasonable to initiate anticoagulant therapy from the beginning of the second trimester, whereas in women with a non-recent history of mild thromboembolism with no residual sequelae anticoagulation could be delayed until the third trimester. It is also known that the risk of deep vein thrombosis during labour increases with maternal age and obstetric complications, justifying peripartum anticoagulation in mothers with a combination of risk factors.

2. Fetal risks of anticoagulation

Heparin, with a molecular weight of 18000, does not cross the placenta and therefore does not damage the fetus directly. Vitamin K antagonists, however, do cross the placenta and their adverse effects on the fetus may arise as a result of their teratogenic and anticoagulant properties.

Teratogenic effects have been observed in mothers who received vitamin K antagonists in the first trimester, especially in the sixth to twelfth week of pregnancy. The commonest malformations [6] are in the head and neck (various anomalies of facial osteogenesis, nasal hypoplasia, frontal hyperplasia and bossing, choanal atresia, short neck, optic atrophy and epiphyseal dysplasia). The exact overall incidence of such malformations is difficult to determine because most studies have been retrospective, but is generally estimated [9] to be between 5 and 10 %. In a study of 418 women who received vitamin K antagonists throughout pregnancy [5] found abnormalities in one out of six infants (17 %). A more recent study [1] found a higher incidence of 29 % (10 affected infants out of 35) but most abnormalities were of a minor nature. In all of these studies the anticoagulants in question were coumarin derivatives. Indanedione derivatives have not been fully assessed.

Because they cross the placenta, vitamin K antagonists, by extension of their therapeutic anticoagulant effect, also expose the fetus to the risk of anticoagulant- related haemorrhages, of which cerebral haemorrhage is the most serious, causing microcephaly, hydrocephaly and mental retardation. These occur much less commonly than abnormalities due to teratogenic effects (less than 1 % of infants at risk). Fresh frozen plasma, the "antidot" of vitamin K antagonists, does not cross the placenta and is therefore of no use in reversing fetal hypocoagulability.

Finally, regardless of the anticoagulant used, there is a substantial risk of premature birth (20 - 30 %)

with its attendant perinatal morbidity and mortality. The perinatal mortality rate was 17 % in a study by Ginsberg [3] and 16 % in Hall's series [5]. Salazar [8] found a higher perinatal mortality rate of 37 % in 128 mothers who had received vitamin K antagonists, but this was at least partly due to the underlying maternal pathology which necessitated anticoagulation in the first place. Even when such pathology is excluded, there is still considerable morbidity and mortality from the teratogenic effects of coumarin derivatives, whereas women who have only received peripartum heparin treatment have a fetal prognosis not too unlike that of the general population (7 % premature birth with no residual sequelae and 2.5 % perinatal mortality) [4].

Neither coumarin derivatives nor heparin are secreted in breast milk and therefore neither contraindicates breastfeeding. Indanedione and derivatives have, however, been found in breast milk and breastfeeding is therefore not advisable in mothers taking this drug [7].

3. Maternal risks of anticoagulation

As in all anticoagulated patients, the main risk is that of anticoagulant-related haemorrhage. Smooth control of anticoagulation in a pregnant woman can be more difficult simply as a result of pregnancy-related physiological changes such as morning sickness and altered hepatic function. This means that more meticulous surveillance of clotting function is required in pregnancy to maintain anticoagulation within a safe therapeutic range. Maternal hypocoagulability caused by heparin can be readily reversed with protamine sulfate. Hypocoagulability due to vitamin K antagonists can be corrected in the mother by fresh frozen plasma but not in the fetus (plasma, as mentioned earlier, does not cross the placenta). This underlines the importance of close surveillance of anticoagulation in order to avoid hypocoagulable states in the fetus, and the superior safety of heparin over vitamin K antagonists for the fetus.

There are two additional risks of prolonged heparin therapy. The first, which may occur only after a substantial amount of heparin has been administered (more than 20000 international units daily for six months) is the risk of maternal osteoporosis and fractures, of which several cases have been reported in pregnancy [2]. The second is the extremely rare but potentially catastrophic syndrome of heparin hypersensitivity. This may develop in susceptible individuals as soon as the fifth day, but usually around the tenth day of heparin administration. The pathophysiology of this syndrome is not fully understood but is thought to be due to the formation of heparin-platelet-immunoglobulin complexes causing widespread intravascular coagulation made up of "white" clots. The syndrome is particularly difficult to recognise because it manifests as hypercoagulability, often leading the unsuspecting clinician to increase the heparin dose. One feature of the syndrome is a sudden drop in the number of platelets in peripheral blood samples (to 50 % or less of previous values). When this happen, heparin therapy should be discontinued while more sophisticated tests are performed to confirm or exclude the diagnosis.

4. Practical guide to anticoagulation in pregnancy

4.1 Anticoagulation for established indications

The diagnosis of pregnancy must be made as early as possible in all women who are receiving long-term treatment with vitamin K antagonists, preferably before the sixth week. This is in order to reduce or eliminate any fetal exposure to these drugs between the sixth and twelfth week, the high risk period for teratogenicity. Thus all anticoagulated women of child-bearing age should be made aware of this risk and encouraged to seek medical opinion as soon as possible whenever pregnancy is suspected. Ideally, pregnancy should, whenever possible, be planned in advance in women receiving anticoagulants.

Women with a mechanical heart valve prosthesis and some women at substantial risk of systemic embolism of cardiac origin (as in mitral valve disease with atrial fibrillation) require lifelong, high level anticoagulation (INR between 3 and 3.5). Treatment with antiplatelets alone is not enough: in one study [8] of 68 women with mechanical heart valves managed with antiplatelets alone the maternal mortality was 4.5 %, a quarter of the women had cerebral emboli half of which left residual deficits and 5 % had other systemic emboli. These patients must be anticoagulated with heparin during the teratogenicity risk period and the doses used must be high enough to maintain a hypocoagulability status equivalent to that achieved on vitamin K antagonists before pregnancy. This is possible with subcutaneous heparin injections three times a day adjusted to maintain an activated clotting time between 1.5 and 2.0 times control (blood sampling should be 6 hours after injection). This treatment is continued until the thirteenth week, when it is replaced by vitamin K antagonists until the end of the eighth month of pregnancy. In the final month heparin treatment is again established as above. This protocol is not without disadvantages: there is still a slight possibility of maternal osteoporosis, teratogenicity may not be totally eliminated and the periods of thrice daily injections can be unpleasant for the mother. In addition, three changes of anticoagulant therapy carry the risk of loss of control of anticoagulation during the alteration. Salazar used this regimen in twelve mothers and found no fetal complications and only one maternal embolic episode. In spite of the disadvantages, this protocol is probably the safest compromise in mothers in whom there is no choice but to maintain high-level anticoagulation throughout pregnancy.

Where the indications for anticoagulation are not absolute, as in mothers with a previous history of deep vein thrombosis with a moderate risk of recurrence, a similar regiment can be adopted but at lower heparin doses to maintain an activated clotting time between 1-1.5 times control. At such doses there is no risk of maternal osteoporosis and heparin therapy can be continue troughout pregnancy, the only disadvantage being that of maternal discomfort due to repeated injections. Low molecular weight heparins have been advocated in such cases of long-term therapy but there are not yet sufficient data confirming their safety in pregnancy.

4.2 Anticoagulation for de novo indications

When a pregnant mother develops pulmonary embolism, deep vein thrombosis or other thromboembolic episode requiring anticoagulation, this tends to occur almost invariably late in the second trimester or in the third trimester because the risk of thromboembolic problems rises with advancing pregnancy. For this reason, the usual treatment is initially by intravenous heparin in sufficient doses and thereafter by subcutaneous heparin to maintain an activated clotting time of 1.5 to 2.0 times control. The use of vitamin K antagonists is delayed until the post-partum period. In the rare cases of de novo thromboembolic episodes arising in the first trimester, a similar regimen of treatment to that in established indications above may be adopted (heparin in the first and third trimesters and vitamin K antagonists in the second).

5. Anticoagulation at the time of labour

Vitamin K antagonists must not be used in the period immediately preceding labour and during labour itself: this is because of the double risk of maternal haemorrhage and fetal cerebral haemorrhage during birth itself. For this reason, and because of the high incidence of premature birth, appropriate heparin therapy must replace vitamin K antagonists during the ninth month regardless of the original indications for anticoagulation. Subcutaneous heparin can be used to maintain an activated clotting time of 1.5-2.0 times normal. Treatment is stopped as soon as labour is diagnosed (or 6 hours before elective caesarian section) and restarted 6 to 12 hours after birth if there are no maternal bleeding complications. For these reasons it is often appropriate to induce labour at a suitable time and to obtain close cooperation between the specialists that may be involved in the management of the patient (haematologist, obstetrician, anaesthetist, cardiologist and cardiac surgeon). In mothers with lifelong absolute indications for anticoagulation, vitamin K antagonists may be restarted as early as the second or third postanatal day, overlapping with heparin treatment until the desired therapeutic effect (INR of 3-4.5) is reached. When lifelong anticoagulation is not required, treatment either by subcutaneous heparin or vitamin K antagonists may be continued for six weeks.

REFERENCES

1. ALESSIO II, FONSECA MC, MUNTCHINK O, SANTOS MA, SAJARIAS A, SALAZAR E. Risks of

anticoagulant therapy in pregnant women with artificial heart valves. N Engl J Med 315, 1390-1393, 1986.

2. GINSBERG JS, HIRSH J. Use of anticoagulants during pregnancy. Chest (Suppl 1) 95, 1595-1605, 1989.

3. GINSBERG JS, HIRSH J, TURNER DC, LEVINE MN, BURROWS R. Risks to the fetus of anticoagulant therapy during pregnancy. Thromb Haemost 61, 197-203, 1989.

4. GINSBERG JS, KOWALCHUCK G, HIRSH J, BRILL-EDWARDS P, BURROWS R. Heparin therapy during pregnancy. Risks to the fetus and mother. Arch Intern Med 149, 2236, 1989.

5. HALL JG, PAULI RM, WILSON KM. Maternal and fetal sequelae of anticoagulation during pregnancy. Am J Med 68, 122-140, 1980.

6. Mc GOLDIN SW, MARTIN JN Jr, MORRISSON JC. Pregnant women with prosthetic heart valves. Clin Obs Gyn 32, 76-88, 1989.

7. Mc KENNA R, COLE ER, VASAN U. Is warfarin sodium contrindicated in the lactating mother? Pediatrics 103, 325-327, 1983.

8. SALAZAR E, ZAJARIAS A, GUTIEREZ N, ITURBE I. The problem of cardiac valve prostheses, anticoagulants and pregnancy. Circulation 70(1), 169-177, 1984.

9. STEVENSON RE, BURTON QM, FERLAUTO GS, TAYLOR HA. Hazards of oral anticoagulants during pregnancy. JAMA 243, 1549-1555, 1980.

14

Anticoagulation in pregnancy

J.J. Leng, P. Delouis

Pregnancy is a hypercoagulable state due to the increased potential for coagulation and thrombosis.

Pulmonary Embolism (PE) during pregnancy is a leading cause of maternal mortality [22, 34, 35, 39, 43, 52]. Although relatively uncommon, accurate estimates of its incidence are hampered by differences in diagnostic techniques and the unreliability of clinical assessment and objective techniques. To a large extent, the location and size of clots and degree of vessel obstruction are also highly variable and make detection more difficult.

1. Incidence

Studies of maternal mortality classifying "pulmonary embolism" do not distinguish venous thromboembolism from amniotic fluid or air embolism [22, 35, 44]. When a distinction has been made, half or more have been found due to thrombotic embolism [22, 23, 34, 39, 46].

Nevertheless, in the United States from 1980 - 1985, 14.3 % of all maternal deaths were due to embolism [44], or approximately 2 deaths per 100,000 live births.

Maternal deaths due to PE declined 50 % from 1970 to 1987 [22]. Black race and older age are both risk factors for PE. The rates changed for black women, from 9.0 down to 4.2 per 100,000 and for white women, from 3.3 to 1.3 per 100,000 [22]. Women age 40 years or older were at nearly ten times greater risk than those under 25 years old in both racial groups [22]. Deep venous thrombosis (DVT) has been reported to occur in 0.018 % to 0.29 % of all deliveries [3, 51]. Thrombi in large veins with few valves and minimal inflammation may be clinically silent and less adherent to the vessel and have the greatest chance of embolization.

The period of greatest risk for thrombosis and embolism appears to be the immediate puerperium, especially after cesarean delivery. Post partum DVT has been reported to be 3 to 5 times more common than antepartum DVT, and 3 to 16 times more common after cesarean compared to vaginal delivery. The risk for PE may be up to 20 times higher in the puerperium. The most important risk factors are a previous history of thromboembolism (5 % - 15 % recurrence risk) (50), operative delivery, immobilization, and inherited deficiencies in the natural inhibitors of coagulation, such as antithrombin III, protein C, or protein S. Additionnally, older age, obesity, lower extremity or pelvic trauma, black versus white race and possibly higher parity add to a woman's risk.

2. Coagulation changes in pregnancy

2.1 Cardiovascular function

The heart increases and changes of electrical axis. The cardiac out-put increases of 1.5 liters within the 10 first weeks. The pulse-rate increases of 15 to 20 beats per minute.

The blood-pressure decreases in the first half of pregnancy.

The peripheral resistances decrease very fast and the peripheral venous blood pressure increases.

2.2 Coagulation

Levels of factors XII, IX, X, VIII, VII, V, and fibrinogen increase and levels of factors XIII and XI decrease during pregnancy [5]. Platelet count remains in the normal range. It appears that there may be an ongoing increase in activation of coagulation during pregnancy, compensated by a concomitant rise in fibrinolytic activity [55]. A low-grade chronic intravascular coagulation results in fibrin deposition in the spiral arteries of the placental bed, gradually replacing the internal elastic lamina and smooth muscle [26].

In addition to tissue factor, an anticoagulant protein has been isolated from human placenta. Decreased fibrinolytic potential, which may return to normal within an hour of delivery, is believed to contribute to hypercoagulability during pregnancy. Increased fibrin splits products and D-dimer, however, suggest an increase in ongoing fibrinolytic activity [55].

Two limited studies suggest that alteration of this carefully balanced system may explain significant disease processes. In one, spontaneous abortion occured when peripheral blood studies showed evidence of a relative increase in coagulation activity over fibrinolytic activity compared to their normal patient population [55]. In another, an autopsy review of pregnancy related deaths, eight of ten cases of intracranial venous thrombosis had associated evidence of disseminated intravascular coagulation [1].

Furthermore, autoimmune disorders may be linked to thrombosis, fetal death, and pregnancy loss through the role of complement in establishing an endothelial membrase-based phase of coagulation [25]. Placental anticoagulant proteins (such as PAP-I) have been identified that have calcium - dependant phospholipid binding properties [122].

Conjecture suggests that the most important key to the problem of pathologic hypercoagulability of pregnancy is the interaction of phospholipids and coagulation factors at endothelial cell membranes. Certain pathologic states elevate risk above that of normal pregnancy. These include inherited deficiencies of natural anticoagulants and antiphospholipid antibodies. Pulmonary thromboembolism complicating recurrent placental abruptio has also been reported [52].

The coagulation becomes normal six weeks after delivery.

2.3 Rheology in pregnancy

The most common of the changes is the increment of erythrocytic aggregation, which decreases after delivery [8]. In the same time blood viscosity, plasmatic viscosity and fibrinogen are increasing; hematocrit, plasmatic osmolarity and fraction albumine over fibrinogen are decreasing. The erythrocytic aggregation can increase the blood viscosity in the veins, especially in the varicose veins.

Plasmatic viscosity decreases between 35 and 40 weeks of gestation; in labour index of erythrocytic rigidity increases and it decreases quickly after the delivery.

2.4 Special considerations

2.4.1 Antithrombin III deficiency

A thromboembolic event may be the first evidence of an inherited antithrombin III (ATIII) defect [40]. Most patients with inherited ATIII deficiency will require therapeutic anticoagulation during their pregnancy. In addition to subcutaneous and intravenous heparin, intravenous administration of ATIII concentrate may be necessary [16, 41]. Without such therapy, maternal morbidity and mortality and fetal loss are extremely high. If untreated during pregnancy, up to 68 % of these women have thromboembolism [11, 28]. Many require lifelong anticoagulation, which is best served by oral anticoagulants when not pregnant and heparin throughout pregnancy.

2.4.2 Protein C or S deficiency

These appear to carry a slightly lower antepartum risk compared to ATIII deficiency [11].

Anticoagulant therapy in the puerperium is strongly recommended. Recommandations for the antepartum period remain to be determinated. If prior thromboembolic events have occured, prophylaxis with heparin is advised. Recurrent thromboembolism or an appropriate family history justifies screening for ATIII, protein C, or protein S deficiencies [21].

2.4.3 Mechanical cardiac valve prostheses

The patients are at unusually high risk for arterial thrombosis, especially if atrial fibrillation is present. Therapeutic anticoagulation is necessary. Adjusted-dose subcutaneous heparin is recommended [37], preferably begun prior to pregnancy.

2.4.4 Septic pelvic thrombophlebitis and ovarian thrombosis

Septic pelvic thrombophlebitis is suspected in patients with endomyometritis who do not respond to antibiotic therapy [33]. Continuous intravenous heparin is the diagnostic test as well as therapy. It is continued until resolution of the patient's symptoms and fever occurs and for as long as 7 to 10 days thereafter. Anticoagulation is then discontinued. For ovarian vein thrombosis, longer period of heparinization should be considered [14].

2.4.5 Preeclampsia

Reduced ATIII levels and possibly reduced protein C levels can be found in women with preeclampsia [15], supporting a possible predisposition to thromboembolic complications, although disseminated intravascular coagulation may be a greater problem. Bed rest is also a risk factor. At this time there is no evidence to suggest that prophylactic heparin should be considered. In any patient with prolonged bed rest, conservative measures to increase venous return from the lower extremities may be considered.

2.4.6 Antiphospholipid antibodies

Lupus anticoagulant and anticardiolipin antibodies are associated with both thrombosis and fetal loss [42, 53]. The incidence of maternal thrombosis is not known however, and there are currently no recommendations for the purpose of avoiding maternal thromboembolism unless a prior event has occured, in which case prophylaxis is appropriate.

2.4.7 Fetal death "in utero"

Most of coagulation factors with a haemorrhagic syndrome are decreasing in case of long retention. The hemorrhagic risk exists when the pregnancy is older than 16 weeks and the retention longer than 4 weeks [6].

3. Drugs

3.1 Anti-aggregating agents (antiplatelet agents)

They can :
- inhibit the platelet adhesion (sulfinpyrazole or ANTURAN)
- inhibit the act of excreting by blockage of the cyclo-oxygenase (aspirin, antiinflammatories)
- inhibit the primary aggregation (ticlopidine or TICLID*)

Their effects are measured by the Duke's test.

3.2 Oral anticoagulants

4.2.1 Mechanism of action and laboratory monitoring

Coumarin derivatives, such as warfarin, function as oral anticoagulants by inhibiting regeneration of active vitamine K in the liver. Vitamine K is required to carboxylate the glutamic acid residues on factors II, VII, IX, X and protein C. These factors otherwise are unable to form complexes on endothelial and platelet membranes using calcium and phospholipid receptors. Measurement of the activity of oral anticoagulants is based on extension of the prothrombin time, which reflects the function of the extrinsic and common pathways of the coagulation cascade. Therapeutic levels may be reached after administration for about 3 days and should yield a value 1.5 to 2.5 times control.

3.2.2 Risks to the fetus

Oral anticoagulants have a molecular weight of about 1000 daltons, cross the placenta into the fetal circulation, and should rarely be considered in a pregnant woman, except when the use of heparin is impossible, such as in hypersensitivity.

Patients receiving coumarin who desire to become pregnant ideally should change to heparin in the preconceptural period.

During the first 6 to 9 weeks's gestation, coumarin is teratogenic. The embryopathy results in defects including nasal hypoplasia, depression of the bridge of the nose, and epiphyseal stippling (Conradi-Hunermann Chondrodysplasia Punctata), which causes abnormal bone shape and growth. Exposure during the second two trimesters is associated with a variety of central nervous system and ophtalmologic abnormalities. It is unknown whether some may be related to fetal hemorrhage and scar tissue formation.

3.2.3 Risks to the mother

In addition to the increased risk to a fetus, there is an increased risk of bleeding in the mother, which occurs more often than with subcutaneous heparin [27]. Oral anticoagulation is also more sensitive to fluxes in clotting factors and plasma volume, and requires more frequent monitoring and adjustement of dose. The use of oral anticoagulants is further complicated by numerous, commonly used medications that augment or inhibit warfarin activity [19]. Nevertheless, use of oral anticoagulants in the post-partum period is favoured by many.

3.3 Heparin anticoagulation

3.3.1 Mechanism of action

Heparin is the anticoagulant of choice in pregnancy. As a mucopolysaccharide, its varying chain lengths give it molecular weight of 4 000 to 40 000 daltons, which are large enough to prevent it from crossing the placenta. Biologic activity may be higher in the lower molecular weight fractions (4 000 to 5 000 daltons) [16, 29]. Heparin exerts its anticoagulant activity by binding to ATIII, causing a conformational change that increases the affinity of ATIII for thrombin and other activated factors including XIIa, XIa, Xa and IXa. The stable complexes of ATIII and the clotting factors release heparin, wich is available to repeat the process with other molecules of ATIII. In the absence of ongoing coagulation, small ammouts of heparin may prevent clotting by inhibiting the initial steps of coagulation. Once the amplification process of the coagulation cascade has developed, however, much larger amounts of heparin are required to prevent extension of the clot [54].

Likewise, as a clot stabilizes and fewer activated factors, especially thrombin, are present, a decreasing requirement for heparin is seen [54].

3.3.2 Laboratory monitoring

A variety of tests can be used, examples include the thrombin time, whole blood clotting time, activated partial thromboplastin time (APTT), and measurement of anti-factor Xa activity or protamine sulfate neutralization.

Therapeutic anticoagulation is associated with prolongation of the APTT to 1.5 to 2 times or possibly 2.5 times the control value. Heparin should achieve levels of 0.2 to 0.4 U/ml for intravenous infusion and 0.2 to 0.3 U/ml 6 hours after subcutaneous injection [6].

The ability of the new antifactor Xa activity tests to detect extremely low levels of heparin is a very important step toward improved management of both therapeutic and prophylactic heparinization.

3.3.3 Complications

Complications of heparin therapy include bleeding, osteoporosis, thrombocytopenia, and hypersensitivity. Drugs that interfere with platelet function, such as aspirin or other nonsteroidal anti-inflammatory agents, are contraindicated because they can double the risk of bleeding.

Doses of at least 20,000 U/day for more than 20 weeks [18] in a pregnant or puerperal woman are likeky to cause bone demineralization. However, patients receiving lower doses for shorter periods of time are not exempt. Reversal of osteopenia does occur and treatment in consecutive pregnancies may not increase a woman's risk [13].

Thrombocytopenia may be attributable to heparin-dependant platelet antibodies and can result in paradoxal thrombosis [9, 10].

Hypersensitivity to heparin may results in urticaria or, rarely, anaphylaxis.

3.3.4 Risks to the fetus

In a review of 97 pregnancies over an approximately 12 years period in which heparin was used, outcomes (such as fetal loss, prematurity...) were found to be comparable to the normal population [24].

3.4 Low-molecular-weight heparin

Using low molecular weight fractions of heparin (LMWH) can be at least potentially useful in pregnant women for certain indications. DAFFOS [12] showed that CY 216 (Fraxiparin) did not cross the placenta in the third trimester of pregnancy but number of cases was too low for allowing LMWH during pregnancy.

4. Recommanded clinical management

4.1 Deep venous thrombosis during pregnancy

An initial intravenous bolus of heparin may be necessary as diagnostic or therapeutic assay [36]. The duration of intravenous therapy may be short, 2 days for example, especially in patients who show a rapid clinical response. Adjunctive measures include bed rest with elevation of the affected extremity to promote venous return. As soon as tolerated, movement and ambulation may be allowed.

The delivery must be induced to stop the anti-coagulation (6 hours before).

4.2 Pulmonary embolism during pregancy

After obtaining baseline laboratory studies and starting an intravenous line, rapid anticoagulation may be achieved with an intravenous bolus of heparin, 70 to 100 U/kg. This is followed by continuous administration of about 15 to 20 U/kg per hour. Laboratory monitoring with the APTT (1.5 to 2.5 times control) or heparin levels (0.2 to 0.4 U/ml) is recommended.

Conversion to subcutaneous heparin requires a stable patient with no evidence of worsening thrombosis. Blood is drawn a midinterval to obtain an APTT 1.5 to 2.0 times control or heparin levels of 0.2 to 0.3 U/ml, which have been show to provide adequate anticoagulation with a low risk of bleeding during 6 or 12 months [38].

Deterioration of hemodynamic status is an indication for pulmonary embolectomy [4].

Recurrent venous emboli originating from the lower extremities and refractory to medical treatment necessitate interruption of the inferior vena cava. Alternatives to complete ligation include Teflon clips or devices inserted transvenously, such as the umbrella filter and Green-filter [31]. A rich supply of collaterals accounts for the ability to tolerate ligation. The use of thrombolytic agents is restricted to life-treatening situations because they may themselves cause life-treatening bleeding complications, particularly in surgical (including obstetric) patients. Fetal death in animals has resulted from bleeding or separation of the placenta [2]. Bleeding from laceration, incision, episiotomy, or the placental bed may be difficult or impossible to control. Streptokinase and urokinase are given as a loading bolus followed by continous infusion for 12 to 72 hours [48]. They are followed by anticoagulant therapy to prevent recurrence.

4.3 Prophylaxis

Thromboembolism in association with a previous pregnancy warrants prophylactic administration of heparin during any subsequent pregnancy and the first 6 weeks post partum.

When a previous thromboembolic event has occured due to surgery, trauma, or oral contraceptives, not all authors agree that antepartum anticoagulant prophylaxis is necessary (maybe an antiplatelet agent must be given). However, the high risk for thrombosis associated with the puerperium makes it reasonable to give heparin or LMWH prophylaxis for the first 6 weeks. Yet other investigators recommend no prophylaxis during pregnancy, dextran during labor, and prophylaxis for 6 weeks post partum [17].

4.4 Duration of therapeutic anticoagulation

The pregnant woman who experiences a thromboembolic episode during her pregnancy is customarly continued on therapeutic anticoagulation for the duration of her pregnancy and 6 weeks post partum.

If a thromboembolism has occured in the post partum period, anticoagulation is generally continued for 3 months unless ongoing risk factor, such as ATIII deficiency, has been discovered, in which case it is continued indefinitely [32].

The newer techniques for monitoring heparin activity, such as measurement of antifactor Xa activity, may allow for more precise adjustment of heparin (or LMWH) doses to the lowest therapeutic level, especially after the initial thrombotic episode is thought to have been resolved (3 months after the event).

The advantage of this approach would be to minimize the risks, such as osteoporosis and bleeding (but the coming of low molecular weight heparin should increase these risks).

4.5 Special considerations

4.5.1 Mechanical heart valves

Subcutaneous heparin in doses adequate to provide therapeutic anticoagulation is preferred over oral anticoagulation because of its greater safety for the fetus [24, 47]. If it is not possible to use heparin, oral agents must be used during the second trimester, and the parents informed, before pregnancy if possible, as to the risks for the fetus.

4.5.2 Perioperative prophylaxis

Early ambulation is key to prevent post cesarean thrombosis. Conservative measures such as intermittent pneumatic compression devices are useful in selected patients.

Women undergoing cesarean delivery who are obese, older, and would be considered at risk for thromboembolism after gynecologic surgery should also be considered or an individual basis for low-dose heparin [3] or LMWH heparin prophylaxis until they are ambulatory. Their risk is higher than for non pregnant women undergoing surgery.

Apparently used more commonly in Great Britain than in the United States, dextran 70,500 to 1000 ml (over a period of 8 to 12 hours) can be started during labour or preoperatively [20].

5. Conclusion

Early diagnosis, treatment, and appropriate prophylaxis may prevent serious maternal sequelae of thromboembolism.

Because of its low fetal risk, heparin is the anticoagulant of choice [45]. Measurement of heparin levels by antifactor Xa activity appears to be more sensitive than the current standard, the APTT.

Although the risks and benefits of prophylaxis during pregnancy are currently debated, it appears most prudent to use subcutaneous heparin in doses larger than for non pregnant patients in women at high risk for recurrence.

REFERENCES

1. ANGELOV A. Intracranial venous thrombosis in relation to pregnancy and delivery. Pathol Res Pract 185, 843, 1989.

2. BARCLAY GR, ALLEN K, PENNINGTON CR. Tissue plasminogen activator in the treatement of superior vena caval thrombosis associated with parenteral nutrition. Postgrad Med J 66, 398, 1990.

3. BERGQVIST A, BERGQVIST D, HALLBOOK T. Acute deep vein thrombosis (DVT) after cesarean section. Acta Obstet Gynecol Scand 58, 473-476, 1979.

4. BLEGVAD S, LUND O, NIELSEN TT, GULDHOL T. Emergency embolectomy in a patient with massive pulmonary embolism during second trimester pregnancy. Acta Obstet Gynecol Scand 68, 267-270, 1989.

5. BOISSEAU MR. Apport actuel de l'étude de l'hémostase au cours des accidents hémorragiques en période obstétricale. J Gynecol Obstet Biol Reprod 2, 745, 1973.

6. BONNAR J. Venous thromboembolism and pregnancy. Clin Obstet Gynecol 8, 455, 1981.

7. BRATT G, TORNEBOHM E, LOCKNER D, BERGSTROM K. A human pharmacological study comparing conventional heparin and a low molecular weight heparin fragment. Thromb Haemost 53, 208-211, 1985.

8. BRUN JF. Modifications physiologiques de la rhéologie sanguine au cours de l'accouchement et de la grossesse. Art et Vein 8(7), 552-557, 1989.

9. CHONG BH, PITNEY WR, CASTALDI PA. Heparin-induced thrombocytopenia : Association of

thrombotic complications with heparin-dependent IgG antibody that induces thromboxane synthesis and platelet aggregation. Lancet 2, 1246, 1982.

10. CINES DB, TOMASKI A. TANNENBAUM S. Immune endothelial-cell injury in heparin - associated thrombocytopenia. N Engl J Med 316, 581, 1987.

11. CONARD J, HORELLOU MH, VAN DREDEN P, LECOMPTE T, SAMAMA M. Thrombosis and pregnancy in congenital deficiencies in AT III, protein C or protein S : Study of 78 women. Thromb Haemost 63, 319-320, 1990.

12. DAFFOS F, FORESTIER F, RAINAUT M, TOULEMONDE F. Low molecular weight heparin (CY 216) does not cross the placenta during the third trimester of pregnancy (letter). Thromb Haemost 57(2), 234, 1987 .

13. DAHLMAN TC, HELLGREN MSE, BLOMBACK M. Thrombosis prophylaxis in pregnancy with use of subcutaneous heparin adjusted by monotoring heparin concentration in plasma. Am J Obstet Gynecol 161, 420, 1989.

14. DALEN JE, BANAS JS Jr, BROOKS HL et al. Resolution rate of acute pulmonary embolism in man. N Engl J Med 280, 1194-1199, 1969.

15. DE BOER K, Ten CATE JW, STURK A, BORM JJ, TREFFERS PE. Enhanced thrombin generation in normal and hypertensive pregnancy. Am J Obstet Gynecol 160, 95-100, 1989.

16. DE STEPHANO V, LEONE G, DE CAROLIS S, FERRELLI R, DI DONFRANCESCO A, MONETA E. Management of pregnancy in women with antithrombin III congenital defect : Report

17. of four cases. Thromb Haemost 59, 193-196, 1988.

18. DE SWIET M, FLOYD E, LETSKY E. Low risk of recurrent thromboembolism in pregnancy. Br J Hosp Med 38, 264, 1987.

19. DE SWIET M, WARD PD, FILDER J, HORSMAN A, KATZ D, LETSKY E, PEACOCK M, WISE PH. Prolonged heparin therapy in pregnancy causes bone demineralization. Br J Obstet Gynaecol 90, 1129-34, 1983.

20. DIXON JE. Pregnancies complicated by previous thromboembolic disease. Br J Hosp Med 37, 449, 1987.

21. DOOUS TW. The clinical significiance of venous thrombosis of the calf. Br J Surg 63, 377, 1973.

22. DUBECQ JP, HOROVITZ S. Déficit en protéine S (de la coagulation) et grossesse. A propos de 3 observations. J Gyn Obst et Biol Reprod 19(5), 637, 1990.

23. FRANKS AL, ATRASH HK, LAWSON HW, COLBERG KS. Obstetrical pulmonary embolism mortality, United States 1970-85. Am J Public Health 80, 720-722, 1990.

24. GABEL HD. Maternal mortality in South Carolina from 1970 to 1984 : An analysis. Obstet Gynecol 69, 307, 1987.

25. GINGSBERG JS, HIRSH J, TURNER C, LEVINE MN, BURROWS R. Risks to the fetus of anticoagulant therapy during pregnancy. Thromb Haemost 67, 197-203, 1989.

26. HAMILTON KK, HATTORI R, ESMON CT, SIMS PJ. Complement proteins C5b-9 induce vesiculation of the endothelial plasma membrane and expose catalytic surface for assembly of the

prothrombinase enzyme complex. J Biol Chem 265, 3809-3814, 1990.

27. HATHAWAY WE, BONNAR J. Perinatal coagulation. New York, Grune & Stratton, 1978.

28. HELLGREN M, NYGARDS EB. Long-term therapy with subcutaneous heparin during pregnancy. Gynecol Obstet Invest 13, 76, 1982.

29. HELLGREN M, TENGBORN L, ABILDGAARD U. Pregnancy in women with congenital antithrombin III deficiency : experience of treatment with heparin and antithrombin. Gynecol Obstet Invest 17, 127, 1982.

30. HIRSH J, BARROWCLIFFE TW. Standardization and clinical use of LMW heparin. Thromb Haemost 59, 333, 1988.

31. HIRSH J, CADE JF, GALLUS AS. Anticoagulants in pregnancy : A review of indications and complications. Am Heart J 83, 301, 1972.

32. HUX CH, WAGNER R, RATTAN P, et al. Surgical treatment of thromboembolic disease in pregnancy (abstract). In proceedings, the society of Perinatal obstetricians. San Antonio, p 62, 1986.

33. HYERS TM, HULL RD, WEG JG. Antithrombotic therapy for venous thromboembolic disease. Chest 89, 265, 1986.

34. JANKY E, CAMBON D, CORMIER P, BASTE JC, LENG JJ. Thrombophlébite des veines ovariennes. A propos d'un cas. Rev Fr Gynecol Obstet 85(11), 615-617, 1990.

35. KAUNITZ A, HUGHES JM, GRIMES DA, SMITH JC, ROCHAT RW, KAFRISSEN ME. Causes of maternal mortality in the United States. Obstet Gynecol 65, 605-612, 1985.

36. LAWSON HW, ATRASK HK, FRANKS AL. Fatal pulmonary embolism during legal induced abortion in the United States from 1972 to 1985. Am J Obstet Gynecol 162, 986, 1990.

37. LENG JJ, BOISSEAU MR, MARTINEZ M, LACLAU-LACROUTS B. Test de sensibilité à l'héparine chez les accouchées suspectes de thrombose. Rev Fr Gynecol Obstet 76(6), 465-468, 1981

38. LEVINE HJ, PAUKER SG, SALZMAN EW. Antithrombotic therapy in valvular heart disease. Chest (Suppl) 89, 36S, 1986.

39. MARKISZ JA. Radiologic and nuclear medicine diagnosis. In : Goldhaber SZ (Ed). Pulmonary Embolism and Deep Venous Thrombosis. Philadelphia, Saunders WB, p 41, 1985.

40. Mc LEAN R, MATTISON ET, COCHRANE NE. Maternal mortality study annual report 1970-1976. NY State J Med 79, 39, 1979.

41. MEGHA A, FINZI G, POLI T, MANOTTI C, DETTORI AG. Pregnancy, antithrombin III deficiency and venous thrombosis : Report of another case. Acta Haematol (Basel) 83, 111, 1990.

42. NELSON DM, STEMPEL LE, BRANDT JT. Hereditary antithrombin III deficiency and pregnancy : Report to two cases and review of the literature. Obstet Gynecol 65, 848, 1985.

43. OUT HJ, KATER L, DERKSEN RHWM. Antithrombolipid antibodies : Risk factors or for thrombosis, fetal loss and thrombocytopenia. Neth J Med 36, 177, 1990.

44. RICHARDS SR, BARROWS H, O'SHAUNESSY R. Intrapartum pulmonary embolus. J Reprod Med 30, 64, 1985.

45. ROCHAT RW, KOONIN LM, ATRASH HK, JEWETT JF. Maternal mortality in the United States : Report from the Maternal Mortality

Collaborative. Obstet Gynecol 72, 91-97, 1988.

46. RUTHERFORD SE, PHELAN JP. Deep venous thrombosis and pulmonary embolism in pregnancy. Obstet Gynecol Clin North Am 18(2), 345-70, 1991.

47. SACHS BP, BROWN DAJ, DRISCOLL SG, SCHULMAN E, ACKER D, RAMSIL BJ, JEWETT JF. Maternal mortality in Massachussetts. N Engl J Med 316, 667-672, 1987.

48. SALAZAR E, ZAJARIAS A, GUTIERREZ N, ITURBE I. The problem of cardiac valve prostheses, anticoagulants and pregnancy. Circulation (Suppl.) 70, 1169-1177, 1984.

49. SHARMA GVRK, CELLA G, PARISI AF, et al. Thrombolytic therapy. N Engl J Med 306, 1268, 1985.

50. TAIT JF, GIBSON D, FUJIKAWA K. Phospholipid binding properties of human placental anticoagulant protein-I, a member of the lipocortin family. J Biol Chem 264, 7944, 1989.

51. TENGBORN L, BERGQVIST D, MATZSCH T, BERGQVIST A, HEDNER U. Recurrent thromboembolism in pregnancy and puerperium : is there a need for thrombo-prophylaxis ? Am J Obstet Gynecol 160, 90-94, 1989.

52. VILLASANTA U. Thromboembolic disease in pregnancy. Am J Obstet Gynecol 93, 142, 1965.

53. VON DADELSZEN P, PEDDIE DJ. Pulmonary thromboembolism complicating reccurent placenta abruptio at 29 weeks' gestation. Aust NZ J Obstet Gynaecol 30, 124, 1990.

54. WANG Y, SCHRIEBER L, COHEN MG, FURPHY L, WEBB J, CHIVERS T, POLLARD K. Antiphospholipid antibodies in systemic lupus erythematosus :

Clinical and laboratory associations in 111 patients. Rheumatol Int 10, 75-80, 1990.

55. WHITE TM, BERNENE JL, MARIÑO AM. Continous heparin infusion requirements : Diagnostic and therapeutic implications. JAMA 241, 2717, 1979.

56. WOODHAMS BJ, CANDOTTI G, SHAW R, KERNOFF PBA. Changes in coagulation and fibrinolysis during pregnancy : Evidence of activation of coagulation preceeding spontaneous abortion. Thromb Res 55, 99-107, 1989.

15

Anticoagulants in pregnancy

I. Iturbe Alessio

The need for anticoagulants during pregnancy is a challenging problem for the clinician. The use of heparin versus coumarin and different intensities of anticoagulation for diverse thrombotic processes along the gestational period have a spectrum of risks for the mother and child and the benefits of various anticoagulant regimens are not well defined.

1. Heparin

Heparin is poorly absorbed via the gastrointestinal tract and therefore needs to be administered by the intravenous or subcutaneous route.

During pregnancy, heparin might be the ideal drug from the baby's view point since it cannot cross the placental barrier, but from the maternal point of view it is less than ideal. The main drawback is the route of administration, making the subcutaneous route the only feasible alternative for long-term use.

Heparin has several side effects, the most common being thrombocytopenia [6, 7, 12], that can be present in up to 15 % of patients despite the dose or route of administration. Usually it manifests during the first

5 to 6 days of use, and seems to be more common with heparin derived from bovine lung than heparin derived from pork gut. Very rarely, in less than 1 % of cases, thrombocytopenia can be associated with arterial thrombosis [2, 19].

A less common complication of long term heparin use that has been well documented during pregnancy is osteoporosis, [7, 9, 11, 12, 14], sometimes associated with fractures, including vertebral collapse. Osteoporosis usually occurs after more than three months of persistent use, and customarily with doses of more than 15 000 U per day. Once heparin is discontinued, the osteoporosis is reversible but the morbidity related to vertebral body compression and other bone fractures needs to be considered.

Less likely side effects of heparin are: alopecia, skin necrosis, hypersensitivity reactions and hypoaldosteronism [8].

Other serious concern is that except for deep vein thrombosis [1, 4], there is no experience in the non-pregnant patient with mechanical heart valves with long-term anticoagulation with subcutaneous heparin, that can be extrapolated to the pregnant patient as is the case with warfarin. In the search for the ideal heparin dose, we have to remember that we are not dealing with one entity but a host of diseases, with multiple etiologies that might require different intensities of anticoagulation and the dose and frequency of heparin administration might need to be tailored for the specific problem. In deep vein thrombosis is accepted to use IV heparin initially, followed by 5000 U subcutaneous twice a day [1, 4]. On the other hand, several studies [17, 29] suggest that the same dose is not effective in preventing valve thrombosis in patients with artificial heart valves. Adjusted doses of heparin in the range of 30000 U per day in divided dose given twice a day, to modify the PTT to 1 1/2 times control 6 hours after administration, has proven effective in DVT [15] and may provide adequate antithrombotic protection in patients with mechanical valve prosthesis, however, until now there is not a large, well designed prospective study that proves this point.

It might even be possible that among the patients with artificial heart valves, the intensity of anticoagulation could vary depending on a number of circumstances like: thrombogenicity of the valve, mitral or aortic position of the prosthesis and other underlaying conditions like atrial fibrillation, auricular and ventricular chambers size and the presence or not of congestive heart failure.

The relative hypercoagulable state of pregnancy manifested by higher fibrinogen levels and higher procoagulant activity of several coagulation factors, [27] might also play a role in the effectiveness of heparin anticoagulation.

2. Anti-vitamin K therapy

Antivitamin-K therapy and specially warfarin provides adequate anticoagulation to the pregnant mother in therapeutic doses to treat deep vein thrombosis, pulmonary embolism, and antithrombotic protection in patients with atrial arrythmias and with mechanical heart valves. The intensity of anticoagulation varies depending on the underlaying condition as has been established and recommended by the American College of Chest Physicians and the National Heart, Lung and Blood National Institute [5] based on prospective and retrospective studies world wide.

The prothrombin time, specially if reported as International Normalized Ratio (INR) [21], can give an accurate reflection of the degree of anticoagulation achieved with the anti-vitamin K therapy.

Coumarin has an excellent gastro-intestinal absorption which makes its administration easier for out-patient, long-term therapy. However, the patient needs to be closely monitored since the progression of pregnancy and other factors, can modify the degree of anticoagulation [13].

In other words, from the maternal point of view seems to be the best option for long term use. The severe drawback is that warfarin and its derivatives cross the placental barrier and the fetus is exposed to the drug and is, in fact, anticoagulated, carrying a series of risks depending on the stage of pregnancy that the baby is exposed.

Use of coumarin during the first trimester and particularly during the sixth to the twelfth week, has the risk of producing certain bone abnormalities that manifest at birth by nasal hypoplasia and depression of the bridge of the nose. Radiographically, there is stippling in uncalcified epiphyseal regions of bones called chondrodysplasia punctata [8]. The whole constellation of findings receive the name of "warfarin embryopathy" [10, 13, 23, 28]. The rate of occurrence is difficult to determine since many times the abnormalities are very subtle and the cases reported are anecdotal, the series published are small and most of them retrospective. Two prospective studies, one from Mexico [17] with 49 pregnancies, report an incidence of warfarin embryopathy of 25 % when the mother was exposed until the seventh week of pregnancy and 29 % when exposed during the first 12 weeks, in contrast, a study from South Africa [26] with 50 pregnancies that received warfarin throughout the pregnancy the incidence of embryopathy was only 4% (2 cases).

Hall [10] reviewed the literature until 1978 and in 418 cases the incidence of embryopathy was 8 %. Gingsberg and Hirsh [8] in their review until 1988 found an incidence of 45 cases in 970 pregnancies or 4%.

There are reports of CNS abnormalities that are thought to be related to warfarin exposure at any time during pregnancy and independent of the warfarin embryopathy syndrome. These defects include dorsal midline dysplasia, Dandy Walker malformation, optic atrophy and eye malformations. Hall [10] compiled 11 patients from 418 pregnancies and Ginsgerg and Hirsh [8] found in their review 26 cases in 970 pregnancies. In the two studies from Mexico, one retrospective [25] with 34 children studied and a second prospective [17] with 54 children studied and a prospective study from South Africa [26] with a total of 50 pregnancies with

32 children born, where all children were exposed to warfarin during the second and third trimester, there were no cases of CNS abnormalities. Other series, also fail to show these neurologic findings [16, 18, 20, 24]. When present the CNS malformations are more devastating than the "warfarin embryopathy".

The controversy of use of oral anticoagulants during the second and third trimester is of extraordinary importance because if, in fact, the risk of CNS abnormalities related to anti-vitamin K therapy is very low or non existent at the present recommended warfarin doses, it means that coumarin can be administered during this period with relative safety for the baby and also means that for 2/3 of the pregnancy an oral anticoagulant can be used with better antithrombotic protection to the mother, this is particularly important when dealing with patients with mechanical valve prosthesis.

At the time of delivery the use of coumarin is contraindicated since it can enhance peripartum related hemorrhage in the mother and more important, because the baby is anticoagulated, has a high risk of internal bleeding as it passes through the birth canal [22]. The issue is complicated by the fact that the fetal coagulation system might take a longer time to correct for the anti-vitamin K effect of warfarin than the mother. In the peri-partum period is recommended to avoid anti-vitamin K therapy.

In labor precipitates when the mother and baby are under the effect of warfarin, it is safer for both to have a cesarean section.

3. Abortion and fetal loss

Another problem that is common to all patients anticoagulated with heparin or coumarin is a higher risk of abortion and fetal loss [3, 8, 10, 16, 17, 20, 25, 26]. How much to blame the anticoagulant therapy for this, is difficult to asses because of comorbid conditions that the mother has. Sometimes for the same underlaying condition for which the patient is being anticoagulated can be a contributing factor for the increase in the abortion rate. The intensity of anticoagulation may also play a role in the increase wastage. For these reasons the literature is not clear in the incidence of abortion for heparin or coumarin. Seems like the rates are similar for both anticoagulants but when prematurity and maternal comorbid conditions are excluded, heparin has a better outcome [8], althouth most of the cases compiled have received lower doses of heparin.

4. Conclusions

With the information today available we can conclude that anticoagulation during pregnancy always carries risks for the mother and child.

Anti-vitamin K therapy provides better antithrombotic protection because the intensity of anticoagulation is the same as in non-pregnant patients.

Warfarin should be avoided during the first trimester of pregnancy to avoid the warfarin embryopathy syndrome.

During the second and third trimester, the best choice of anticoagulant is not yet been defined, coumarin might give better protection to the mother, and heparin is less risky to the fetus. With our current knowledge, both are valid alternatives.

The incidence of CNS abnormalities related to warfarin is small and not reported in the prospective studies, suggesting that warfarin is safer than initially thought during the second and third trimester.

Long-term subcutaneous heparin administration with doses in the range of 30.000 U per day in divided doses might provide adequate anticoagulation for patients with prosthetic heart valves but further studies are needed to delineate better the incidence of thrombosis and possible side effects like osteoporosis, abortion and prematurity. For DVT smaller doses of heparin have proven to be effective.

Coumarin should be avoided in the peripartum period to prevent fetal internal bleeding and vaginal hemorrhage.

Biologic prosthesis should be considered when undergoing valve replacement in the fertile woman to avoid the use of anticoagulants.

REFERENCES

1. An International Multicenter Trial. Prevention of fatal postoperative pulmonary embolism by low dose heparin. Lancet 45-51, 1975.

2. ARTUR CK, ISBISTER JP, ASPERY EM. The heparin induced thrombosis-thrombocytopenia syndrome (H.I.T.T.S.): A review. Pathology 17, 82-86, 1985.

3. BUXBAUM A, AYGEN MM, SHAHIN W et al. Pregnancy in patients with prosthetic heart valves. Chest 59, 639-642, 1971.

4. BYNUM LJ, WILSON JE. Low-dose heparin therapy in long-term management of venous thromboembolism. Am J Med 67, 553-556, 1979.

5. DALEN JE, HIRSH J. American College of Chest Physicians and the National Heart, Lung and

Blood Institute National Conference on Antithrombotic Therapy. Arch Intern Med 146, 462-472, 1986.

6. DEREK JK, KELTON JG. Heparin-associated thrombocytopenia. Ann Intern Med 100, 535-540, 1984.

7. GERVIN AS. Complications of heparin therapy. Surg Gynecol Obstet 140, 789-796, 1975.

8. GINSBERG JS, HIRSH J. Anticoagulants during pregnancy. Ann Rev Med 40, 79-86, 1989.

9. GRIFFITH GC, NICHOLS G Jr, ASHER JD et al. Heparin osteoporosis. JAMA 193, 91-94, 1965.

10. HALL JG, PAULI RM, WILSON KM. Maternal and fetal sequelae of anticoagulation during pregnancy. Am J Med 68, 122-140, 1980.

11. HELLGREN M, HYGARDS EB. Long-term therapy with subcutaneous heparin during pregnancy. Gynecol Obstet Invest 13, 76-89, 1982.

12. HIRSH J. Heparin. N Engl J Med 324, 1565-1574, 1991.

13. HIRSH J. Oral anticoagulant drugs. N Engl J Med 324, 1865-1875, 1991.

14. HOWELL R, FIDLER J, LETSKY E, DE SWEIT M. The risk of antenatal heparin prophylaxis: a controlled trial. Br J Obstet Gynecol 90, 1124-1128, 1983.

15. HULL R, DELMORE T, CARTER C, HIRSH J, GENTON E, GENT M, TURPIE G, McLAUGHLIN D. Adjusted subcutaneous heparin versus warfarin sodium in the long-term treatment of venous thrombosis. N Engl J Med 306, 189-194, 1982.

16. IBARRA-PEREZ C, AREVALO-TOLEDO N et al. The course of pregnancy in patients with

artificial heart valves. Am J Med 61, 504-512, 1976.

17. ITURBE-ALESSIO I, FONSECA MC, MUTCHINIK O, SANTOS MA, ZAJARIAS A, SALAZAR E. Risks of anticoagulant therapy in pregnant women with artificial heart valves. N Engl J Med 315, 1390-1393, 1986.

18. JAVARES T, COTO EO, MAIQUEZ V, RINCON A, SUCH M, CAFFARENA JM. Pregnancy after heart valve replacement. Int J Cardiol 5, 731-746, 1984.

19. KING DJ, KELTON JG. Heparin-associated thrombocytopenia. Ann Intern Med 100, 535-540, 1984.

20. LARREA JL, NUNEZ L, REQUE JA, GIL AGUADO M, MATARROS R, MINGUEZ JA. Pregnancy and mechanical valve prostheses: a high risk situation for the mother and fetus. Ann Thorac Surg 36, 459-463, 1983.

21. LOEGHER E, ICSH/ICTH. Recommendations for reporting prothrombin time in oral anticoagulant control. Thromb Haemost 53, 155-156, 1985.

22. OAKLEY C. Valve prosthesis and pregnancy. Br Heart J 58, 303-305, 1987.

23. PAULI RM, HALL JG. WILSON KM. Risks of anticoagulation during pregnancy. Am Heart J 100, 761-762, 1980.

24. PRIDMORE BR, MURRAY KH, Mc ALLEN PM. The mamangement of anticoagulant therapy during and after pregnancy. Br J Obstet Gynaecol 82, 740-744, 1975.

25. SALAZAR E, ZAJARIAS A, GUTIERREZ N, ITURBE I. The problem of cardiac valve prosthesis, anticoagulants and pregnancy. Circulation 70(1), 169-177, 1984.

26. SARELI P, ENGLAND MJ, BERK MR, MARCUS RH, EPSTEIN M, DRISCOLL J, MEYER T, McINTYRE J, Van GELDEREN C. Maternal and fetal sequelae of anticoagulation during pregnancy in patients with mechanical heart valve prosthesis. Am J Cardiol 63, 1462-1465, 1989.

27. SCHAFFER AT. The hypercoagulable states. Ann Intern Med 102, 814-828, 1985.

28. SHAUL WL, HALL JG. Multiple congenital anomalies associated with oral anticoagulants. Am J Obstet Gynecol 127, 191-198, 1977.

29. WANG RYC, PUI KEE LEE et al. Efficacy of low-dose, subcutaneously administered heparin in treatment of pregnant women with artificial heart valves. Med J Aust 2, 126-128, 1983.

16

Anticoagulant therapy and myocardial infarction

Ph. Le Métayer, V. Puel, M. Haissaguerre, J.F. Warin

Anticoagulant therapy for patients with acute myocardial infarction (AMI) aims at reducing early and long term mortality and at decreasing morbidity by preventing deep venous thrombosis (DVT) and pulmonary embolism (PE), left ventricular mural thrombus (LVMT) formation and systemic embolism (SE), coronary reocclusion after successful thrombolysis, early recurrence or extension of AMI and late reinfarction [2].

The incidence of DVT in patients with AMI ranges from 17 to 38 percent [27] and PE occurs in 5 percent of patients without anticoagulants [46]. The risk is increased in patients with large AMI, heart failure, cardiogenic shock, patients over than 70 years or with previous history of DVT and PE [27]. Low dose subcutaneous heparin (5.000 units every 8 to 12 hours) started on admission to hospital and early mobilization give adequate prophylaxis with no hemorrhagic risk. Thus, in three randomized trials, the incidence of DVT was reduced to 4 percent in a low-dose heparin group compared with 23 percent in untreated controls [30, 48, 14]. In three other large randomized placebo controlled trials, heparin reduced PE incidence from 5 to 6 percent in the control group to 2 to 4 percent in the anticoagulated group [46, 32, 13]. The low molecular weight heparin fraction may be proposed as an alternative therapy to unfractionated heparin [34], but platelet inhibitor agents are not effective in preventing DVT and PE.

LVMT is easely and accurately detected by two-dimensional echocardiography with a diagnosis sensitivity and specificity of about 90 percent [47, 37]. Thrombus usually occurs during the first 10 days and its location is generally apical with attachment to a dyskinetic or akinetic segment of the left ventricular cavity [19]. Its early occurence during the first 48 hours is frequent in large AMI and has a pejorative significance [12]. The incidence of LVMT is 20 percent in AMI, lower than 5 percent in inferior AMI, 40 percent in anterior AMI and exceeds 50 percent in large AMI, producing peak serum creatine kinase concentrations > 2000 units/liter [29]. Two randomized double-blind studies found that high-dose subcutaneous heparin (12.500 units every 12 hours) reduced the incidence of echo-detected LVMT [44, 39]. In the Canadian study [44] the incidence of echo-detected LVMT at 10 days of anterior AMI was reduced by 69 percent in the high-dose heparin group compared with the low-dose heparin control (5.000 units every 12 hours). The benefits of high-dose heparin were associated with an activated partial thromboplastin time (APTT) between 50 and 60 seconds, but were achieved without increasing the incidence of bleeding. In the Italian study SCATI [39], LVMT incidence was reduced by 52 percent in the high-dose heparin group compared with untreated controls. The risk of SE is clearly increased in patients with LVMT. Thus, Johannessen and al [23] documented SE in 27 percent of patients with echo-detected LVMT and in only 2 percent of patients without it. Risk factors for embolization are echocardiographic mobility, protrusion of the thrombus within the ventricular chamber and the presence of adjacent myocardial hyperkinesia [26]. The risk of embolic events is great in the first 10 days and persists for 2 to 3 months [29]. Anticoagulant agents may hasten thrombus resolution [43] and reduce SE. Thus, initial treatment with heparin followed by administration of an oral anticoagulant agent resulted in a significant relative risk reduction of SE in two large randomized-controlled trials [46, 32]. Therefore, it seems reasonable [36] to administer high-dose subcutaneous heparin (12.500 units every 12 hours) to patients with anterior AMI during the early phase. Before discharge, when echocardiography shows persistent LVMT or a large akinetic region, heparin should be delayed by an oral anticoagulant at a dose sufficient to obtain an International Normalized Ratio (INR) of 2.0 - 3.0. After 3 months, anticoagulants may be discontinued except in patients with echocardiographic evidence of mobile thrombus, ventricular aneurysm, ischemic cardiomyopathy with severe left ventricular dysfunction, atrial fibrillation or pervious history of SE. Platelet inhibitors are not an alternative therapy : aspirin alone [15] or combined with dipyridamole [24] has proven no effect on the incidence and the embolic potential of LVMT in anterior AMI.

Coronarography performed within 6 hours following the onset of symptoms shows coronary occlusion in 80 percent of patients with AMI [11]. Intravenous thrombolytic therapy produces reperfusion of the infarct related artery, early recanalization allows myocardial salvage, improvement of ventricular function and reduction of early and late mortality [45]. Coronarography performed 90 minutes following thrombolytic therapy shows that recombinant-tissue plasminogen activator (rtpA) induces a higher patency rate than streptokinase [41]. Nevertheless, because of reocclusion, the patency rate is identical and is from 75 percent for streptokinase and 81 percent for rtpA when control angiography is performed at 1 to 3 weeks after initial successful thrombolysis [9].

Persistent coronary artery stenosis and/or disrupted plaque with residual non-occlusive thrombus are predisposing factors for reocclusion [16]. Several therapeutic approaches have been proposed for preventing rethrombosis; immediate percutaneous transluminal coronary angioplasty has not proven to be of additional benefit [42], and prolonged administration [25], combination [6] and improvement [9] of thrombolytic agents have been evaluated or are presently being explored. At present, the use of antiplatelet and anticoagulant medication is the common therapy. In the Second International Study of Infarct Survival (ISIS-2), the combination of intravenous streptokinase with oral aspirin (160 mg per day) given on admission and continued for 1 month reduced the incidence of reinfarction, stroke and early mortality without increased hemorrhagic risk [21]. Furthermore, the higher rate of infarction associated with the use of streptokinase alone was entirely avoided by the addition of aspirin, and this benificial effect persisted after 15 months of follow-up [21]. These data have served to recommend the administration of aspirin (160 to 250 mg per day) in patients receiving thrombolysis immediately on admission and daily thereafter [36]. The role of heparin as an adjunctive treatment during and after thrombolytic therapy of AMI is highly controversial [31]. The second Gruppo Italiano per la Studio della Sopravivenza nell'Infarto Miocardico (GISSI-2) [18], the third International Study of Infarct Survival (ISIS-3) [22] and their combined experience have demonstrated a small but significant reduction in both reinfarction and early mortality in patients receiving subcutaneous heparin (12.500 units every 12 hours) started 12 hours (GISSI-2) and 4 hours (ISIS-3) after the onset of thrombolytic therapy. However, this beneficial effect was significant in patients treated with streptokinase but not in patients who received rtpA. Many authors argue that timing, dosage and route of heparin administration in these studies were suboptimal for rtpA. Indeed, when full-dose intravenous heparin (bolus of 5.000 units followed by 1.000 U/hour and adjusted to an APTT ratio of 1.5 to 2 times normal) was started simultaneously with rtpA, coronarography performed 18 to 84 hours after the acute event showed that heparin improved patency of the infarct-related artery (20, 5, 10). The potential benefit of full-dose intravenous heparin as adjunctive treatment to thrombolysis on 1-month mortality is not yet demonstrated. It is being investigated in the Global Utilization Streptokinase and tpA for Occluded Coronary Arteries (GUSTO) trial [17]. Adjunctive heparin therapy is associated with an increase in the risk of intercranial and systemic hemorrhage. Thus in the GISSI-2 [18] and ISIS-3 [22] studies, the risk of major bleeding requiring transfusion was augmented from 0.5 percent to 1 percent and 0.8 percent to 1.1 percent respectively, and intracranial hemorrhage from 0.4 to 0.6 percent. This increase is modest but it should be remembered that both major and minor bleeding episodes were more common with the more intense heparin group in the ISIS-2 trial [9]. We are waiting further information one full-dose intravenous heparin risk from the GUSTO trial.

For the moment, it would be reasonable [31] to delay heparin treatment for 4 hours when thrombolysis is achieved with streptokinase or anistreplase, which have a long plasma half-life and a significant systemic anticoagulant effect. One the other hand, full-dose intravenous heparin may be used in conjunction with rtpA, which has a short plasma half-life and only rarely a systemic anticoagulant effect. A recent study suggests that this adjunctive heparin therapy may be discontinued after 24 hours and replaced with an oral antiplatelet regimen without any adverse effects on chest pain, reinfarction, coronary patency or left ventricular function [40].

In experimental models, newer specific thrombin antagonists and antiplatelet agents have shown superiority over heparin and aspirin [4]. Combined Administration of Aspirin and argatroban have been used in normal male volunteers [8] but not yet in the prevention of coronary reocclusion.

Despite efforts to widen the indications and to increase the number of patients who can benefit from thrombolysis, a significant proportion of infarct arteries are not opened by thrombolytic therapy [33]. In these patients, the benefit of anticoagulant agents in preventing early recurrence and extension of AMI is controversial. In a review of several trials of subcutaneous and intravenous heparin, Mac Mahon et al [28] showed reduction of early mortality by 16 ± 7 % and a decrease in subsequent reinfarction by 22 ± 10%. In a metaanalysis of 6 randomized controlled trials, Chalmers et al found that anticoagulants gave a significant 21 % reduction in mortality and 30 % decrease in reinfarction [7], and concluded that "all patients who present no contraindication should receive anticoagulants during hospitalisation for infarction". However, these data must be compared with those of the ISIS-2 study which demonstrated that aspirin alone (without any fibrinolytic agent) reduced early cardiovascular mortality by 23% and non-fatal reinfarction by about 50% without any increase in bleeding episodes [9].

Two recent studies [35,1] have demonstrated that long-term oral anticoagulant agents are effective in secondary prevention after AMI : in the Warfarin Reinfarction Study (WARIS) [35] 1214 patients (mean age 61.4 years) who had recovered from AMI were randomized to warfarin (at a dose sufficient to obtain an International Normalized Ratio 2.8 - 4.8) or placebo. The mean interval from the onset of AMI was 27 days and the follow-up was 37 months. The authors concluded that long-term therapy with warfarin had an important beneficial effect with reduction in risk of mortality, reinfarction and cerebrovascular accidents by 24 percent, 34 percent and 55 percent respectively.

The Sixty Plus Reinfarction Study [1] is a double-blind trial limited to 878 patients over 60 years (mean age 67.6 years) and on anticoagulant therapy for at least 6 months and for a median of 6 years after an AMI. Half the patients were given placebo instead of the anticoagulant and the other half continued on anticoagulant therapy (INR 2.7 - 4.5). After a follow-up of 24 months, mortality was reduced by 26 % and reinfarction by 55 % in the anticoagulant group.

However, in both studies, there was a significant increase in bleeding in the treated patients and the incidence of bleeding was clearly related to the intensity of treatment. A recent study demonstrated that lower levels of anticoagulant therapy (INR 1.5 - 2.7) were effective in the prevention of systemic embolism associated with non-valvular AF (38), but these data cannot be extrapolated to secondary prevention after AMI. Furthermore, beneficial effects of long-term oral anticoagulant agents after AMI must be compared with data observed with antiplatelet inhibitor agents.

In a metaanalysis of several trials, long-term platelet inhibitor therapy reduced cardiovascular mortality by 13 % and non-fatal reinfarctions by 31 %, with a risk of bleeding much lower than with anticoagulants [3].

REFERENCES

1. A double-blind trial to assess long term oral anticoagulant therapy in elderly patients after myocardial infarction : report of the Sixty Plus Reinfarction Study Research Group. Lancet 2, 989-994, 1980.

2. ACC / AHA Task Force. Guidelines for the early management of patients with myocardial infarction. J Am Coll Cardiol 16, 249-292, 1990.

3. ACHESON J, ARCHIBALD B, BARNETT H et al. Secondary prevention of vascular disease by prolonged antiplatelet treatment. Antiplatelet trialist's collaboration. Brit Med J 296, 320-331, 1988.

4. BECKER RC. Thrombin antagonists and antiplatelet agents. Am J Cardiol 69, 39A-51A, 1992.

5. BLEICH SD, NICHOLS T, SCHUMACHER R, COOKE D, TATE D, STEINER C, BRINKMAN D. The role of heparin following coronary thrombolysis with tissue plasminogen activator (t-PA) (Abstr.). Circulation 80 (Suppl.II), 113 , 1989.

6. CALIFF RM, TOPOL ES, STACK RS et al for the TAMI Study Group. Evolution of combination thrombolytic therapy and timing of cardiac catheterisation in acute myocardial infarction. Results of thrombolysis and

angioplasty in myocardial infarction. Phase 5 randomized trial. Circulation 83, 1543-1556, 1991.

7. CHALMERS TC, MATTA RS, SMITH H Jr, KUNZLER A. Evidence favoring the use of anticoagulants in the hospital phase of acute myocardial infarction. N Engl J Med 297, 1091-1096, 1977.

8. CLARKE RJ, MAYO G, FITZGERALD GM, FITZGERALD DJ. Combined administration of aspirin and specific thrombin inhibitor in man. Circulation 83, 1510-1518, 1991.

9. COLLEN D. Designing thrombolytic agents : focus on safety and efficiency. Am J Cardiol 69, 71a-81a, 1992.

10. DE BONO DP, SIMOONS ML, TIJSSEN J, ARNOLD AE, BETRIU A, BORGERSDIJK C, LOPEZ BESCOS LL, MUELLER E, PFISTERER M, VAN DE WERF F et al. The effect of early intravenous heparin on coronary patency infarct size and bleeding complications after alteplase thrombolysis : results of a randomized double blind European Cooperative Study Group Trial. Br Heart J 67(2), 122-128, 1992.

11. DE WOOD MA, SPORES J, NOSTKE R, MOUSER LT, BURROUGHS R, GOLDEN MS, LANT HT. Prevalence of total coronary occlusion during the early hours of transmural myocardial infarction. N Engl J Med 303, 897-902, 1980.

12. DOMENICUCCI S, CHIARELLA F, BELLOTI P, LUPI G, SCARSI G, VECCHIO C. Early appearance of left ventricular thrombi after anterior myocardial infarction : a marker of higher in hospital mortality in patients not treated with antithrombotic drugs. Eur Heart J 11, 51-58, 1990.

13. DRAPKIN A, MERSKEY C. Anticoagulation therapy after acute myocardial infarction. Relation

of therapeutic benefit to patient's age, sex and severity of infarction. JAMA 222, 541-548, 1972.

14. EMERSON PA, MARKS P. Preventing thrombosis after myocardial infarction. Brit Med J 1, 18-21, 1977.

15. FUNKE KUPPER AJ, VERHEUGT FWA, PEELS CH, GALETA TW, den HOLLANDER W, ROOS JP. Effect of low dose acetylsalicylic acid on the frequency and hematologic activity of left ventricular thrombus in anterior wall acute myocardial infarction. Am J Cardiol 63, 617-620, 1989.

16. FUSTER V, STEIN B, AMBROSE JA, BADIMON L, BADIMON JJ, CHESEBRO JH. Atherosclerotic plaque rupture and thrombosis. Evolving concepts. Circulation 82 (Suppl.II), 47-59, 1990.

17. GRANGER C, KALBFLEISCH J, CALIFF A, WOODLIEF L, KARNASH S, TOPOL F for the GUSTO Pilot Investigators. The global utilization of streptokinase and tissue plasminogen activator for occluded coronary arteries (GUSTO) pilot study : combined streptokinase and tPA. Circulation 84 (Suppl.II), 573, 1991.

18. Gruppo Italiano per la Studio della Sopravivenza nell'Infarto Miocardico GISSI-2. A factorial randomized trial of alteplase versus streptokinase and heparin versus no heparin among 12,490 patients with acute myocardial infarction. Lancet 336, 65-71, 1990.

19. GUTTERMAN DD. Characterization of the acute left ventricular thrombus : Hermit or nomad ? J Am Coll Cardiol 13, 565-566, 1989.

20. HSIA J, HAMILTON WP, KLEIMAN N, ROBERTS R, CHAITMAN BR, ROSS AM for the heparin-aspirin

reperfusion trial (HART) investigators. A comparison between heparin and low-dose aspirin as adjunctive therapy with tissue plasminogen-activator for acute myocardial infarction. N Engl J Med 323, 1433-1437, 1990.

21. ISIS-2 (Second International Study of Infarct Survival) Collaborative Group. Randomized trial of intravenous streptokinase, oral aspirin, both or neither among 17,187 cases of suspected acute myocardial infarction : ISIS 2. Lancet i, 349-361, 1988.

22. ISIS-3. Unpublished but reported at a press conference preceding the American College of Cardiology meeting in Atlanta. 1991.

23. JOHANNESSEN KA, NORDREHAUG JE, VON DER LIPPE G, VOLLSET SE. Risk factors for embolization in patients with left ventricular thrombi and acute myocardial infarction. Br Heart J 60, 104-110, 1980.

24. JOHANNESSEN KA, STRATTON JR, TAULOW E, OSTERUD B, VON DER LIPPE G. Usefulness of aspirin plus dipyridamole in reducing left ventricular thrombus formation in anterior wall acute myocardial infarction. Am J Cardiol 63, 101-102, 1989.

25. JOHNS JA, GOLD HK, LEINBACH RC, YASUDA T, GIMPLE LW, WERNER W, FINKELSTEIN D, NEWELL J, ZISKINDA A, COLLEN D. Prevention of coronary artery reocclusion and reduction in late coronary artery stenosis after thrombolytic therapy in patients with acute myocardial infarction. A randomized study of maintenance infusion of recombinant human tissue-type plasminogen activator. Circulation 78, 546-556, 1988.

26. JUGDUTT BI, SIVARAM CA. Prospective two-dimensional echocardiographic evaluation of left ventricular thrombus and embolism after

acute myocardial infarction. J Am Coll Cardiol 13, 554-564, 1989.

27. KAKKAR VV. Prevention of venous thrombosis and pulmonary embolism. Am J Cardiol 65, 50C-54C, 1990.

28. MAC MAHON S, COLLINS R, KNIGHT C, YUSUF S. Reduction in major morbidity and mortality by heparin in acute myocardial infarction (Abstr.). Circulation 78 (Suppl.II), 389, 1988.

29. MELTZER RS, VISSER CA, FUSTER V. Intracardiac thrombi and systemic embolization. Ann Intern Med 104, 689-698, 1986.

30. NICOLAIDES AN, KAKKAR VV, RENNEY JT, KIDNER PH, HUTCHINSON DC, CLARKE MB. Myocardial infarction and deep vein thrombosis. Brit Med J 1, 432-435, 1971.

31. PRINS MH, HIRSH J. Heparin as an adjunctive treatment after thrombolytic therapy for acute myocardial infarction. Am J Cardiol 67, 3A-11A, 1991.

32. Report of the working party on anticoagulation therapy in coronary thrombosis to the medical research council. Assessment of short-term anticoagulation administration after cardiac infarction. Brit Med J 1, 335-342, 1969.

33. RUTHERFORD JD, BRAUNWALD E. Thrombolytic therapy in acute myocardial infarction. Chest 97(4), 1365-1455, 1990.

34. SCALA PJ, THIOLLET M, MIDAVAINE M, KHER A, FUNCK BRENTANO C, JAILLON P, ROBERT A, VALTY J. Prevention of deep vein thrombosis and left ventricular thrombosis by a low molecular weight heparin in acute myocardial infarction. Haemostasis 20, 368-369, 1990.

35. SMITH P, ARNESEN H, HOLME I. The effect of warfarin on mortality and reinfarction after myocardial infarction. N Engl J Med 323, 147-152, 1990.

36. STEIN B, FUSTER V. Antithrombotic therapy in acute myocardial infarction : prevention of venous, left ventricular and coronary artery thromboembolism. Am J Cardiol 64, 33B-40B, 1989.

37. STRATTON JR, LIGHTY GW, PEARLMAN AS, RICHTIE JL. Detection of left ventricular thrombus by two dimensional echocardiography : sensitivity specificity and causes of uncertainty. Circulation 66, 156-166, 1982.

38. The Boston Area Anticoagulation Trial for Atrial Fibrillation Investigators. The effect of low-dose warfarin on the risk of stroke in patients with non-rheumatic atrial fibrillation. N Engl J Med 323, 1505-1511, 1990.

39. The SCATI Group. Randomized control trial of subcutaneous calcium-heparin in acute myocardial infarction. Lancet 2, 182-186, 1989.

40. THOMPSON PL, AYLWARD PE, FEDERMAN J, GILES RW, HARAIS PJ, HODGE RL, NELSON GIC, THOMPSON A, TONKIN AM, WALSH WF for the National Heart Foundation of Australia Coronary Thrombolysis Group. A randomized comparison of intravenous heparin with oral aspirin and dipyridamole 24 hours after recombinant tissue-type plasminogen activator for acute myocardial infarction. Circulation 83, 1534-1542, 1991.

41. TIEFENBRUNN AJ, SOBEL BE. The impact of coronary thrombolysis on myocardial infarction. Fibrinolysis 3, 1-15, 1989.

42. TOPOL ES, CALIFF RM, GEORGE BS, KEREIAKES DJ, ABBOTT-SMITH CW, CANDELA RJ, LEE KL, PITT B,

STACK RS, O'NEIL L. A randomized trial of immediate versus delayed elective angioplasty after intravenous tissue plasminogen activator in acute myocardial infarction. N Engl J Med 517, 581-588, 1987.

43. TRAMARIN R, POZZOLI M, FEBO O, OPASICH C, COBELLI F, SPECCHIA G. Echocardiographic assessment of therapy efficacy in left ventricular thrombosis post-myocardial infarction (Abstr.). Circulation 68 (Suppl.III), 331, 1983.

44. TURPIE AGG, ROBINSON JG, DOYLE DJ, MULJI AS, MISHKEL GS, SEALEY BJ. Comparison of high dose with low-dose subcutaneous heparin to prevent left ventricular mural thrombosis in patients with acute transmural anterior myocardial infarction. N Engl J Med 320, 352-357, 1989.

45. VERSTRAETE M. Thrombolytic treatment in acute myocardial infarction. Circulation 82 (Suppl.II), 96-109, 1990.

46. Veterans Administration Cooperative Clinical Trial. Anticoagulants in acute myocardial infarction. JAMA 225, 724-729, 1973.

47. VISSER CA, KANG, DAVID KG, LIE KI, DURRER D. Two dimensional echocardiography in the diagnosis of left ventricular thrombus. Chest 83, 228-232, 1983.

48. WARLOW G, TERRY G, BEATTIE AG, OGSTON D, DOUGLAS AS. A double-blind trial of low doses of subcutaneous heparin in the prevention of deep vein thrombosis after myocardial infarction. Lancet 2, 936-937, 1973.

17

Anticoagulant therapy and atrial fibrillation

Ph. Le Métayer, V. Puel, M. Haissaguerre, J.F. Warin

Atrial fibrillation (AF) is one of the most common cardiac arrhytmias but the only one known to be associated with an increased risk of systemic embolism (SE).

In a review of several studies [10], Fisher found that the site of 43 to 82 percent of SE associated with AF was localized in the cerebral arteries; in a retrospective study [11], Harrisson and Marshall noted that emboli from the fibrillating atrium, probably because of their size, cause usually "long" transient ischemic attacks (TIAs) or completed strokes. In a review of cardiogenic brain embolism [6] Dyken and al found that about 50 percent of presumed cardiogenic embolic strokes resulted from valvular or non-valvular AF, and that stokes associated with AF were often large, functionally devasting and usually unheralded by warning TIAs. Therefore, an effective therapy obviously appears essential for the prevention of these severe complications.

However, the incidence of SE in AF varies with different predisposing factors associated with the dysrythmia itself. Thus, the annual rate of SE ranges from below 1 percent in patients with lone AF and younger than 60 years [14] to about 17 percent in those with AF and a previous history of SE [19]. Added to that, adverse effects are not uncommon in long term anticoagulant therapy. With conventional levels of anticoagulation, risk of brain haemorrhage is about 1 percent per year and risk of severe haemorrhage is 2 percent per year [6]. This risk is increased in patients over 65 years, with renal insufficiency, hypertension, history of previous stroke and with the intensity of anticoagulation [16]. Consequently, while an aggressive antithrombotic therapy is justified in patients with high risk of SE, in those at lower risk the expected benefit of therapy should always be balanced against haemorrhagic complications.

Furthermore, blood stasis by releasing the activation of the coagulation system and the generation of fibrin induces thrombus formation in the left atrial chamber (or in the atrial appendage) which constitute the main source of SE [22]. Visualisation by transesophageal echocardiography of spontaneous contrast echoes within the left atrium and the atrial appendage [5] and the increase of plasma D-dimer levels [15] in patients with AF seem to confirm this mechanism. However, the presence of AF does not necessarily mean that an ischemic event is or will be due to cardiogenic embolism [6]. In non-valvular AF and especially in elderly patients, concomittant cerebrovascular or atherosclerotic ascending aortic diseases must be sought [7]. Thus, the prevalence of carotid artery stenosis is two-fold higher in patients with non-valvular AF [25], and it seems likely that at least 20 to 30 percent of strokes in patients with non-valvular AF are not due to cardiogenic embolism [12]. Consequently, in some cases, the use of antiplatelet agents should be considered as an alternative therapy to anticoagulant medication.

It is acknowledged that the risk of SE in patients with AF varies with the underlying heart disease. Thus, there is a 17-fold increase in stroke associated with AF and rheumatic mitral valve disease [13], and the annual rate of SE is estimated to be about 6 percent in patients with AF and mitral stenosis [16]. Therefore, despite the lack of randomized placebo controlled trials, anticoagulant therapy at a dose sufficient to obtain an International Normalized Ratio (INR) 2.0 to 3.0 has been used in these patients for many years and with an acceptable benefit risk ratio [16].

In non-valvular AF, the importance of SE risk and the benefit of anticoagulant therapy have long been controversial. In the Framingham study [13], patients with non-valvular AF had a more than 5-fold increase in stroke incidence.

Several studies [3, 18] have produced conflicting results about the predisposing effect to embolism of left atrial size, type of AF (paroxysmal versus chronic), duration of arrhytmia, age and sex of patients. However, there is general agreement that the rate of SE is significantly increased to about 4 to 6 percent per year in AF with coronary artery disease, to 6 percent per year in uncontrolled thyrotoxicosis and in AF with heart failure of any cause [16]. This risk is even higher when patients with non-valvular AF have a previous history of SE: risk of recurrent stroke is about 17 percent in the first year and remains at this level in subsequent years [19]. In sinoatrial disease (SAD), Fairfax et al [9] found that the prevalence of SE was about 16 percent, whereas it was only 1.3 percent in patient with auriculoventricular block. Several studies have shown that VVI pacing in SAD favors SE through various mechanisms including retrograde ventriculo-atrial conduction and AF induction [4]. Conversely, physiologic stimulation allows a significant reduction in risk from 13 percent in VVI pacing to 1.6 percent in AAI pacing [24]. In a recent study [20] Santini et al found that stroke mortality was higher in patients with SAD treated with VVI pacing (8 %) compared to that in patients paced with AAI mode (2 %) ($p<0.01$), and this difference was statistically very significant in patients over 70 years (17 percent versus 3 percent $p<0.001$).

The danger of embolic complication in cardioversion of AF is small but not unimportant. Thus, in a study of 348 patients and 454 cardioversions, Bjerkellund found that long-term anticoagulant therapy before electrical cardioversion reduced embolism from 6.5 percent in the control group to 1.1 percent in the anticoagulated group [1].

Catheter-induced ablation of the atrioventricular junction is indicated in some patients with chronic AF which are not controlled by medication. It implies destruction of the His bundle, the AV node or both and the insertion of a permanent pace maker [21]. As the atrial dysrythmia itself persists, this procedure probably does not modify the risk of SE.

In lone or idiopathic AF which is defined as AF in the absence of any demonstrable heart disease, the risk of SE appears lower. At the Mayo Clinic, Kopecky found that patients under 60 years with lone AF had an annual rate of SE below 1 percent [19]; however, in the Framingham study [2], in a group of older patients (mean age 70 years) the risk was evaluated at 2.4 percent per year.

On the whole, data of numerous studies suggest that the risk of SE is significantly increased in patients with non-valvular AF, except for patients with lone AF and under 60 years.

The benefits of antithrombotic preventive therapy in non-valvular AF have long been discussed. Since 1989, we have had further information with the data from four randomized and controlled trials [2, 17, 23, 26]. The Copenhagen Atrial Fibrillation Aspirin Anticoagulation Study (AFASAK) [17] was a 2-year controlled randomized trial which compared the effects of warfarin (at a dose adjusted to obtain an INR 2.8 to 4.2), oral aspirin (75 mg per day) and placebo in 1007 patients (mean age 74.2 years) with non-valvular chronic AF. After a mean follow-up of 11 months, yearly incidence of SE was the same in placebo and aspirin groups (5.5 percent) but was reduced to 2.0 percent in the warfarin group. Bleeding was more frequent with warfarin (6.9 percent) than with aspirin (2.4 percent) and placebo (1.8 percent). Therapy was discontinued in 6.2 percent of patients with warfarin and in 0.6 percent of patients taking aspirin. The only fatal bleeding was one brain haemorrhage with an INR 3.7.

The Stroke Prevention in Atrial Fibrillation Study (SPAF) [23] included 1244 patients (mean age 67 years) with non-valvular AF (34 percent with paroxysmal AF) who were assigned in two groups. In group 1, patients (without contra-indication for anticoagulation) were randomized to warfarin (at a dose adjusted to obtain INR 1.8 - 3.4) or, in a double-blind, to oral aspirin

(325 mg per day) or placebo. In group 2, patients (with warfarin contra-indication) were double-blind randomized to oral aspirin (325 mg per day) or placebo. The endpoints were ischemic stroke and systemic embolism. After a follow-up of 1.13 years, in group 1 patients with active therapy (warfarin or aspirin) had a reduction in risk of 81 percent compared to the placebo group (1.6 percent vs 8.3 percent yearly).

In groups 1 and 2, aspirin decreased the annual risk of stroke and SE by 49 percent (3.2 percent vs 6.3 percent in placebo group p = 0.014) but this benefit of aspirin was not significant in patients over 75 years.

Discontinuation of therapy was 10.9 percent in warfarin group, 4.2 percent in aspirin group and 6.3 in placebo group.

The Boston Area Anticoagulation Trial for Atrial Fibrillation (BAATAF study) [26] was a controlled randomized trial which compared the effects of low-dose warfarin (adjusted to obtain INR 1.7 to 2.7) with a control group without therapy or aspirin. End points were ischemic stroke, death and bleeding. Four hundred and twenty patients (mean age 68 years) with non-valvular AF (17 percent with paroxysomal type) were included. After a follow-up of 2.2 years, there was an 86 percent reduction in risk of stroke in the warfarin group (0.41 percent per year vs 2.98 percent per year in the control group p=0.0022); the death rate was markedly lower (2.21 percent per year in the warfarin group versus 5.97 percent in the control group p=0.005). There was one fatal haemorrhage in each group, a higher rate of minor haemorrhage in the warfarin group, but the frequency of severe bleeding events was the same in both groups. Only 10 percent of the patients assigned to receive warfarin discontinued the therapy permanently.

The stroke prevention in non-rheumatic atrial fibrillation (SPINAF) study [8] was a randomized double-blind prospective study comparing low-dose coumarin to placebo in 538 male veterans with persistent non-valvular fibrillation and no clinical evidence of stroke. Primary endpoint was stroke and secondary endpoints were cerebral haemorrhage and death. There was a 73 percent reduction in risk of stroke in the coumarin group without increased haemorrhagic risk. This benefit was seen with advancing age, even for patients between 70 and 80 years.

In summary, it is reasonable to propose in non-valvular AF an antithrombotic therapy with warfarin which maintains its efficacy even with low anticoagulation level (INR 1.7 - 2.7). Aspirin (325 mg/day) may be an alternative therapy when patients with non-valvular AF have a warfarin contraindication, although its efficacy has not been proven in all studies.

REFERENCES

1. BJERKELUND CJ, ORNING OM. The efficacy of anticoagulant therapy in preventing embolism related to DC electrical conversion of atrial fibrillation. Am J Cardiol 23, 208-216, 1969.

2. BRAND FN, ABBOTT RD, KANNEL WB, WOLF PA. Characteristics and prognosis of lone atrial fibrillation: 30 - year follow up in the Framingham study. JAMA 254, 3449-3453, 1985.

3. CABIN HS, CLUBB KS, HALL C, PERLMUTTER RA, FEINSTEIN AR. Risk for systemic embolization of atrial fibrillation without mitral stenosis. Am J Cardiol 65, 1112-1116, 1990.

4. CAMM AJ, KATRITSIS D. Ventricular pacing for sick sinus syndrome: a risky Business? Pace 13, 695-699, 1990.

5. CASTELLO R, PEARSON AC, LABOVITZ AS, LENZEN P. Prevalence and clinical implication of atrial spontaneous contrast in patients

undergoing transesophageal echocardiography. Am J Cardiol 65, 1149-1153, 1990.

6. Cerebral Embolism Task Force. Cardiogenic brain embolism. Arch Neurol 43, 71-84, 1986.

7. CHESEBRO J, FUSTER V, HALPERIN JL. Atrial fibrillation. Risk marker for stroke. N Engl J Med 323, 1556-1558, 1990.

8. EZEKOWITZ MD, BRIDGERS SL, JAMES KE and SPINAF Investigators. Interim analysis of VA cooperative study. Stroke prevention in non-rheumatic atrial fibrillation. (SPINAF). Circulation II, 450, 1991.

9. FAIRFAX AJ, LAMBERT CD, LEATHAM A. Systemic embolism in chronic sinatrial disease. N Engl J Med 295, 190-192, 1976.

10. FISHER CM. Embolism in atrial fibrillation. In: Kulbertus HB, Olson SB, Schlepper M (Eds). Atrial Fibrillation. Hassle AB, Molndal, Sweden, 1982.

11. HARRISSON MJG, MARSHALL J. Atrial fibrillation, TIAs and completed strokes. Stroke 15, 441-442, 1984.

12. HART RG, COULL BM, HART D. Early recurrent embolism associated with non-valvular atrial fibrillation: a retrospective study. Stroke 14, 688-693, 1983.

13. KANNEL WB, ABBOTT RD, SAVAGE DD, Mc NAMARA PM. Epidemiologic features of chronic atrial fibrillation: the Framingham Study. N Engl J Med 306, 1018-1022, 1982.

14. KOPECKY SL, GERSH BI, Mc GOON MD, WHISNANT JP, HOLMES Dr Jr, ILSTRUP DM, FRYE RL. The natural history of lone atrial fibrillation: a population based study over three decades. N Engl J Med 317, 669-674, 1987.

15. KUMAGAI K, FUKUNAMI M, OHMORI M, KITABATAKE A, KAMADA T, HOKI N. Increased intracardiovascular clotting in patients with chronic atrial fibrillation. JACC 16, 377-380, 1990.

16. LANDEFELD CS. Major bleeding in outpatients treated with warfarin: incidence and prediction of factors known at the start of outpatient therapy. Am J Med 87, 144, 1989.

17. PETERSEN P, BOYSSEN G, GODTFREDSEN J, ANDERSEN ED, ANDERSEN B. Placebo controlled randomized trial of warfarin and aspirin for prevention of thromboembolic complications in chronic atrial fibrillation: the Copenhagen AFASAK study. Lancet 1, 175-179, 1989.

18. PETERSEN P, KASTRUP J, HELWEG-LARSEN S, BOYSSEN G, GODTFREDSEN S. Risk factors for thromboembolic complication in chronic atrial fibrillation. The Copenhagen AFASAK Study. Arch Intern Med 150, 819-821, 1990.

19. SAGE JL, VAN UITERT RL. Risk of recurrent stroke in patients with atrial fibrillation and non-valvular heart disease. Stroke 14, 537-540, 1983.

20. SANTINI M, ALEXIDOU G, ANSALONE G, CACCIATORE G, CINI R, TURITTO G. Relation of prognosis in sick sinus syndrome to age, conduction defects and modes of permanent cardiac pacing. Am J Cardiol 65, 729-735, 1990.

21. SCHEINMAN MM, MORADY F, HESS DS, GONZALEZ R. Catheter - induced ablation of the atrioventricular junction to control refractory supraventricular arrhytmia. JAMA 248, 851-855, 1982.

22. STEIN B, FUSTER V, HALPERIN JL, CHESEBRO JH. Antithrombotic therapy in cardiac disease. An emerging approach based on pathogenesis and risk. Circulation 80 1501-1513, 1989.

23. Stroke prevention in atrial fibrillation study group investigators. Preliminary report of the stroke prevention in atrial fibrillation study. N Engl J Med 3322, 863-868, 1990.

24. SUTTON R, KENNY RA. The natural history of sick sinus syndrome. Pace 9, 1110, 1986.

25. TEGELER CH. Stroke prevention in atrial fibrillation study: Carotid Stenosis Study Group. Carotid stenosis in atrial fibrillation. Neurology 39(1), 159 (Abstr.), 1989.

26. The Boston Area-Anticoagulation Trial for Atrial Fibrillation Investigators. The effect of low-dose warfarin on the risk of stroke in patients with non-rheumatic atrial fibrillation. N Engl J Med 323, 1505-1511, 1990.

18

Anticoagulation and venous thrombosis

G. Sassout, P.M. Garcia, F. Hayek

Anticoagulants take up a dominant place in the preventive treatment of deep venous thrombosis (DVT), in every situation in which this risk is present, and especially in the context of a surgical act, prolonged immobilization or in the event of diseases which disturb the biological mechanisms of coagulation. Anticoagulants are also the base of a curative treatment of compound deep veinous thrombosis, possibly linked with surgical intervention or a fibrinolytic treatment.

Venous thrombosis remain a warryng disease due to their progressive forms marked by two formidable complications:

- pulmonary embolism which can be revealing, often recurring, and sometimes fatal.
- post-phlebetic disease caused by an obstacle in the venous blood flow or by the distal blood reflux, essentially in orthostatism following valval destruction.

The use of low molecular weight heparin (LMWH) has come to modify the findings of the preventive treatment, and the most recent studies, which are still to be confirmed, show an interest in the curative treatment of DVT.

The unfractionnated heparin (UFH) still holds an important role in the curative treatment.

The oral anticoagulants are used at an earlier stage, to take over from the heparin treatments.

The indisputable effectiveness of these anticoagulant treatments goes hand in hand with a, not inconsiderable, risk of complications, dominated by hemorrhagic accidents.

The appearance of LMWH has brought the hope of considerably reducing these risks. Research carried out in test tubes and with animals have brought to light [42]:

- a large bioavalibility for subcutaneous injections allowing the reduction of the number of daily injections
- a reduction in bleeding time
- a lesser effect on the activation of platelet functions
- the hope of reducing the risk of hemorrhage and at the same time keeping the same level of effectiveness
- the hope of reducing the frequency of thrombopenia caused by the heparin

However, these hopes have been partially dashed because, even though the heparins have proved that in the sphere of prevention a level of effectiveness at least equivalent to that of the UFH, the frequency of hemorrhagic accidents is not always reduced in a statistically significant manner.

The risk of thrombopenia has not been eliminated and the problem of the biological monitoring of the treatment remains open.

Oral anticoagulants used in the long time, as a relief treatment from heparins, are also responsible for hemorrhagic accidents. However, since a system of surveillance of the treatment was created, based on the INR (International Normalized Ratio), one tends to use weaker doses of oral anticoagulants on the grounds of fundamental biological findings, backed up well run clinical tests [15].

One must pay particular attention with prescribing anticoagulant treatments to pregnant women and be especially aware of its repercussions on the fetus.

1. Heparins and venous thrombosis

Nowadays, heparins are the most widely selected drugs for the prevention and treatment of venous thromboembolic disease.

From now, on this cases, non fractionned heparin will be competiny against heparins of low molecular weight.

1.1 Unfractionated heparin

Heparin was discovered in 1916 by Mac LEAN. The first pharmaceutical preparation of heparin was extracted from hepatic tissues (hepar = liver in Greck). The first patient to be successfully treated with heparin in 1938 was suffering from recurring venous thrombosis which resisted against all other treatments [51].

1.1.1 UFH can be administered intra-venously or subcutaneously

- continuous perfusion with an electric syringe remains the standard method of reference. This must be preceeded by a starting dose (50 UI/kg) of intra-venous bolus. Without the bolus, one would have to wait 4-6 hours before reaching an effective level of hypocoagulability [1].
- discontinuous intra-venous perfusion is possible, but it must be carried out every 2 hours due to the half-life of heparin which is from 60-90 minutes. More spaced out injections (every 4 hours for example) expose the patient to a significant hemorrhagic risk in connection with the relative overdose during the first two hours after the injection.

- subcutaneous perfusion can also be used at the rate of two or three injections a day. Its effectiveness is comparable with that of the intra-venous method, subject to the extension of the activated partial thromboplastin time corresponding to the levels of effectiveness biologically required.

It is not adviseable to exceed 15 000 UI per injection. The total dose for 24 hours is comparable or slightly superior to that injected intra-venously (20 % max).

In the curative treatment of DVT, the effectiveness depends on the hypocoagulability obtained effect. HULL [37] demonstrated this by showing that out of 113 patients (DVT carriers) treated with heparin either intra-venously or subcutaneously, 63 % of patients receiving heparin subcutaneously still had insufficiently anticoagulated blood after the first 24 hours, whereas only 29 % of these treated intravenously suffered from this state of insufficient anticoagulation after time. This study brought to light the ineffectiveness of the subcutaneous treatment with an insufficient dose. DOYLE [14] confirmed this hypothesis and adapted the dose of heparin from the second injection onwards in order to obtain a comparable hypocoagulability in both groups. The frequency of embolic accidents and hemorrhagic complications become the same in both groups (regardless of the type of injection used).

On the grounds of these findings, some physicians advocate the injection of an intra-venous bolus of 50 UI/kg before the first subcutaneous injection.

Furthermore, an untreated and inadequately treated venous thrombosis at the calf, runs a 20 to 30 % risk of spreading which is virtually eliminated by an anticoagulant treatment for the duration of at least six weeks [30-45].

1.1.2 The posology is variable according to whether the treatment is curative or preventive

There exists a connection between administered dose and the biological effect between the phlebographic evolution (when there is a phlebitis) and, to a lesser degree, hemorrhagic complications [32-33].

When the treatment is preventive, one must distinguish between prevention of low risks and the prevention of high risks (orthopedic surgery or patients with other factors of risk: old age, obesity, neoplasia, previous history of thromboembolic disease, abnormal blood crasis).

- the prevention of high risks : the daily dose must be adapted to produce a moderate extension of the activated partial thromboplastin time (1.2 to 1.3 times the control) when the blood sample is taken in the middle of the interval between the two injections.

- the prevention of low risks: among adults 5000 UI of Un-Fractionated-Heparin (UFH), 2 to 3 times daily relatively reduces the risk of thrombosis by 60-70 % [10].

- the curative treatment of DVT: the normal initial dose is 500-600 UI/kg/24 h; whatever the type of injection administered. This dose will be adapted according to the biological monitoring and varies in practice from 400-800 UI/kg/24 h.

1.1.3 The biological monitoring of the treatment

This is based essentially on the control of the activated partial thromboplastin time (global test), but can also concern the activity of anti-factor X (STUART Factor).

The activated partial thromboplastin time must be normal before the treatment in order to be interpretable. Likewise, among patients with a circulating anticoagulant, antithromboplastin type, or those deficient in factor XII (Hageman): two circumstances in which a thrombotic risk is associated with a spontaneous extension of the activated partial thromboplastin time, this test does not reflect the effectiveness of the heparin. Conversly, a significant inflammatory syndrom can bring about a minor extension of the activated partial thromboplastin time for an identical heparinemia [1].

The extension of the activated partial thromboplastin time also varies according to the reagent used and according to the time at which the blood sample is taken in relation to the heparin injection.

- during the continuous perfusion, the time at which sample is taken is of no importance. The activated partial thromboplastin time is to be maintained between two to three times the control (0.3 to 0.6 UI/ml anti Xa).

- during the discontinuous subcutaneous or intravenous injections, if the blood sample is taken half way between the two injections, the activated partial thromboplastin time should be two to three that of the control. On the other hand, if the blood sample is taken just before the following injection, one then controls the residual anticoagulant effect the activated partial thromboplastin time should be 1.5 times that of the control (0.15 UI/ml anti Xa).

1.1.4 The duration of the treatment

- in the case of preventive treatment, the treatment will be followed until the resumption of activity after surgical intervention or for as long as there is still a significant risk factor.

- the traditional duration of curative treatments of DVT is from 7 to 10 days. Some physicians suggest, with equivalent clinical results, a shorter treatment with the joint administration of oral anticoagulants right from the start. The total duration of the heparin treatment is therefore roughly five days. However, the effectiveness of such treatments, determined by the phlebographic score, has not yet been established [21-38].

The need to carry on with an anticoagulant treatment has been confirmed by the studies of Lagerstedt and Hull [45-36]. The effectiveness of unfractionated heparin or of oral anticoagulants is identical as to the prevention of recurrence [35-36].

1.1.5 Thrombopenia caused by heparin

Hemorrhagic complications linked to heparinotherapy have been known for a long time, but thrombopenia induced by heparin was discover much later on.

In order to call to mind the diagnosis of thrombopenia induced by heparin, it is necessary to check the normality of the platelet count before any kind of treatment, and then set up a control of the platelets at least twice a week until the 21th day if the treatment is prolonged. After this length of time thrombopenia become very rare.

One must distinguish between two types of thrombopenia however [24]:

- transitory and benign thrombopenia
- severe thrombopenia

1.1.6 Transitory and benign thrombopenia

They arise before the 5th day of treatment with a moderate reduction of platelets of which the count varies from 100 and 150000/mm^3.

They are not accompanied by any form of complication, in particular thrombotic, and may often disappear in spite of the continuation of the treatment.

The frequency of thrombopenia arising varies according to different findings, form 1 % to 30 %

[18]. The highst level of incidence being observed among patients who had already received the heparin of bovine origin. The mechanism of the thrombopenia has not yet been clearly established.

1.1.7 Severe thrombopenia induced by heparin

They are exceptional during preventive medical treatments (incidence lower than 1/1000). They concern above all the curative treatment of DVT or some surgical acts at risk: 3.4 % after a total hip prothesis [46].

Sometimes, a myeloproliferative disorder pre-exists (primary hemorrhagic thrombocythemia or primary polyglobulia) [43].

The diagnosis is called to mind in the event of a thrombopenia sometimes linked to thrombotic sight. Arterial thrombosis are responsible for a high level of mortality and significant morbidity.

Thrombopenia occurs in more than 80 % of cases between the 5th and 15th day of treatment, irrespective of the way of administration of the treatment or of the posology of heparin. The platelet count is lower than 50 000/mm^3 in more than 80 % of cases, linked to coagulation anomalies among 25 % of patients (increase of fibrin split products or a full picture of consumption coagulopathy) [44].

The clinical picture is dominated by thrombotic complications (65 % of cases). Arterial thrombosis tend to touch the abdominal aorta and its division branches (the iliac arteries), but the coronary or cerebral arteries are not spared. These lesions can be responsible for distal arterial embolisms. Painful prodroms in the lower limbs and in the abdomen may occur 24 to 48 hours before the appearance of the thrombosis. These prodroms could be connected with distal micro-embolism [3]. The thrombus surgically extracted has a whitish colouring (white clot syndrom) [54].

Venous thrombosis or pulmonary embolisms are observed in approximately 30 % of cases [24]. Signs of hemorrhage are more rare (20 % of cases) and are on the whole benign: purpura, cutaneous-mucors hemorrhages.

The diagnosis can be affirmed by thrombopenia, the correction obtained after stopping heparin therapy, and at last biological tests seeking an heparin-dependant antibody in serum or plasma.

The mechanism of severe thrombopenia is immunological but may also imply the role of the endothelial cell.

The treatment of these thrombopenia is based on the stoppage of heparin. A substitute treatment of oral anticoagulants is generally necessary. The platelet inhibiting drugs, although inhibiting in vitro dumping of induced platelets, has an inconstant clinical effectiveness. The usefulness of prostacyclin remains debatable.

1.1.8 The neutralization of heparin by protamine

The neutralization of heparin can become necessary in the event of a hemorrhagic accident, be it as a result of an overdose of heparin or irrespective of the anticoagulant treatment but worsened by the latter. The frequency of serious hemorrhagic accidents is at about 5 %.

After an intravenous injection of heparin (using the normal therapeutic doses) the time taken for the half-disappearance of the unfractioned heparin is about an hour. After the subcutaneous injection, this time lapse is doubled. These findings are useful when evaluating the heparinemia according to the injected dose and the time lapse from the time of the injection awards.

1 mg of protamine sulfate neutralises 100 UI of unfractionated heparin.

The injection of protamine sulfate can bring about 2 types of reaction:

- the well known anaphylactic reaction

- and more recently other reactions have been pointed out which appear to be more frequent and dominated by severe pulmonary hypertension [47].

Protamine administered intra-venously can bring about systemic hypotension. A simple vascular filling suffices in order to restore a normal hemodynamic.
The anaphylactic reaction entails, in various degrees: urticaria, bronchospasm, hypertension, even circulatory collapse. These reactions are unforseeable.
The last type of heparin-protamine reaction is marked by severe pulmonary hypertension which leads rapidly to heart failure (on the right hand side). The incidence of this reaction is 1.5 % in a sample group of 1000 patients after extracorporeal circulation (ECC) [48].
This reaction could be due to a very significant release of thromboxane from the pulmonary vascular bed.

1.2 Low molecular Weight Heparins (LMWH)

LMWH were discovered in 1976. Their discovery brought the hope of reducing the risk of hemorrhage without changing the therapeutic effectiveness. The hypothesis discussed was the following [52]:

- the antithrombotic effect is characterised by the anti-Xa activity.
- the risk of hemorrhage is connected with the anti-II a activity.

The activity relationship between anti-Xa/ anti-IIa is from 2 to 5 for the different LMWH, whereas it is near to 1 for unfractionated heparin [51], the risk of hemorrhage for LMWH should theoretically be much lower than that of the UFH.
However, clinical trials have not clearly confirmed this hypothesis. Initially, these studies headed towards the prophylaxis of thrombo-embolic accidents,

an area in which numerous studies have shown a level of effectiveness for the LMWH which is at least equal to that of the UFH in general and orthopedic sugery [23].

The interest of LMWH in the curative treatment of DVT is less well researched [16, 26]. In 1990, only 6 studies bringing together about a hundred patients had been carried out in this type of indication [30].

There has not been a marked reduction in the frequency of hemorragic complications, other than in Albada's studies [2]. The risks of thrombocytopenia have been for from eliminated.

However, for Duroux [17], the standards of Arn essen's phlebographic index go up significantly after a 10 days treatment of DVT by LMWH in comparison with a treatment of the same length using LMWH. The encouraging phlebographic evolution, eventhough the activated partial thromboplastin time remains normal, seems to show a dissociation between the anti-thrombotic effect and the anticoagulant effect, furthermore, numerous studies fail to bring to light the close relationship between the activated partial thromboplastin time and the risk of hemorrhage [4-9].

However, inspite of several dasked hopes, LMWH have already often replaced the UFH in the prophylaxis of post-operation thromboembolic accidents, and will may be replaced, in the short time, UFH in the curative treatment of DVT. Their success is explained by their real effectiveness linked to a significant bioavalibility, allowing the limitation of their administration to only one subcutaneous injection daily in the prophylaxis of thromboembolic accident and by a simplification of the biological surveillance (this is not however an unanimous view).

1.2.1 The practical use of LMWH

- In the context of prophylactic treatment of thrombo-embolic disease

LMWH are used at the rate of 1 subcutaneous injection daily.

Every speciality exists under 3 different posologies, corresponding to a low, medium, or high risk as to be occurence of DVT. The minor risk is represented by general surgery and the high risk by orthopedic and gynecological surgery. The doses used in the latter form of surgery are greater than those used in general surgery.

With regard to the prophylaxis of thrombotic accidents in the medical field, the posology of LMWH is still not perfectly defined. The posology can be an intermediary between that used in general surgery and that used in orthopedic surgery.

- In the context of curative treatment of DVT

To have 2 subcutaneous injections daily is in that case necessary. The posology, based on many studies, is from 3 to 6 times-upper than those used in prophylactic treatment, according to weight of patients.

1.2.2 The surveillance of the treatment by LMWH

LMWH currently available, have been developed in the absence of standardisation, according to different procedures and their properties are not strictly identical. The unity systems used are distinctive in each preparation.

An international standard of LMWH has consequently been suggested in order to determine the equivalences between the different LMWH. This standard, the object of numerous controverties, has far from brought about a feeling of unanimity in medical circles [6], because the international unities are based on the anti-Xa activity but neither takes into account the differences of anti-IIa activity, nor the anti-thrombotic effect, nor prohemorrhagic activity, nor the bioavailability when using subcutaneous injections. The conversion into international unities of anti-Xa of LMWH doses have however the great advantage by reducing the apparent difference of posologies of the varying LMWH.

The surveillance method of a treatment using LMWH, in practice, is the determination of the activity of the circulating anti-Xa Factor. However, this measure is not the exclusive and faithful therapeutic reflection of the anti-thrombotic activity of the LMWH [51] but it consists at a good biological indication of the presence of products in the plasma.

It is standard practice to control the anti Xa Factor activity from 3 to 4 hours after the subcutaneous injection.

When preventivy for low or high risk, it is useless to measure the anti-Xa Factor activity, as no clinical test has fareseen the adaptation of the preventive doses in accordance with these results, while prooving at the same time the safety of LMWH.

There are exceptions which concern some patients who are exposed to a particular risk of hemorrhage, who have a heavy body weight, and those prove to renal failure, whom the best equation benefit/risk would be obtained for a heparinemia between 0.3 and 0.45 UI anti Xa-Factor.

As in the case of UFH, a twice weekly control of the platelets until the 21th day is necessary.

For the surveillance in a curative treatment of DVT, several clinical studies have adjusted the posology according to the results of the heparinemia anti-Xa Factor. Whereas in other studies, there has been no further adjustment and therefore the initial determination of the posology according to weight, remains standard.

Anti-Xa activity seems to have to be maintained between 0,3 and 1 UI/ml when the blood sample is taken 3-4 hours after the injection. The posology adjustments are however more rare than with UFH, because of the lesser importance of individual variability of the biological effect. A control within the first 48 hours of treatment and when the oral anticoagulants take over are usually sufficient.

1.2.3 Secondary accidents due to the LMWH treatment

These accidents are common in both UFH and LMWH treatments:

- induced thrombopenia. The stoppage of LMWH is necessary and oral anticoagulants should be used as a substitute if possible

- hemorrhagic accident. The time of the half-life of the LMWH is about 4 hours after the subcutaneous injection. The protamine sulfate completely neutralises the anti-IIa activity but incompletely the anti-Xa activity of the LMWH (50-60 % of which persist even with high doses of protamine sulfate). It is consequently more difficult to neutralise a LMWH based treatment then by UFH. The recommanded doses of protamine sulfate are the same as those recommanded for the UFH.

2. The treatment by oral anticoagulant (AVK)

AVK appeared 2 years after heparin. Their principal interest is to be able to used oraly as a substitute for heparin treatment.

These drugs provoke a reduction in the biological activity of certain coagulation factors II (prothrombin), VII (stable factor), IX (Christmas Factor), X (Stuart Factor), C and S proteins.

They are used as a long term treatment, the risk of which is the still too frequent occurence of hemorrhagic accidents [53]: 22 hemorrhagic accidents, 9 of which were fatal, out of 100 patients a year. These accidents are related to an overdose, drug interference or a disregard of the contra-indications.

The biological monitoring of oral anticoagulant treatments has benefited recently from a better standardisation with the definition of therapeutic zones, the consequence of which is the prescription of weaker doses of oral anticoagulants, permitting the antithrombotic activity to go on with little risk of hemorrhage [28].

Furthermore, the fear of thrombopenias induced by heparin favours the substitution of AVK at an earlier stage (less than 5 days after the beginning of the heparin therapy).

Experimentally, the antithrombotic effect of heparin appears greater than that of AVK at the severe stage of venous thromboembolic accident [29]. These indications have recently been questioned by a study by Gallus [21], which demonstrates that a period of 9 days of heparin treatment is not superior to a 4 days treatment with an early take over by the AVK.

The AVK indications for venous pathology are deep venous thrombosis, its extension, the prevention of recurrences and embolic complications.

2.1 Chosing an oral anticoagulant

There are 2 categories of AVK: one has a short life span (or medium), and the other has a long life span.

Several studies [15, 27] show that it is recommandable to prescribe AVK of long half-lives, to be taken once daily, in the evening. The AVK reduce the biological activity of the coagulation factors, vitamin-K dependent, which all interfer in the phase of hemostasis, but not with the same relative importance. The short life span factors will first break down (VII factor: 5 hours) whilst the long life span factors will only diminish secondarily (II factor: 60 hours). The break down of the factors of the life span of which is shorter will bring about a risk of hemorrhage, but their rapid build up as soon as the AVK ceases to be active will bring about a thrombotic risk.

These fluctuations spaced out of the rate of drugs and of the vitamin-K dependent factor, make the equilibration of the treatment difficult with the succession of risks of hemorrhage and thrombosis.

When using short life AVK, the difficulties of equilibration lead to fractionning the daily dose 2 or 3 times over 24 hours and prescribing different doses every other day which would make the treatment very difficult.

2.2 Posology of AVK

The necessary dose in order to obtain a balanced anticoagulant treatment varies from person to person.

The balance can be obtained at the end of 3 to 4 half-lives (7 days in practice) [12].

Load doses at the beginning of the treatment are dangerous and injustified for the reasons exposed in the above paragraph about the varying half-lives of varied vitamin-K dependent factors.

2.3 Contra-indications of AVK

An oral anticoagulant treatment must only be prescribed among patients likely to understand the risks and to assume the regular surveillance.

This treatment is not recommanded in certain pathological circumstances [12]:

- non controled serious hypertension (diaslotic pressure higher than 120 mm/Hg)
- grave renal failure (creatinine clearance under 20 ml/min)
- recent cerebral vascular disease
- intracranial sugery, recent cranial traumatism; in these 2 cases, the AVK can be prescribed as soon as the cerebral scanner is normal or shows scar-tissue as

a low density lesion non opacified by contrast product.
- an evolutionnal gastro-duodenal ulcer, proven by fiber optic endoscopy
- esophageal varix
- decompensated hepatic cirrhosis
- hemorrhagic diathesis

With old aged patients, a surveillance precautions and a weak posology are recommanded.

2.4 Drug interaction

Certain drugs are responsible for a potentialisation of the AVK, or for an increase of hemorrhagic risk. Amongst these products which increase the risk of hemorrhage, are must especially remember the non steroidal anti-inflammatories, the acetyl salicylic acid, and more generally platelet inhibiting drugs.

Other drugs, on the contrary, reduce the AVK's effects. They are mostly hepatic enzyme inducers.

Furthermore, the diet can modify the action of the AVK: fasting potentializes this action, whereas diet rich in K1 vitamins reduce it.

2.5 Resistances to oral anticoagulant

It is a frequent problem which calls for the necessity to ascertain drugs interaction, diet, as well as insuring the effective taking of the drugs or no laboratory error. In the absence of one of these causes, one can increase the dose up to 3 pills a day under the strict INR surveillance.

2.6 Biological surveillance

The reference for the surveillance of AVK treatment is the "Quick's Test", expressed as a percentage in relation to the normal reading. An international standardisation recommands the usage of INR (International Normalized Ratio) which is a form of "Quick's Test", inespective of the reagents used for its determination.

The activated partial thromboplastin time is a test which does not really take into account the deficit of vitamin-K dependent factors. Therefore this test is of little interest of the AVK's treatment apart from in 2 situations [12]:

- in the event of a relay from the heparins therapy
- the significant zones of anticoagulation (INR 4-4.5) for which it can provide complementary information about the hemorrhagic risk.

The INR measures recommanded for the prevention of venous thromboembolic accidents, in a high risk situation, or for the treatment of thromboembolic accidents are between 2 and 3.

In practice, during the take over period from the heparin therapy, a INR control and a activated partial thromboplastin time test are necessary every other day, until a therapeutic balance is obtained. The heparin can be stopped when the INR is in the designated therapeutic zone, but both therapies will be linked together for at least 4 days.

2.7 Duration of the AVK's treatment

For Coon [11], a 12th weeks anticoagulant treatment reduces by 2/3 the frequence of the recurrence of venous thrombosis.

In Holmgren [34] opinion, this frequence is at 17 % for the year, irrespective if the AVK treatment has lasted one month or six months. On the contrary, in the Hull findings [35, 36], the incidence of recurrence after 12 weeks of treatment was held a 5 %.

This underlines that the risk of recurrence and consequently the duration of the treatment must be based on the etiology of the thrombosis. Sural thrombosis, which is a complication of plaster immobilisation, will be treated for 3 months. A thrombosis linked to an antithrombin III deficit may necessitate an indefinate treatment.

2.8 Hemorrhagic complications during AVK treatment

- in the event of a minor accident (gingivorrhagia), one should stop treatment for 24 hours, then recommence it with weak doses. This procedure is in general sufficient.

- in the event of more serious signs of hemorrhage

  * slow intra-venous injection of K1 vitamin, without exceeding 5 to 10 mg, corrects the hemorrhagic tendance in 6 to 8 hours but might induce an ulterior resistance against AVK.

  * an intra-venous injection of PPSB (dose=20 units of IX factor/kg) allows the "Quick's Test" to go up by about 30 %.

Surgical intervention is in principle possible, without significant hemorrhagic risk, when the INR has gone down to under 2.

3. Deep venous thrombosis and pregnancy

The indication of an anticoagulant treatment during pregnancy is always aired at the mother, be it for the prevent of a DVT or a curative treatment of DVT linked or not to a pulmonary emboly.

The hemorrhagic risk among pregnant woman is equivalent to that of an adult in general, but the main problem is that of the mother-child relationship.

The essential therapeutic principles in this situation can be brought to light thanks to the 186 publications about 1325 pregnancies which put forward the incidences of an anticoagulant treatment on the fetus or newly born infant [20].

3.1 AVK

They are not recommanded because of their teratogenic effect: nasal hypoplasia, punctuated epiphysis, asplenia syndrom, central nervous system anomalies, hydrocephaly, microcephaly, optical atrophia

Between the 6th and the 12th week of pregnancy, the AVK are responsible for 28.6 % of embryofetopathy [33].

Fetal or natal mortality is 16,8 % for Ginsberg [22].

On the other hand, AVK are not a contra-indication when breast feeding [50].

3.2 Heparins

UFH and LMWH do not reach the placenta barrier. No teratogenic effect is reported, but the problem posed by long term treatment is that of the risk of thrombocytopenia.

Peri natal mortality is 6 times lower with UFH and LMWH than with AVK's treatment [22].

UFH and LMWH are not released in the milk.

The risk of recurrence of a thromboembolic accident among pregnant women who have already had a DVT during a previous pregnancy is from 4 to 12 % [20].

In this case, the preventive treatment by heparin is possible during the last trimester of pregnancy or during the entire pregnancy when there is certain deficits (C or S protein). LMWH promised in these situations the comfort of a superior usage to that of UFH.

For compounded DVT, a 7 days heparin treatment using venous injects is usual, followed by the taking over by LMWH until labour.

4. Conclusion

The anticoagulant treatment of thromboembolic disease has undergone these last years many significant modifications, the main one of which is the introduction of Low molecular Weight Molecule Heparin which tends to replace the unfractionated heparin in the prophylactic treatment of phlebitis, and more recently, in the curative treatment.

Their effectiveness in all these areas seems to be at least the same to that of the UFH, but the case of using then is much greater for the patient as for the prescribing physician, because of the excellent bioavability.

However, the problems induced by such treatments are not completely resolved and a biological test remains to be created which would reflet simultaneously the antithrombotic activity and the hemorrhagic risk of LMWH.

At last, for long term anticoagulant treatment, the AVK, administered orally remains the essential part of the therapy, but their posologies tend to be reduced thanks to the use of the INR for regular biological controls. The effectiveness of the low doses of oral anticoagulants, as demonstrated by recent studies, deserves however to be confirmed by more significant and more numerous studies.

REFERENCES

1. AIACH M, BONEU B, POTRON G. Utilisation des héparines en pratique médicale courante. STV n° spécial 4-10, 1991.

2. ALBADA J, NIEUWENHUIS HK, SIXMA JJ. Treatment of acute venous thromboembolism with low molecular weight heparin (Fragmin). Results of a double kind randomized study. Circulation 80, 935-940, 1989.

3. BAIRD RA, CONVERY FR. Arterial thromboembolism in patients receiving systemic heparin therapy. A complication associated with heparin induced thrombocytopenia. J Bone Joint Surg 59A, 1061-1068, 1977.

4. BASU D, GALLUS A, HIRSH J, CADE J. A prospective study of the value of monitoring heparin treatment with the activated partial thromboplastin time. N Engl J Med 17, 324-327, 1972.

5. BELL WR, TONASULO PA, ALVING BM, DUFFY TP. Thrombocytopenia occuring during the administration of heparin. A prospective study in 52 patients. Ann Int Med 85, 155-160, 1976.

6. BONEU B, GOUDABLE C, ROSTIN M, BAYROU B, D'AZEMAR P, HOUIN G. Pharmacokinetics of CY

216 (Fraxiparine*) after bolus intravenous injection to patients affected with chronic renal insufficiency of increasing severity. Thromb Heamost 62, 524 (Abstr.), 1989.

7. BONEU B. Heparines de bas poids moléculaire: polémiques autour du standard international. STV 2, 233-235, 1990.

8. BRATT G, TORNEBOHME E, GRANQUIST J, ABERG W, LOCKNER D. A comparison between low molecular weight heparin (Kabi 2165) and standard heparin in the treatment of deep vein thrombosis. Thromb Haemost 54, 813-817, 1985.

9. CARPINI JA, VAGHER JP, RABIDI SI, MITCHELL JE. Laboratory monitoring of continuous intravenous heparin therapy. Thromb Res 29, 91-94, 1983.

10. COLLINS R, SCRIMGEOUR A, YUSUF S, PETO R. Reduction in fatal pulmonary embolism and venous thrombosis by peri-operative administration of subcutaneous heparin. N Engl J Med 318, 1162-1173, 1988.

11. COON WW, WILLIS PW. Recurrence of venous thromboembolism. Surgery 73, 823-827, 1973.

12. DERLON A, FIESSINGER JN. Utilisation des antivitamines K en pratique médicale courante. STV n° spécial 11-15, 1991.

13. DOUTREMEPUICH C, FERNANDEZG, PEREIRA F, de SEZE O, DOUTREMEPUICH F. Les héparines de bas poids moléculaire en réanimation post-chirurgicale. Ann Biol Clin 46, 190-194, 1988.

14. DOYLE DJ, TURPIE AGG, HIRSH J. Ajusted subcutaneous heparin or continuous intravenous heparin in patients with acute vein thrombosis. Ann Intern Med 107, 441-445, 1987.

15. DROUET L, SCROBOHACI ML. La logique derrière la prescription d'AVK à faible dose. STV 5(1) 313-316, 1989.

16. DUROUX P. Treatment of proximal deep vein thrombosis of the lower limb by CY 216 versus unfractionated heparin. Thromb Heamost 58, 122 (Abstr.), 1987.

17. DUROUX P et al. Traitement curatif des thromboses veineuses profondes : Fraxiparine * versus héparine non fractionnée. Premier symposium international. Paris. Cité des Sciences 20, 1987.

18. EIKA C, GODAL HC, LAAKE K, HAMBORG T. Low incidence of thrombocytopenia during treatment with hog mucosal end beef lung heparin. Scand J Haematol 25, 19-24, 1980.

19. Etude multicentrique française. Traitement des thromboses veineuses profondes constituées. Etude comparative d'un fragment d'héparine de bas poids moléculaire (Fragmine) administré par voie sous-cutanée, et de l'héparine standard administrée par voie intraveineuse continue. Rev Med Int 10, 375-381, 1989.

20. FORESTIER F. Anticoagulants, femme et enfant. STV 2, 119-120, 1990.

21. GALLUS A, TILLETT J, JACKAMAN J, MILLS W, WYCHERLEY A. Safety and efficacy of warfarin started early after submassive venous thrombosis or pulmonary embolism. Lancet 11, 1293-1296, 1986.

22. GINSBERG JS, HIRSH J. Use of anticoagulants during pregnancy. Chest 95, 156-160, 1989.

23. GUISEPPE G, NENCI and GIANCARLO AGNELLI. Clinical experience with low molecular weight heparins. Thromb Res (Suppl.) XI, 69-87, 1990.

24. GRUEL Y. Les thrombopénies induites par l'héparine. Notions actuelles. STV 1, 233-236, 1989.

25. HALL JAG, PAUL RM, WILSON KM. Maternal and fetal sequelae of anticoagulation during pregnancy. Ann J Med 68, 122-140, 1980.

26. HARENBERG J, HUCK K, BRATSCH H, STEHLE G, DEMPFLE CE, MALL K, BLAUTH M, USADEL KH, HEENE DL. Therapeutic application of subcutaneous low molecular weight heparin in acute venous thrombosis. Haemostasis (Suppl.) 20, 205-219, 1990.

27. HEMKER HC, FRANCK HLL. The mechanism of action of oral anticoagulants and its consequences for the practise of oral anticoagulation. Haemostasis 15, 203-270, 1985.

28. HIRSH J, POLLER L, DEYKIN D, LEVINE M, DALEN JE. Optimal therapeutic range of oral anticoagulants. Chest 95, 55s-115s, 1989.

29. HIRSH J. Anticoagulant therapy in venous thromboembolism. BAILLIERE's Clinical Haematology 3, 685-692, 1990.

30. HIRSH J. From unfractionated heparins to low molecular weight heparins. Acta Chir Scand (Suppl.) 556, 42-50, 1990.

31. HOLM HA. Amidolytic heparin assay and correlation to clinical effects in heparin treatment of deep venous thrombosis. Acta Chir Scand (Suppl.) 509, 115-116, 1982.

32. HOLM HA, ABILDGAARD W, KALVENES S. The antithrombotic effect of heparin in deep venous thrombosis relation to four heparin assay. Acta Med Scand 216, 287-293, 1984.

33. HOLM HA, ABILDGAARD W, KALVENES S. Heparin assays and bleeding complications in

treatment of deep venous thrombosis with particular references to retroperitoneal bleeding. Thromb Haemost 53, 278-281, 1985.

34. HOLMGREN K, ANDERSSON G, FAGRELL B, JOHNSSON H, LJUNGBERG B, NILSSON E, WILHELMSSON S, ZETTERQUIST S. One month versus six-months therapy with oral anticoagulants after symptomatic deep vein thrombosis. Acta Med Scand 218, 279-284, 1985.

35. HULL R, DELMORE T, GENTON E. Warfarin sodium versus low dose heparin in the long-term treatment of venous thrombosis. N Engl J Med 301, 855-858, 1979.

36. HULL R, HIRSH J, JAY R. Different intensities of oral anticoagulant therapy in the treatment of proximal vein thrombosis. N Engl J Med 307, 1676-1681, 1982.

37. HULL RD, RASKOB GE, HIRSH J. Continuous intravenous heparin compared with intermittent subcutaneous heparin in the initial treatment of proximal vein thrombosis. N Engl J Med 315, 1109-1114, 1986.

38. HULL RD, RASKOB GE, ROSENBLOOM D. Heparin for 5 days as compared with 10 days in the initial treatment of proximal venous thrombosis. N Engl J Med 322, 1260-1264, 1990.

39. ITURBE-ALESSIO I, del CARMEN FONSECA M, MUTCHINIK O et al. Risks of anticoagulant therapy in pregnant women with artificial heart valves. N Engl J Med 315, 1390-1393, 1986.

40. KAKKAR V. Prevention of venous thrombosis and pulmonary embolism. Am J Cardiol 65, 50c-54c, 1990.

41. KAPSCH DN, SILVER D. Heparin induced thrombocitopenia with thrombosis and hemorrhage. Arch Surg 116, 1423-1427, 1981.

42. KHER A, BARA L, SAMAMA M. Les héparines de bas poids moléculaire. Path Biol 34(1), 61-69, 1986.

43. KITZIS M, HUISSE MG, HANNOUN L, COUFFINHAL KC, PARMENTIER G, ANDREASSIAN B. La thrombopénie induite par l'héparine. A propos de 6 cas et de leurs complications vasculaires. J Mal Vasc 5, 277-280, 1980.

44. KLEIN HG, BELL WR. Dessiminated intravascular coagulation during heparin therapy. Ann Int Med 80, 477-481, 1974.

45. LAGERSTEDT C, FAGHER BO, OLSSON CG, OQVIST BW, ALBRECHTSSON W. Need for long-term anticoagulant treatment in symptomatic calf-vein thrombosis. Lancet II, 515-518, 1985.

46. LEROY J, LECLERC MH, DELAHOUSSE B, GUEROIS C, FOLOPPE P, GRUEL Y, TOULEMONDE F. Treatment of heparin associated thrombo- cytopenia and thrombosis with low molecular weight heparin (CY 216). Semin Thromb Haemostas 11(3), 326-329, 1985.

47. LOWENSTEIN E, JOHNSTON WE, LAPPAS DG, D'AMBRA MN, SCHNEIDER RC, DAGGETT WM, AKINS CW, PHILBIN DM. Catastrophic pulmonary vasoconstriction associated with protamine reversal of heparin. Anesthesiology 59, 470-473, 1983.

48. LOWENSTEIN E, LYNCH K, ROBINSON DR, FITZGIBON CM, ZAPOL WM. Incidence, severity and causation of cardiomulmonary response to protamine reversal of heparin anticoagulation in man. Am Rev Resp Dis 137, 245 (Abstr), 1988.

49. MONTALESCOT G. Reactions gravissimes après neutralisation de l'héparine par la protamine. STV 1, 101-105, 1989.

50. ORME LE, LEWIS M, DE SWIET M et al. May mothers given warfarin breast-feed their infant? Brit Med J 1, 1564-1565, 1977.

51. SAMAMA MM, BARA L, CHAPPEY O. Les héparines de bas poids moléculaire. STV 1, 107-117, 1989.

52. SAMAMA MM, KHER A. Le traitement des thromboses veineuses profondes constituées par les héparines de bas poids moléculaire. STV 1, 353-357, 1989.

53. TOBELEM G. Les nouvelles normes d'expression de surveillance des traitements anti-vitamine K. STV 1, 59, 1989.

54. TOWNE JB, BERNHARD VM, HUSSEY C, GARANCIS JC. White clot syndrom: peripheral vascular complications of heparin therapy. Arch Surg 114, 372-377, 1973.

55. VITOUX JF, AIACH M, RONCATO M, FIESSINGER JN. Should thromboprophylactic dosage of low molecular weight heparin be adapted to patient's weight. Thromb Haemost 59, 120, 1988.

19

Antithrombotic post-operative treatment in recontructive arterial surgery

J.C. Baste - D. Midy

Conserving permeability of the different procedures in reconstructive arterial surgery is the main aim of the vascular surgeon. Yet in spite of care taken during these different procedures, thromboendarteriectomy, venous graft and synthetic or biosynthetic prosthesis have a rate of failure which is certainly variable but which may irreversibly compromise the clinical result. For example, although permeability five years later of an aortobifemoral prosthesis is about 85 % in the literature, the distal femoropopliteal synthetic prosthesis is only 12 % after four years in the multicentric study reported by VEITH [26].

Understanding the causes of these failures and the suitable preventive therapeutic answers are necessary areas of research for the surgeon. Therefore, anticoagulant long-term treatment was proposed and more recently antiaggregant treatment, of which the former was largely empirical.

The results of these various propositions and therapeutic practices must be appreciated both on a strictly surgical basis in terms of maintaining permeability and in widening the point of view, ie examining the consequences on prognosis in other locations in atherosclerosis, since it is so widespread, in particularly in coronary and cerebral areas.

1. Facts of the problem

Failure factors in reconstructive vascular surgery have been studied for a long time, but the intimate mechanism of a few still remain unknown. Analysis of these failures can be made in a chronologically as proposed Bergqvist [2] and Rutherford [21]. Their classification is certainly arbitrary but allows logical reflection as regards the use of antithrombotic medicine. Thus the following are envisaged:

- early failures during the first week after restoration,
- secondary failures during the two years after restoration,
- subsequent failures (after two years).

1.1 Early Failures

These can be either a technical or an indicational error: poor appreciation of haemodynamic level conditions regarding both the upstream and downstream vascular bed levels. However the following may also be involved:

- thrombogenecity of the prothesis: Found when establishing of a synthetic prosthesis, this is also noted in the thromboendarteriectomied zones. An increase in the aggregation of platelets and activation of the humoral factors of coagulation (VIII) and a decrease in antithrombinic activity have been demonstrated in vivo [11].

- Rheologic modification: Blood fibrinogen rates after vascular surgery increase during the early post-operative period. These higher levels persist for about one week and are the origin of blood hyperviscosity. This can be noted as an increase in the fibrin degradation products persisting for several months after intervention.

- Central haemodynamic factors leading to low cardiac flow: All of these factors justify the numerous efforts to limit the thrombogenicity of the prothesis: impregnation of the prosthetic surface with heparin, attempt at endothelialisation, research for new components and the use of heparin during the operation and the early post-operative period.

1.2 Secondary failures (during the two years after restoration)

Secondary failures are the consequences above all of fibro-intimal hyperplasia (FIH). This complex process essentially concerns the anastomotic zones, in particular the distal ones, reduces the diameter of anastomosis and induces upstream thrombosis by stasis.

This FIH explains the difference in permeability between supra-inguinal restorations with a high flow performed with a large caliber prosthesis (from 8 to 10 mm and above) and infra-inguinal restorations with lower flow performed with a reduced caliber prosthesis (from 5 to 6 mm). It occurs both with synthetic prosthesis and with vein by-pass or thromboendarteriectomy zones. In carotid thromboendarteriectomies, the rate of asymptomatic recurrence of stenosis is from about 7 to 25 % in the two years following operation [8]. FIH interferes also in the mid-term results of endoluminal angioplasties and represents the main secondary complication. Thus,

Levine [17] in 1985 underlined that in his experience fibro-intimal hyperplasia was responsible partially or completely for 42 % of all failures in "in situ" vein by-pass and for 62 % of those occurring in the first two years.

The different pathogenic hypothesis involve mediators such as the proliferating factor of platelet origin (PDGF) that interferes in the proliferation of smooth muscle cells of the vascular wall. It is the essential element of fibro-intimal hyperplasia [4].

Although the intimate mechanism of this fibro-intimal hyperplasia is not yet well known, the above facts do nevertheless justify the start of platelet antiaggregant treatment. Others factors of arterial restoration failures also intervene during this interval: persistence of increased thrombogenicity in the prosthesis, structural alteration of a vein graft, trauma on removal or during the valvular destruction in the "in situ" vein by-pass.

Moreover, persistence of prosthetic thrombogenicity is the main justification for anticoagulant treatment during this progressive phase.

1.3 Subsequent failures

These are also plurifactorial and concern the structural alteration of the prosthesis, anastomotic FIH and progression of atherosclerotic lesions on the upstream and downstream vascular bed. During this phase antithrombotic treatments seem to have only a minor value compared with monitoring of the risk of atherosclerotic progression.

However whatever analysis is made of the thrombotic causes of arterial restorations, it is to be noted that the most occur during the year following restoration both in supra- and sub-inguinal surgery.

2. Therapeutic answers

Various answers have been proposed as a response to these failures:

2.1 Technical improvement of removal and preservation conditions in vein grafts; search for less thrombogenic synthetic prosthesis.

2.2 Pharmacological

In particular long-term anticoagulant and antiaggregant treatments.

These drugs differ not only in their modes of action and effectiveness but also in their modes of administration, cost, and secondary effects.

2.2.1 Dextran 40

Dextran 40 has been proposed during and immediately after operation [3]. The haemodilution and increase in plasmatic volume resulting from its activity causes blood viscosity to decrease. It might also reduce platelet adhesivity.

Rutherford [22], in a randomised multicentric study, reports a decrease in thrombosis rate during the first week with distal prosthetic by-pass (6.3 % versus 22 %) using posologies of Dextran 40 at 10 % from 500 ml to 750 ml per hour. Filling was poorly tolerated by unstable cardiac or renal insufficiency patients. This limited its use so much that prosthetic thrombosis occured after one month with no difference in permeability being found in the groups with and without Dextran.

Nevertheless, the rheologic consequences of haemodilution obtained by Dextran 40 could depend on its concentration. Recent work by G. Janvier (not yet published) using Dextran 40 at 3 % seems to demonstrate a stronger action on platelet and corpuscular aggregability with this concentration.

2.2.2 Anticoagulants

Standard heparin, either as sodium heparinate by venous patchway or as calcium heparinate by subcutaneous patchway is widely used during the intervention with variable posologies (average 10 U.I./kg), and during the immediate period after, to treat hypercoagulation, prosthetic thrombogenicity and to combat low flow consequences of clamping. Its prolonged use is limited owing to its necessary parenteral administration and haemorrhagic risk.

Low weight molecular heparins (fragmented heparins) have not often been used in repairing arterial surgery, so cannot be appreciated in this indication. However one should not here the experimental studies in long-term administration of heparin not to use its global anticoagulant action, but, rather its antiproliferative action described about ten years ago on growing smooth muscle cells of the vascular wall, an action which would conserve the fractions of the polysaccharidic complex.

2.2.3 Antivitamins K

These interfere with vitamin K in the synthesis of coagulation factors II, VII, IX, X. Long-term anticoagulant treatment aims at depressing these factors and obtaining global hypocoagulation appreciated by INR. Therefore this represents primary answer for thrombosis in arterial restoration. The use of antivitamins K needs regular and tight surveillance to limit therapeutic accidents (particularly hematoma) in the long-term.

2.2.4 Platelet antiaggregant treatment [20]

These are heterogeneous owing to the diversity of action and posologies used in the various clinical reports.

Their aim is to limit platelet aggregation on the thrombogenic interfaces, prosthesis or thromboendarteriectomy zones/blood, but also to limit the secretion of PDGF by the aggregated platelets, therefore leading to FIH.

2.2.4.1 Acetylsalicylic acid (aspirin)

Used in doses varying from 300 to 1 500 mg per day, this irreversibly inhibits cyclooxygenase and therefore the formation of thromboxane A_2, a platelet aggregant and vaso-constricting agent.

Initially used in high doses, aspirin posologies were progressively reduced:

- for theoretical reasons: high doses inhibit not only platelet cyclooxygenase but also cyclooyigenase of endothelial cells which secrets vasodilative prostacyclin;

- for clinical reasons: on the one hand the complications observed, in particular forms of digestive haemorrhage are dose-dependent [12]; on the other, clinical studies on the prevention of recurrence of cerebral ischaemic accidents due to atherosclerosis report no difference between high and low posologies of 1 000 mg and 300 mg per day, respectively [25].

2.2.4.2 Dipyridamole

With posologies varying from 150 to 400 mg a day this inhibits platelet phospho- diesterase and increases the plasmatic adenosine rate by blocking inhibition by blood cells, adenosine being a vasodilatator and platelet antiaggregant. Mainly used after aorto-coronary vein by-pass, most are often associated with aspirin.

2.2.4.3 Ticlopidine

Used at a posology from 250 mg to 500 mg a day, this significantly inhibits platelet aggregation induced by ADP from 24 to 48 hours after the beginning of the treatment, and persisting 4 to 8 days after the end. This inhibition leads to longer bleeding time. Ticlopidine may cause secondary effects: minor digestive problems, nausea, diarrhea, but these do not require the treatment to be stopped. Exceptional but severe can haematologic complications may occur: neutropenia may even become agranulocytosis, thrombopenia or even medullary, aplasia occuring in the 3 months following the beginning of treatment. Haematologic surveillance is therefore necessarly.

Other antiaggregants can be used: Sulfinpyrazone, Ibuprofen, from time to time.

3. Clinical facts

Appreciating the results of anticoagulant or platelet antiaggregant treatment must be performed in comparison with the natural course, without any adjuvant treatment for arterial restoration.

Therefore, it is particularly in sub-inguinal restoration that one may best appreciate the effects which are eventually favorable for maintaining permeability.

In the literature, the results appear contradictory, with studies often being performed in comparison with historic series which are difficult to interpret.

3.1 Results of long-term anticoagulant treatments

These seem to improve the permeability of femoro-popliteal vein by-pass with a poor vascular bed. In a prospective study by Kretschner [15] on 88 patients randomised into two groups regarding the risk factors, the permeability rate at thirty months of the group with antivitamin K was improved in comparison with the control group, but only in clinical sub-groups III and IV and not in less advanced clinical stages II. However, the same team studying retrospectively the influence of antivitamin K treatment on whole vein by-pass performed from 1970 to 1985 (including the prospective study) did not find any significant improvement in permeability even in the stages III and IV.

Long-term anticoagulant treatments with antivitamin K also improved the permeability of sub-inguinal prosthetic by-pass; the study of Baxter [1], reported in 1990 at the Vascular Surgery Congress in Los Angeles supports this and complements that Flinn [9] in 1988. Both find an increased permeability calculated with the Kaplan Meier method of 58 % at 2 years and 47 % at 4 years, compared to historic studies [26] with antivitamin K (Warfarine). The permeability rate was significantly increased ($p<0.026$).

3.2 Long-term platelet antiaggregant treatments

Results of these studies are difficult to assess owing to the heterogeneity of protocols used. One point seems certain: the inefficiency of Sulfinpyrazone to prevent peripheral arterial restoration obstruction or reobstruction, whatever its nature.

The potential benefit of an association of Aspirin/Dipyridamole at a posology of 600 mg and 300 mg a day respectively has been studied in a prospective study by Clyne [7]; benefit is found only with femoropopliteal prosthetic by-pass at one year follow-up, but not in vein by-pass (table I).

TABLE I

Femoro-popliteal by-pass	Patients	Permeability 1 year follow up	
VEIN			
ASPIRIN + DIPYRIDAMOLE	49	83 %	NS
PLACEBO	44	72 %	
PROSTHESIS			
ASIRIN + DIPYRIDAMOLE	29	85 %	S
PLACEBO	26	53 %	

NS = Not significant
S = Significant, $p<0.01$

This same finding is made in the English multicentric prospective study by Collum [18], in Goldman's 10 and Koller's [14]. No improvement in femoro-popliteal vein by-pass permeability was found by using the association Aspirin/Dipyridamole. Only prosthetic by-pass permeability seemed favorably influenced.

The effectiveness of Ticlopidine in preventing post-operative thrombosis in peripheral arterial surgery has been studied by Shionaya [23], comparing Ticlopidine 300 mg per day versus placebo. In supra-

surgery has been studied by Shionaya [23], comparing Ticlopidine 300 mg per day versus placebo. In supra- or sub-inguinal surgery no difference was found overall, but the analysis of sub-groups does indicate a favorable trend which is just significant for stages III and IV of sub-inguinal surgery and is significant for patients presenting hypercholesterolemia and/or hypertriglyceridemia (100 % of permeability at 3 years against 72.6 %).

As for comparative and respective benefits of these treatments, Aspirin/Dipyridamole and antivitamins K have been studied by Bollinger (6) for 90 patients. There was no significant difference between these drugs.

The side effects of these different antithrombotic therapies cannot be neglected in the perspective of long-term treatment. During prolonged treatment with antivitamins K, 5 of the 42 (12 %) patients in Krestner's study [15] had to interrupt their treatment because of complications: 1 epistaxis, 2 gastro-intestinal tract haemorrhage, 1 cerebral haemorrhage, 1 unspecified complication. In Baxter's study [1] 11 % of haemorrhagic complications (5/47) needed surgical draining for hematoma. Scott underlines that secondary effects in elderly people may counterbalance the eventual favorable effects of antivitamins K.

During platelet antiaggregant treatment the side effects have been well analysed in multicentric studies regarding the prevention of cerebral and myocardic ischaemic accidents i.e:

- European stroke prevention study (Aspirin/Dipyridamole versus placebo) 1987 [24].
- United Kingdom transient ischaemic attack (Aspirin/Dipyridamole versus placebo) 1988 [13].
- Ticlopidine/Aspirin stroke study (TASS) (Ticlopidine) versus Aspirin) 1989 [16].

Gastralgia, nausea, dyspepsia and bleeding are found in about 17 % requiring aspirin treatment to be stopped in the United Kingdom study. Diarrhea, gastralgia and exceptionally neutropenia (< 1 %) required treatment to be stopped in the TASS study in 12 %.

4. Conclusion

Reflection concerning the indications for antithrombotic treatment after reconstructive arterial surgery must take an essential element into account i.e diffusion of the atheromatous process and results obtained in preventing cerebral and myocardic ischaemic attacks with platelet antiaggregants [13, 16, 24]. In Mc Collum's study [18] although no advantage was found for the permeability of vein by-pass by using the association Aspirin/Dipyridamole the same was not true for the occurence of cardiac and neurologic events. The difference during an average follow-up of 34 months was 8.2 % in favour of antiaggregant treatment versus placebo.

Current indications

In peripheral vascular surgery the appropriate antithrombotic treatment must be selected by taking into account:

- the topography of vascular restoration and its specificity
- the quality of the vascular bed
- the first of recurrent restoration type
- the presence or not of ischaemic involvement of the myocardial or cerebral areas.

The following proposals may then be suggested
- during intervention, heparin is suitable before any clamping. In our center sodium, heparin (50 U.I./kg) is infused, excepted in thoracoabdominal reconstructions in which heparin is not indicated
- during the post-operative period heparinization is continued either intravenously or subcutaneously for 7 days in average.

Dextran 40 (500 ml daily for 5 days) is used only in distal prosthetic by-pass.

Afterwards antithrombotic treatment either with antivitamin K or antiaggregant drug is begun as early as the 72nd hour, thus ensuring an overlap between heparin and oral antithrombotic agents.

The choice between antivitamin K and antiaggregant platelet drugs is governed by the following:

- the possible side effects of each treatments according to the clinical profile.
- the possible need for anticoagulant treatment for an associated cardiac pathology.
- the beneficial effect of antiaggregant drugs to prevent ischaemic accident of atherosclerotic disease.

The choice between antiaggregant drugs is to be made by taking into account the side effects and cost of each.

The length of treatment depends on the little improvement expected in the long-term permeabililty rate in aorto-iliac surgery or in venous femoro-popliteal by-pass with a good distal bed. In such procedures antithrombotic treatment is to be reduced to 12 months unless incidents occur since the risk of thrombosis is statistically the highest as is time. Subclavian reconstructions such as carotido-subclavian reimplantation are treated in the same manner.

In other procedures including carotid reconstructive surgery as well as the reconstructions mentionned above, after a previous failure, the antithrombotic treatment is to be indefinitely. Whatever the procedure in the event of an ischaemic occurrence in the myocardial or cerebral areas, it is to be treated in the same manner.

REFERENCES

1. BAXTER BT, BERGMAN RT, Mc CARTHY WJ et al. Prospective accessment of antithrombotic therapy following primary below knee prothetic by pass. American Society of Vascular Surgery, Los Angeles, 1990.

2. BERGQVIST D. Pharmacologic prevention of graft occlusion. Acta Chir Scand (Suppl.) 529, 107-114, 1985.

3. BERGQVIST D, BERGENTZ SE. The role of Dextran in severe ischemie chronic disease and arterial reconstructive surgery. A review. VASA 12, 213, 1983.

4. BIRINYI LK, LOGERFO FW. Intimal hyperplasia: evoluing concepts of pathophysiology and therapy. In: Quality Medical Publishing. Inc. St. Louis Missouri (Ed). Perspective in vascular surgery 2, 97-111, 1989.

5. BLAKELY JA, POGORILER G. A prospective trial of Sulfinpyrazone after peripheral vascular surgery. Thromb Haemost 38, 238, 1977.

6. BOLLINGER A, BRUNNER H. Antiplatelet drugs improve the patency after femoro-popliteal endarterectomy. VASA 12, 172-178, 1983.

7. CLYNE CA, ARCHER TJ, ATUHAIRE LK, CHANT AD, WEBSTER JH. Random control trial of short course Aspirine and Dipyridamole (Persantin) for femoro-distal graft. Br J Surg 74, 246-248, 1987.

8. DE GROOTE RD, LYNCH TG, JAMIL Z, HOBSON RW. Carotid restenosis: long term non invasive follow up after carotid endarteriectomy. Stroke 18, 1031-1036, 1987.

9. FLINN WR, ROHRER MJ, YAO ST. Improved long term patency of infragenicular polytetrafluoroethylene graft. J Vasc Surg 7, 685-690, 1988.

10. GOLDMAN M, Mc COLLUM L. A prospective randomized study to examin the effect of Aspirin and Dipyridamole on the patency of prosthetic femoro-popliteal grafts. Vasc Surg 18, 217-220, 1984.

11. GOLDMAN MD, SIMPSON D, HAWKER RJ, NORCOTT HC, McCOLLUM CN. Aspirin and Dipyridamole reduce platelet deposition on prothetic femoropopliteal grafts in man. Ann Surg 198, 713-716, 1983.

12. GRAHAM DY, SMITH JL. Aspirin and the stomach. Ann Intern Med 104, 390-398, 1986.

13. HASS WK, EASTON JD, ADAMS Jr et al for the ticlopidine aspirine stroke study group. A randomized trial comparing Ticlopidine hydrochloride with Aspirin for the prevention of stroke in high risk patients. N Engl J Med 321, 501- 507, 1989.

14. KOLHER TR, KAUFMAN JL, KACOYANGIS G, CLOWES A, DONALDSON MC, KELLY E, SKILLMAN J, COUCH NP, WHITTEMORE AD, MANNICK JA et al. Effects of Aspirine and Dipyridamole on the patency of lower extremity by pass grafts. Surgery 96, 462-466, 1984.

15. KRETSCHMER G, WENZLE E, PIZA F, POLTERAUER P, EHRINGER H, MINAR E, SCHEMPER M. The influence of anticoagulant treatment as the probability of function in femoropopli-tealvein by pass surgery: analysis of clinical series (1970 to 1985) and interim evaluation of a controlled clinical trial. Surgery 3, 453-459, 1987.

16. LEPANTALO MAURI. Adjuvant medical therapy to improve patency rate following reconstruction

for atherosclerosis obliteration. Acta Chir Scand (suppl). 555, 51-58, 1990.

17. LEVINE AW, BANDYK DF, BONIER PH, TONNE JB. Lesions learned in adopting the in situ saphenous vein by pass. J Vasc Surg 2, 145-153, 1985.

18. McCOLLUM C, ALEXANDER C, KENCHINGTON G, FRANKS PJ, GREENHALGH R. Antiplatelets drugs in femoro-popliteal vein by passes: a multicenter trial. J Vasc Surg 13, 150-161, 1991.

19. McDANIEL MD, PEARCE WH, YAO JS, ROSSI EC, FAHEY VA, GREEN D, FLINN WR, BERGAN JJ. Sequential changes in coagulation and platelet function following tibial by pass. J Vasc Surg 1, 261- 268 1984.

20. Recommandations du groupe d'études sur l'hémostase et la thrombose sur l'utilisation des traitements antithrombotiques en pratique médicale courante. STV: John Libbey (Ed). Paris, numéro spécial, mai 1991

21. RUTHERFORD RB. Role of Antithrombotic drugs in maintening graft patency. In Current therapy in vascular surgery, 2nd edition, Ernst Stanley, BC Decker Inc. 1991.

22. RUTHERFORD RB, JONES DN, BERGENT SE et al. The efficacity of Dextran 40 in preventing early thrombosis following difficult lower extremity by-pass. J Vasc Surg 1, 765-773, 1984.

23. SHIONOYA S, SAKUKAI T. Influence de la Ticlopidine sur les résultats de la chirurgie artérielle périphérique - Etude prospective multicentrique de 3 ans. STV (Suppl) 2(4), 12-16, 1990.

24. The European stroke prevention study - ESPS - Principal end point. Lancet 2, 1351-1354, 1987.

25. U.K.T.I.A. Study group (United Kingdom transcent Ischaemic Attack). Aspirin trials: Interim results. Brit Med J 296, 316-320, 1988.

26. VEITH FJ, GUPTA SK, ASCER E, WHITE-FLORES S, SAMSON RH, SCHER LA, TOWNE JB, BERNHARD VM, BONIER P, FLINN WR et al. Six years prospective multicenter randomized comparaison of autologous saphenous vein and expanded polytetrafluoroethylene graft in infrainguinal reconstructions. J Vasc Surg 3, 104-113, 1986.

20

Anticoagulant therapy and heart valve prosthesis

C. Deville, F. Madonna, S.A.M. Nashef, C. Doutremepuich

The success of current heart valve surgery is largely due to the development of valve prostheses to replace damaged native valves. Since 1960, when Starr performed the first successful mitral valve replacement with a caged ball prostheses [2], some 60 different prosthesis have been developed in 30 years. Most prostheses fall within two broad categories: mechanical (ball, disc or bileaflet valves) and biological (porcine, pericardial and homografts). There is no perfect replacement valve and different complications may develop in patients in whom artificial valves are implanted, regardless of their type. Among the so-called valve-related complications, thrombo-embolic events associated with mechanical valves represent an ever-present risk which requires lifelong meticulous anticoagulation with its attendant risk of anticoagulation-related haemorrhage. Thrombo-embolic complications can present in two ways: either as systemic embolism (cerebral, brachial, femoral) or as thrombosis of the valve itself. The mortality of systemic embolism is in the region of 25%, whereas valve thrombosis leads to sudden catastrophic cardiac failure which is fatal in 80% of cases [1]. The rates of thromboembolic complications and anticoagulant-related haemorrhage in anticoagulated patients with mechanical valves are detailed in tables I and II.

Table I : Thromboembolic complications by valve position in patients with mechanical valves (number of events per 100 patients/years) [1]

Implant site	Systemic embolism (25% fatal)	Valve thrombosis (80% fatal)
Aortic	2	0.75
Mitral	2	2.80

Table II : Anticoagulant-related haemorrhage (number of events per 100 patient/years)

Total	10
Major	2.2
Fatal	0.5

(Major events are defined as those requiring hospitalisation or transfusion.)

1. Indications for anticoagulation

Anticoagulation is recommended for the first three months after valve replacement with a biological valve. Beyond that period, the presence of the valve itself does not require anticoagulation, but there may be other indications in some patients to continue long-term anticoagulation such as atrial fibrillation and preoperative history of thrombo-embolic episodes.

By contrast, anticoagulation must be continued for life after valve replacement with a mechanical valve. This clearly has implications on the choice of prosthesis in individual patients.

2. Monitoring anticoagulant therapy

Except for the immediate postoperative period, anticoagulation is normally achieved using vitamin K antagonists. The level of anticoagulation should be monitored by periodic blood sampling at three-weekly or four-weekly intervals. Adequate anticoagulation is defined as any of the following :

- prothrombin index between 25% and 35% of control
- international normalized ratio (INR) of 3 to 4.5 times control
- thrombotest between 6% and 12%.

Two to four times a year a full coagulation screen is carried out. The activated cephalin clotting time (ACCT) should be 1.5 times control. Finally, yearly blood counts and erythrocyte sedimentation rates are measured.

3. Stopping anticoagulation

In the absence of other indications, anticoagulation may be stopped at three months postoperatively in patients with biological valves. In patients with mechanical valves, however, any interruption of anticoagulation for whatever reason (dental or other surgery, pregnancy) must be performed under strict supervision and a rigourous treatment protocol in order to prevent valve thrombosis. The protocol can be summarised in three important points:

- substitution of intravenous or subcutaneous heparin for vitamin K antagonists during the period in question
- overlap of the two modes of treatment to prevent any rebound hypercoagulation states
- continuation of heparin therapy during the reintroduction of vitamin K antagonists until the latter are again effective.

4. Conclusion

In patients with artificial heart valves careful monitoring of anticoagulation with vitamin K antagonists is essential for an uneventful outcome. This can only be achieved by close cooperation between patient, physician and cardiologist.

REFERENCES

1. KIRKLIN JW, BARRATT-BOYES BG. Acquired valvular heart disease. Wiley Medical New York. Cardiac Surgery III, 323-490, 1986.

2. STARR A, EDWARDS ML. Mitral replacement : clinical experience with a ball-valve prosthesis. Ann Surg 154, 726-740, 1961.

21

Anticoagulation and coronary bypass grafts

X. Roques, S.A.M. Nashef, E. Baudet,

C. Doutremepuich

Early studies have suggested that anticoagulation reduces mortality and myocardial infarction rates after coronary artery bypass surgery. As a result, anticoagulants were routinely used in the past for the purpose of maintaining the patency of aortocoronary bypass grafts. More recent studies, however, have shown that any benefit from such treatment was small and largely outweighed by the risks of universal anticoagulation in these patients. Routine long-term anticoagulation of patients with coronary grafts has therefore fallen out of favour, to be replaced by antiplatelet drugs as soon as the immediate postoperative period has passed. There is, however, still a role for anticoagulation in the peri-operative period and, in selected patients, in the long term.

1. Therapeutic principles

In general, there are two purposes of anticoagulation in patients with coronary grafts: the first is to prevent graft thrombosis and the second is favourably to influence the progression of coronary disease. The most commonly used conduits for coronary grafting are autologous veins (such as the long saphenous) and arteries (such as the internal mammaries). We shall consider these separately.

1.1 Vein conduits

Early thrombosis occurs in 10-20 % of all coronary grafts and its aetiology is multifactorial. Contributing causes include technical anastomotic errors, technical errors in graft lay-out (such as inappropriate length or a tendency to kink) and damage to the endothelium of the conduit by over-distension or surgical manipulation. With accumulating experience in coronary surgery, the occurence of such causative factors is probably minimised and the majority of graft thromboses nowadays may be stagnation due to low flow within the graft leading because of poor "run-off" in the native coronary bed. The quality of "run-off" in coronary vascular beds cannot be readily measured on preoperative arteriograghy. In addition to these physical, flow-related causes of graft thrombosis, there are metabolic and haematological contributory factors such as platelet and coagulation disorders, postoperative inflammatory states and the intravascular presence of suture lines and disrupted endothelial surfaces which may form the initial focus for thrombus formation.

Anticoagulant therapy cannot influence any physical, flow-related causes of thrombosis such as a badly constructed graft, but can reduce the likelihood of thrombosis due to haematological and endothelial disturbances. For this purpose, heparin therapy is ideal in that it possesses both anticoagulant and anti-inflammatory activity, has a rapid action with a relatively short half-life and can be easily monitored, maintained within the desired therapeutic range and readily reversed when necessary. Heparin treatment should be started in the first few hours postoperatively (once the risk of surgical bleeding has receded) and continued for the period of anticipated platelet dysfunction and inflammatory reaction and until the conduits and anastomoses have been endothelialised, usually for three to four weeks.

Late graft thrombosis occurs at an annual rate of 5 % in vein grafts that have remained patent in the postoperative period. A contributing factor to this thrombosis is the development, in the first two years, of intimal hypersplasia in the wall of the vein graft, possibly as a result of subjecting the vein wall to systemic arterial pressure. Intimal hyperplasia begins with sub-adventitial fibrosis which may be due to vein wall ischaemia or trauma secondary to harvesting. This fibrosis reduces the elasticity of the vein and thus renders it more susceptible to the barotrauma of systemic arterial pressure, resulting in reactive intimal hypersplasia, more thickening and loss of elasticity, which establishes a vicious cycle leading either to a stabilised, thick-walled graft or to eventual graft occlusion. Several studies have confirmed that, as would be expected, intimal hyperplasia cannot be prevented by anticoagulation. The other factor in the development of late graft thrombosis is the progressive natural history of atheromatous disease which, in due course, will lead to stenoses in the coronary arterial bed supplied by the graft, thus reducing the "run-off" and risking graft thrombosis from low flow. Anticoagulation has a minimal effect on the progression of atherosclerosis but antiplatelet therapy and attempts to modify other risk factors for coronary disease may play an important role in the prevention of graft thrombosis due to this cause.

1.2 Arterial conduits

Current coronary surgery is relying more on arterial conduits than ever before, and some centers attempt coronary revascularisation by the exclusive use of arterial conduits whenever possible. The most commonly used arterial conduit is the left internal mammary artery which has given long-term patency rates that are distinctly superior to those obtained with saphenous veins: internal mammary patency at ten years of 90 % versus 35 % for veins. The causes of this superiority are not fully understood but may be at least partly related to the absence of intimal hyperplasia and the better caliber concordance between the internal mammary and the coronary arteries. Another factor is the preservation of the physiological ability of the arterial conduit to respond to changes in flow requirements with appropriate vasodilatation and constriction and its proven ability to grow in caliber over the years to provide increased flow if necessary. This has led several institutions to explore the use of other arterial conduits of which the right internal mammary artery, the right gastro-epiploic artery, the radial arteries and the inferior epigastric arteries have all been in clinical use. For all the above reasons, it can be seen that there is little use for long-term anticoagulation in the "protection" of the internal mammary arterial conduit from thrombosis: it is unlikely that any long-term anticoagulation will improve the already excellent patency results of internal mammary artery grafts. Anticoagulation will therefore only serve in the postoperative period to prevent thrombosis which may originate on disrupted endothelium and intravascular suture lines. Further data are needed on the long-term performance of other, non-mammary, arterial conduits before we can be certain that their long-term behaviour and patency rates will match that of the internal mammary artery.

2. Prevention of early graft thrombosis

Three groups of drugs may be used to prevent early thrombosis: heparin and derivatives, vitamin-K antagonists and antiplatelet drugs.

2.1 Heparin is the treatment of choice in the immediate postoperative period because of its dual antithrombotic anti-inflammatory actions and the ease of its therapeutic manipulation. Immediate postoperative treatment may be by continuous intravenous infusion or by four-hourly injections. Where calcium or magnesium heparins are available, intravenous therapy may be replaced by intermittent eight-hourly subcutaneous injections from 48 hours after operation. Treatment should be aimed at obtaining a serum concentration of 0.2 units/ml or (ACT: Activated Cephalin Time) of one and a half times control. The advantage of subcutaneous treatment is the ability to continue therapy after discharge from hospital and thus maintain antithrombotic protection for a whole postoperative month, covering the entire theoretical risk period.

2.2 Vitamin-K antagonists are the alternative to heparin therapy in the early stages: they can be administered from 48 hours postoperatively instead of heparin and

Table I: Randomized comparative studies of early permeability of aorto-coronary bypass by grafts saphenous vein between treated and non-treated patients with anticoagulants.

Authors	Total grafts	Angio control	Rate of permeability AVK control
GOHLKE* [2]	219	2 months	81 % 67 % **
Mc ENANY [4]	64	3 to 24 months	83 % 69 % **

* : Debit<90 ml/mn
** : p<0.02

therapy should be adjusted to maintain a prothrombin time of 25 - 35 % or an international normalised ratio of 2.5 to 3.5 times control. Golke [2] and McEnany [4] have reported 80 % vein graft patency respectively at two months and a mean of 4 months postoperatively using such a treatment regimen (table I).

2.3 Antiplatelets represent an entirely different approach to anticoagulation. Several studies have reported favourable graft patency rates in patients treated with antiplatelets; four of these studies are summarised in table II. Patency rates obtained with antiplatelet drugs has been at least as good as that obtained by anticoagulation with vitamin-K antagonists, but several unresolved controversies remain.

Table II: Randomized comparative studies of early permeability of aorto-coronary by-pass by grafts saphenous vein between treated and non-treated patients with antiaggregants.

Authors	Total grafts	Angio control	Rate of permeability AAG control
MAYER, 1980 ATS	113	3td,4th months	92 % 77 % p<0.02
Mc ENANY 1982 JTCS	106	0-24 months	80 % 69 %
CHESEBRO 1982 N Engl J Med	260	6 months	92 % 63 % p<0.02
GOLDMAN 1988 CIRCUL.	555	2 months	91 - 93 % 84 % p<0.5

Most studies used either low-dose aspirin (320 mg per day) or a combination of aspirin and dipirydamole. Goldman [3] and Sharma [5] found no difference in graft patency between patients receiving aspirin alone and those receiving various aspirin-dipyridamole combinations, but Sharma [5] found no significant difference between patency rates after antiplatelet regimens and placebo, but antiplatelet treatment in that study was not started until three to five days after surgery. Chesebro [1] emphasised the need to start antiplatelet therapy with two days before surgery. Goldman found significantly higher patency rates with antiplatelets only for grafts to small (<2 mm) coronary arteries. The field remains controversial and a definitive study is needed to assess the efficiency of antiplatelets and to determine the optimal time for the commencement and duration of therapy.

3. Prevention of late thrombosis

McEnany [4] found no difference between graft patency rates in patients who received anticoagulants and those who received antiplatelets for three years postoperatively (table III). This, and the higher haemorrhagic risk from anticoagulation with vitamin-K antagonists, leads us to conclude that the prevention of graft thrombosis is not an indication for the maintenance of anticoagulation beyond two months after operation. Thus the only therapy which may be useful at that stage is the administration of antiplatelet drugs. Chesebro [1] has found a higher long-term patency rate with antiplatelet treatment over placebo but this was not confirmed by others [3, 4]. It may be that antiplatelets have little effect beyond the early postoperative month on the patency

Table III: Randomized comparative studies of tardy permeability of aorto-coronary by pass by grafts saphenous vein between treated and non-treated patients with anticoagulants or antiaggregants.

Authors	Total	Delay month	Rate of permeability due to graft		
			AAV (%)	AAG (%)	control (%)
CHESEBRO 1984 N. ENGL. J. MED	407	36	-	89	75 p<0.2
Mc ENANY 1982 JTCS	41	46	73	68	62 NS
SHARMA 1983 CIRCUL	176	12-24	-	83	80 NS
GOLDMAN 1988 CIRCUL.	406	12-18	-	84	78 NS
		ϕ<2mm		80	68 p=0.008

of the graft itself. They may, however, play a role in the prevention of atheromatous progression and its complications, but this role is outside the scope of this chapter.

4. Summary and practical guide

The current state of knowledge does not allow for hard-and-fast rules about the prophylaxis of coronary graft thrombosis using various therapeutic approaches, but what we do know can be summarised in a longitudinal time figure (table IV).

In the first 48 to 72 hours, anticoagulation is maintained by continuous or intermittent intravenous heparin. Thereafter, this treatment may be replaced by intermittent subcutaneous heparin, antiplatelet drugs or both. The former is stopped at 1 month, the latter may be continued for up to six months. Beyond that time limit antiplatelet therapy may be continued if it is seemed necessary for prophylaxis because of the underlying coronary disease, because of particularly severe multivessel disease or to protect small grafts with limited flow. It is unlikely to benefit patients with a single arterial graft and otherwise normal coronary vasculature. For patients between these two extremes, the clinician should exercise individual judgment. It should be remembered that attempts to reduce or remove coronary disease risk factors may be more important for long-term survival than whether antiplatelet therapy is continued or not.

Table IV: Actual therapeutic scheme

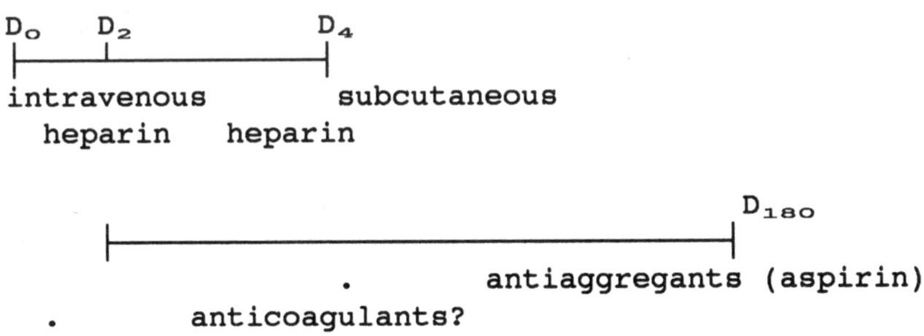

REFERENCES

1. CHESEBRO JH, FUSTER V, ELVEBACK LR, CLEMENTS IP, SMITH HC, HOLMES DR Jr, BARDSLEY WT, PLUTH JR, WALLACE RB, PUGA FJ et al. Effect of dipyridamole and aspirin on late vein graft patency after coronary bypass operations. N Engl J Med 310, 209-214, 1984.

2. GOHLKE H, GOHLKE-BARWOLF G, STURZENHOFECKER P, GORNANDT L, RITTER B, REICHELT M, BUCHWALSKY R, SCHMUZIGER M, ROSKAMM H. Improved graft patency with anticoagulant therapy after aortocoronary bypass surgery: a prospective randomized study. Circulation 64(Suppl II), 22-27, 1981.

3. GOLDMAN S, COPELAND J, MORITZ T, HENDERSON W, ZADINA K, OVITT T, DOHERTY J, READ R, CHESLER E, SAKO Y, LANCASTER L, EMERY R, SHARMA GVRK, JOSA M, PACOLD I, MONTOYA A, PARIKH D, SEHTI G et al. Saphenous vein graft patency 1 year after coronary artery bypass surgery and effects of antiplatelet therapy. Circulation 80, 1190-1197,1989.

4. McENANY MT, SALZMAN EW, MUNDTH ED, DE SANCTIS RW, HARTHORNE JW, WEINTRAUB RM, GATES S, AUSTEN WG. The effect of antithrombotic therapy on patency rates of saphenous vein coronary artery bypass grafts. J Thorac Cardiovasc Surg 83, 81-89, 1982.

5. SHARMA GVRK, KHURI SF, JOSA M, FOLLAND ED, PARISI AF. The effect of antiplatelet therapy on saphenous vein coronary artery bypass graft patency. Circulation 68 (Suppl II), 218, 1983.

22

Anticoagulants and orthopedic surgery

A. Planes, N. Vochelle

In orthopedic surgery the risk of thromboembolic disease has been recognized as high and anticoagulant drugs have been found effective in reducing this risk. Their level of efficacy has been demonstrated only when properly designed, prospective, randomized, controlled trials were performed based on objective criteria assessed by independent observers.

Fatal pulmonary embolism was the first outcome of thromboembolic disease studied [68] It is certainly the most important and relatively easy to assess if a systematic autopsy is performed. It needs to be demonstrated in a large number of patients. For example halving the deaths due to pulmonary embolism from 0.8 % to 0.4 % would require 20,000 patients in each group. [11]. If based on the total mortality (fatal pulmonary embolism + pulmonary embolism contributing to death) 10,000 patients in each group would be necessary for a decrease from 4 % to 3.6 % [11].

Pulmonary embolism (PE) may also form the basis for research. Clinical pulmonary embolism is not in itself a good end point. Signs and symptoms are unreliable and clinical manifestations only the visible tip of the iceberg. Detection of silent pulmonary embolisms, which are the majority, would need a systematic examination of all patients by perfusion ventilation scanning, confirmed, if indicated, by pulmonary angiography.

Deep vein thrombosis (DVT) of the lower limbs may preferably be considered as a useful, simplified marker of the disease [1]. In orthopedic surgery, only deep vein thrombosis demonstrated by a systematic bilateral venographic examination between day 10 and 14 post operatively should be considered. [13, 36, 67, 81]. Because of a substantially high incidence of DVT, prophylactic treatments can be evaluated in smaller trials. For example, a reduction from 20 % to 10 % of DVT would require only 500 patients in each group. The effectiveness of this approach is based on the assumption that a reduction in DVT is followed by a reduction in pulmonary embolism (but the relationship is not necessarily a linear one).

1. What is the level of risk in various groups of orthopedic patients?

1.1 Elective hip replacement

A natural venographic pattern of DVT after total hip replacement has been defined in a number of control studies [19, 32, 35, 39, 45, 60]. For 908 patients, 459 DVT were observed (50.5 %) - 95 % confidence interval 47.2 % - 53.7 %. Of these DVT, 222 were proximal (24.4 %), - 95 % confidence interval 22.7 % - 28.4 % [65]. Incidence is the same in trials reported from Europe and North America. Proximal DVT were reported to be responsible for about 75 % of the cases of fatal pulmonary embolism in the autopsy study of Havig [33].

The natural history of pulmonary embolism (PE) is still unknown. No large study has screened the patients of the placebo group by mandatory scintigraphic ventilation and perfusion scans confirmed by a pulmonary angiographic assessment. The observed rates of fatal PE varied between 1.4 % [40] and 3.4 % [12]. Recently, in patients protected by standard heparin, Eriksson et al [17] found a true incidence of PE of 30.6 % and of 12.3 % in patients receiving a low molecular weight heparin.

It also seems that the risk of DVT persists for several weeks after surgery [40].

1.2 Acute hip surgery

There is no reason to think that the patient received and treated soon after fracture of the hip is at higher risk of DVT than after elective hip arthroplasty. Often, though, the patient is seen several hours after the fracture. In studies on patients without prophylaxis the pre operative prevalence of phlebographic DVT was about 12 to 15 %, depending on the time elapsed since the injury [23, 70]. In a more recent study the preoperative frequency of phlebographic DVT was 9 % [66]. In all of these studies most of the thrombi were proximal.

1.3 Knee surgery

A number of studies in which patients received a mandatory venographic examination have been performed [29, 52, 54, 69, 72]. All the results of these studies are consistent and show a higher risk of total DVT than after hip surgery. The best trial designed to define the case history after knee surgery is that of Stringer et al [71].

312 consecutive patients without prophylaxis, received a systematic ipsilateral venography 7 to 10 days post operatively, with the following results:

- Total knee arthroplasty	Total DVT : 60 % Proximal DVT : 9.1 % Symptomatic PE : 1.8 %
- Arthrodesis of the knee	Total DVT : 99 % Proximal DVT : 33 % Symptomatic PE : 16.7 %
- Arthrotomy	Total DVT : 25 % Proximal DVT : 2 %
- Open menisectomy	Total DVT : 25 % Proximal DVT : 2 %
- Synovectomy	Total DVT : 50 % Proximal DVT : 0 %
- Patellectomy	Total DVT : 50 % Proximal DVT : 0 %

1.4 Traumatology

The study by Geerts et al [26] is of particular interest. 395 consecutive trauma patients received a bilateral venographic assessment at day 21 or prior in cases of earlier discharge from hospital or if clinical or impedance plethysmographic signs and symptoms of DVT or PE occurred. They observed an overall incidence of DVT of 47 %, 12 % being proximal.

Prevalence was high in all the localisations of trauma.

- Face - chest- abdomen	40 %
- Head injury	47 %
- Spinal cord injury	60 %
- Lower limb injury	
- pelvis	44 %
- acetabulum	49 %
- femur	66 %
- tibia	61 %

1.5 Lower limb and plaster cast

Kujath et al [44] compared a low molecular weight heparin versus placebo in 200 consecutive patients. The diagnostic of DVT was suboptimal. They used real time ultrasonography confirmed by venography when positive. In the placebo group they observed a 12.1 % prevalence of DVT in ligamental ruptures and 26.5% in fractures. This study is probably an underestimation of the true prevalence of the disease.

1.6 Conclusion

The natural prevalence of DVT in orthopedic surgery is high and all patients must be protected.

2. What is the role of oral anticoagulants (vitamin K antagonists) in this context?

The first demonstration of their efficacy was given by Sevitt and Gallagher [68]. They performed the first prospective, randomized, controlled trial in orthopedic surgery. Since then, intensive research has been performed. The findings are as follows:

2.1 Oral anticoagulants were found effective when the dosage was adjusted.

Sevitt and Gallagher [68] used warfarin post operatively and observed that protected patients with fractured neck of the femur developed significantly less clinical DVT, clinical or fatal PE, than unprotected patients.

Conventry et al [12] used warfarin and observed that when begun post operatively on 2,012 consecutive total hip replacements, a reduction from 3.4 % to 0.05 % in fatal PE was obtained. (According to our preliminary definition the sample is too small to be demonstrative, but the trend is impressive).

A number of authors used warfarin begun the night before surgery. Amstutz et al [3] observed a rate of clinical PE of 0.5 % on 3000 total hip replacements. Using mandatory venographies, Harris et al [31] observed a rate of 19.5 % of total DVT for 55 patients, Paiement et al [63], a rate of 16.6 % of total DVT for 72 patients and Bailey et al [4], a rate of 26.6 % of total DVT for 45 patients.

Francis et al [22] described the two step warfarin therapy begun 10 to 14 days pre operatively. They adjusted a low pre operative dosage which was increased post operatively. Using mandatory venographic examination, they observed an incidence of 21 % of total DVT for 53 patients.

2.2 Fixed mini-doses of oral anticoagulants were found ineffective by Fordyce et al [21].

148 patients received a fixed dose of 1 mg of warfarin or a placebo daily for one week before and three weeks after surgery. DVT diagnosed by the fibrinogen uptake test occurred in 34 % of the patients given warfarin and 26 % of the controls (NS).

3. What is the role of unfractionated standard heparin?

Standard heparin has been used alone, or in combination with dihydroergotamine, or when dosages were adjusted.

3.1 Fixed doses of unfractionated heparin have been widely used, with contradictory results [2, 7, 15, 25, 30, 53, 55, 59, 60, 78-80].

The diagnostic of DVT in these trials was suboptimal. Patients were screened by a fibrinogen-uptake test which if positive was confirmed by a venography. The results were pooled and a meta analysis realized by Collins et al [11]. He showed that a reduction in the incidence of DVT was observed in elective hip surgery. ($p<0.0001$) and traumatic orthopedic surgery ($p<0.001$). Although the focus in orthopedic trials was restricted to proximal thrombi for which confirmation venographies were available, the overall totals were still 32 patients assigned to the heparin group and 63 control patients ($p<0.001$).

The duration of treatment was similar in all trials - 7 to 10 days or until the patient was ambulatory - and the frequency of subcutaneous injections was always either every 8 or every 12 hours. There was no apparent difference in the efficiency of different regiments in the orthopedic surgery trials. The Collins's meta analysis also showed a significant reduction in fatal pulmonary embolism and in total mortality. There was clear and consistent evidence of an increased risk of bleeding after subcutaneous administration of heparin, but even if "excessive bleeding" or "need of transfusion" appeared to be increased by about one half to two thirds, the absolute excess was small (about 2 per cent).

Subsequently three studies were performed where the patients were protected by subcutaneous fixed doses of standard heparin and received a mandatory venographic assessment [17, 48, 64]. For 465 patients, 26 % of DVT (95 % confidence interval 22 % - 30 %) was observed. Among them, proximal DVT was defined for 387 patients, the observed incidence being 18.3 % (95 % confidence interval 14.4 % - 22.11 %) [65].

3.2 The association with dihydroegotamine 5000 IU of standard heparin with 0.5 mg of dihydroergotamine mesylate administered three times daily has been demonstrated to be more effective in a number of trials which were performed with or without a control group [6, 18, 24, 42, 45, 50]. Considered together, these studies show that for 925 patients an incidence of 17.3 % of total DVT was observed (95 % confidence interval 14.8 %-19.7 %). Proximal DVT was described in 104 patients with an incidence of 11.2 % (95 % confidence interval 9.2 % - 13.2 %). Dihydroergotamine does possibly afford a better protection against proximal DVT [65].

3.3 Adjusted doses of standard heparin to the APTT have been used in a number of trials. [5, 15, 49-51]. Considered together, 370 patients were studied in these trials with an incidence of total DVT of 17.0 % (confidence interval 9.7 % - 16.6 %). Adjusted doses were more effective in reducing the rates of total and proximal DVT than fixed doses of unfractionated heparin. But frequent adjustment of the heparin dose is very labour intensive and is not precisely defined at that time.

4. What is the role of low-molecular-weight heparins (LMWH) and heparinoïd?

These new drugs have been intensively investigated because they exhibit a number of potential advantages over standard unfractionated heparin. These advantages include after subcutaneous administration, an almost complete bioavailability, a prolonged half-life in the circulation which makes a single daily injection sufficient and also, experimentally, an increased safety margin between hemorrhagic and antithrombotic doses [20, 37, 61, 62, 74].

4.1 In elective hip surgery

4.1.1 Low molecular weight heparins have been assessed versus placebo. Five studies have been performed [36, 45, 46, 75, 76]. In all these studies a high efficiency was observed. When based on trials by Turpie et al [76] and Hoek et al [36] where mandatory venographic examinations were performed, the metaanalysis demonstrates a reduction in the observed rates of venographically demonstrated DVT from 51.6 % to 13.6 %, a relative risk reduction of 73 % [65].

4.1.2 Low molecular weigt heparins have been assessed against Dextran by Ericksson et al [16], Matzsch et al [56, 57], and the Danish Enoxaparin study group [14]. In all these studies low molecular weight heparins were found significantly superior to Dextran by statistical analysis. Based on a mandatory venographic examination, the Danish trial showed a reduction in total DVT from 24 of 111 patients in the Dextran group to 7 of 108 patients in the Enoxaparin group (p=0.0013).

4.1.3 Low molecular weight heparins have been assessed versus fixed doses of standard unfractionated heparin three times daily in seven studies [5, 15, 48, 51, 64]. A significantly higher antithrombotic efficiency of low molecular weight heparins was found [48, 51, 64]. Transfusion requirements were less in the LMWH group in the study by Planes et al [64] and Levine et al [48].

4.1.4 Low molecular weight heparins have been assessed versus low dose heparin dihydro- ergotamine twice daily by Lassen et al [45], Haas et al [28]. Both regimens were found equally effective but the patients did not receive a mandatory venographic examination.

4.2 In acute hip surgery

4.2.1 Low molecular weight heparins have been assessed versus placebo [41, 46]. Both studies used fibrinogen isotopic screening confirmed by venographic examination. The results were in favor of LMWH.

4.2.2 Low molecular weight heparins have been assessed versus low dose heparin twice or three times daily [8, 43, 46, 58]. The results was a trend in favor of LMWH. An heparinoïd (Org 10172) was found significantly more effective than Warfarin [27].

5. Recapitulation and conclusions

- Oral anticoagulants in orthopedic surgery have been demontrated to be more effective than aspirin [31], than dextran [22, 31], and as effective as external pneumatic compression [4, 63]. The low dose regimen popularized by the Mac Master University [38] is certainly an attractive method for reducing the bleeding risk. The international sensitivity index (ISI) of the reagent must be clearly defined, and the results expressed with the international normalized ratio (INR) to obtain and maintain the range of INR between 2 and 3 [34]. Oral anticoagulants have also been demonstrated to be effective in reducing the incidence of fatal pulmonary embolism [3, 12, 68].

- Unfractionated heparin in standard doses have been demonstrated by Collins et al [11], to be effective in preventing DVT and PE. Analysis of trials performed later, and venographically controlled, confirm this finding. But the protection remains inferior in comparison to the other methods. The increased risk of bleeding is small (about 2 %).

- Association of dihydroergotamine to fixed doses of unfractionated heparin does possibly afford a better protection against proximal DVT. Yet the associated but rare problems of ergotism [77] have led to this drug being rejected in some countries (France, USA, UK).

- Adjusted doses of standard unfractionated heparin have been demonstrated to be more effective in reducing the rates of total and proximal DVT than fixed doses, as effective as Kabi 2165 (Fragmin[R] LMWH) [5, 15], and CY 216 (Fraxiparine[R] LMWH) [51]. A significant superiority of LMWH in preventing proximal DVT was observed, but it is difficult to obtain and maintain the adjustment on a day to day basis.

- Low molecular weight heparins reduced absolute risk of total DVT by 73 % in elective hip surgery with the added benefit of simplicity of administration by eliminating the need for laboratory adjustments. They were found superior to unfractionated heparin, to dextran, to fixed doses of unfractionated heparin plus dihydroergotamine. Theses trials were conducted with PK 10169 (Lovenox[R], Clexane[R]) [14, 48, 64, 76], with Kabi 2165 (Fragmin[R]) [5, 15, 56, 57], CY 216 (Fraxiparin[R]) [51], an association of LMWH and dihydroergotamine [28, 45], an heparinoïd, Organon 10172 (Lomaparan[R]) [27, 36], and Logiparin[R] [47]. In

North America there are used post operatively [48, 76]. The question of the superiority of a pre-operative administration is still debatable. With the recommended dosage tolerance was demonstrated to be better than fixed doses of unfractionated heparin [48, 64] but this finding is still disputed [73]. They are now the treatment of choice. At present each LMWH is considered as a different entity, so each drug must be assessed separately in independent trials. It is important to evaluate the clinical documentation of the efficacy and safety of a compound before using it. Administration must conform to the recommendations of the manufacturers and to legal accreditations.

REFERENCES

1. American Consensus Conference on the Prevention of venous thrombosis and pulmonary embolism. JAMA 256, 744-749, 1986.

2. ABRAHAM - INPIJN L, VREECKEN J. Effect of low dose heparin on incidence of post operative thrombosis in orthopedic patients. Arch Chir Neerl 27, 63-68, 1975.

3. AMSTUTZ HC, FRISCIA DA, DOREY F, CARNEY BT. Warfarin prophylaxis to prevent mortality from pulmonary embolism after total hip replacement. J Bone Joint Surg (Am) 71, 321-326, 1989.

4. BAILEY JP, KRUGER MP, SOLANO FX, ZAJKO AB, RUBASH HE. Prospective randomized trial of sequential compression devices vs low-dose warfarin for deep venous thrombosis prophylaxis in total hip arthroplasty. J of Arthroplasty S6, 29-35, 1991.

5. BARRE J, PFISTER G, POTRON G, DROULLE C, BAUDRILLARD JC, BARBIER P, KHER A. Efficacité et tolérance comparée du Kabi 2165 et de l'héparine standard dans la prévention des thromboses veineuses profondes au cours des prothèses totales de hanche. J Mal Vasc (Suppl B) 12, 90-95, 1987.

6. BEISAW NE, COMEROTA AJ, GROTH HE, MERLI GJ, WEITZ HH, ZIMMERMAN RC, DISERIO FJ, SASAHARA AA. Dihydroergotamine / heparin in the prevention of deep vein thrombosis after total hip replacement. J Bone Joint Surg (Am) 70, 2-10, 1988.

7. BERGVIST D, EFSING HO, HALLBOOK T, HEDLUND T. Thrombolism after elective and post traumatic hip surgery: a controlled prophylactic trial with dextran 70 and low dose heparin. Acta Chir Scand 145, 213-218, 1979.

8. BREYER HG, AL-THERIB J, BACHER P, WERNER B. Thrombosis prophylaxis with low molecular weight heparin in trauma surgery. Thromb Res S6, 167, 1986.

9. CADE JF, BUCHANAM MR, BONEU B, OCKELFORD P, CARTER CJ, CERSKUS AL, HIRSH J. A comparison of the anti thrombotic and hemorrhagic effects of low molecular weight heparin fractions: the influence of the method of preparation. Thromb Res 35, 613-625, 1984.

10. CARTER CJ, KELTON JG, HIRSH J, CERSKUS A, SANTOS AV, GENT M. The relationship between the hemorrhagic and antithrombotic properties of low molecular weight heparin in rabbits. Blood 59, 1239-1245, 1982.

11. COLLINS R, SCRIMGEOUR A, YUSUF S, PETO R. Reduction in fatal pulmonary embolism and venous thrombosis by perioperative administration of subcutaneous heparin. N Engl J Med 318, 1162-1170, 1988.

12. COVENTRY MB, NOLAN DR, BECKENBAUGH RB. "Delayed" prophylactic anticoagulation: a study of results and complications in 2012 total hip arthroplasties. J Bone Joint Surg (Am) 55, 1487-1492, 1973.

13. CRUICKSHANK MK, LEVINE MN, HIRSH J, TURPIE AGG, POWERS P, JAY R, GENT M. An evaluation of impedance plethysmography and ^{125}I Fibrinogen leg scanning in patients following hip surgery. Thromb Hemost 62, 830-834, 1989.

14. Danish Enoxaparin study group. Low Molecular Weight Heparin (Enoxaparin) vs Dextran 70. Arch Int Med 151, 1621-1624, 1991.

15. DECHAVANNE M, VILLE D, BERRUYER M, TREPO F, DALERY F, CLERMONT N, LERAT JL, MOYEN B, FISHER LP, kher a, BARBIER P. Randomized trial of a low molecular weight heparin (Kabi 2165) versus adjusted dose subcutaneous standard heparin in the prophylaxis of deep-vein thrombosis after elective hip surgery. Haemostasis 1, 5-12, 1989.

16. ERICKSSON BI, ZACHRISON BE, TEGER-NILSSON AC, RISBERG B. Thrombosis prophylaxis with low molecular weight heparin in total hip replacement. Br J Surg 75, 1053-1057, 1988.

17. ERICKSSON BI, KALEBO P, ANTHYMYR BA, WADENVIK H, TENGBORN L, RISBERG B. Prevention of deep vein thrombosis and pulmonary embolism after total hip replacement. J Bone Joint Surg (Am) 73, 484-493, 1991.

18. ESTOPPEY D, HOCHREITER J, BREYER HG, JAKUBEK H, LEYVRAZ PF, HAAS S, STIEKEMA JCJ. Org 10172 (Lomaparan) versus heparin - DHE in prevention of thromboembolism in total hip remplacement. A multicentre trial. Thromb Hemost 62, 356 (Abstr), 1989.

19. EVARTS CM, FEIL EJ. Prevention of thromboembolic disease after elective surgery

of the hip. J Bone Joint Surg (Am) 53, 1271-1280, 1971.

20. FERNANDEZ J, N'GUYEN P, VAN RYN J, OFOSU FA, HIRSH J, BUCHANAN MR. Hemorrhagic doses of heparin and other glycosaminoglycans induce a platelet defect. Thromb Res 43, 491-495, 1986.

21. FORDYCE MJF, BAKER AS, STADDON GE. Efficacy of fixed minidose warfarin prophylaxis in total hip replacement. Brit Med J 303, 219-220, 1991.

22. FRANCIS CW, MARDER VT, EVARTS CM, YAUKOOLBODI S. Two step warfarin therapy. JAMA, 249, 374-378, 1983.

23. FREEARK KJ, BOSWICK J, FARDIN R. Post-traumatic venous thrombosis. Arch Surg 95, 567, 1967.

24. FREDIN HO, ROSBERG B, ARBORELIUS JRM, NYLANDER G. On thrombo-embolism after total hip replacement in epidural analgesia: a controlled study of dextran 70 and low dose heparin combined with dihydroergotamine. Br J Surg 71, 58-60, 1984.

25. GALLUS AS, HIRSH J, TUTLE RJ et al. Small subcutaneous doses of heparin in prevention of venous thrombosis. N Engl J Med 288, 545-551, 1973.

26. GEERTS WH, CADE KI, JAY RM, SZALAI JP. Venous thrombosis in trauma. A prospective study. Thromb Haemost 65, 703 (Abstr), 1991.

27. GERHART TN, YETT HS, ROBERTSON LK, LEE MA, SMITH M, SALZMAN EW. Low molecular weight heparinoïd compared with warfarin for prophylaxis of deep-vein thrombosis in patients who are operated on for fracture of the hip. A prospective randomized trial. J Bone Joint Surg S. (Am) 73, 494-502, 1991.

28. HAAS S, STERNBERGER A, FRITSHE HM et al. Prophylaxis of deep vein thrombosis in high risk patients undergoing total hip replacement with low molecular weight heparin plus dihydroergotamine. Arzneimittelforschung, 37, 839-843, 1987.

29. HAAS SB, INSALL JN, SCUDERI GR, WINDSOR RE, GHELMAN B. Pneumatic sequential compression boots compared with aspirin prophylaxis of deep-vein thrombosis after total knee arthroplasty. J Bone Joint Surg (Am) 72, 27-31, 1990.

30. HAMPSON WGJ, HARRIS FC, LUCAS HK et al. Failure of low dose heparin to prevent deep-vein thrombosis after hip replacement arthroplasty. Lancet 2, 795-797, 1974.

31. HARRIS WH, SALZMAN EW, ATHANASOULIS CA et al. Comparison of Warfarin, low molecular weight dextran, aspirin, and subcutaneous heparin in prevention of venous thromboembolism following total hip replacement. J Bone Joint Surg (Am) 56, 1552-1562, 1974.

32. HARRIS WH, SALZMAN EW, ATHANASOULIS CA, WALTMAN AC, DESANCTIS RW. Aspirin prophylaxis of venous thromboembolism after total hip replacement. N Engl J Med 297, 1246-1249, 1977.

33. HAVIG O. Deep vein thrombosis and pulmonary embolism. Acta Chir Scand S478, 1-120, 1977.

34. HIRSH J, POLLER L, DEYKIN D, LEVINE L, DALEN JE. Optimal therapeutic range for oral anticoagulants. Chest S95, 5-11, 1989.

35. HOEK JA, LENSING AWA, TEN CATE JW, BORM JJ, NURMOHAMED MT, COGO A, COURANT A, PRANDONI P, LING E. The clinical utility of objective diagnostic tests for diagnosing deep vein thrombosis of the legs. Br J Clin Pract Symp (Suppl) 65, 26-35, 1989.

36. HOEK J, NURMOHAMED MT, TEN CATE H, TEN CATE JW, BULLER HR. Prevention of deep vein thrombosis following total hip replacement by a low molecular weight heparinoïd. (Org 10172). Thromb Haemost 62, 520 (Abstr), 1989.

37. HOLMER E, MATTSSON C, NILSON S. Anticoagulant and antithrombotic effects of heparin and low molecular weight heparin fragments in rabbits. Thromb Res 25, 475-485, 1982.

38. HULL R, HIRSH J, JAY R, CARTER CJ, ENGLAND C, GENT M, TURPIE agg, McLOUGHLIN D, DODD P, THOMAS M, RASKOB G, OCKELFORD P. Different intensities of oral anticoagulant therapy in the treatment of proximal-vein thrombosis. N Engl J Med 307, 1676-1681, 1982.

39. HULL RO, RASKOB GE, GENT M, McLOUGHLIN D, JULIAN D, SMITH FC, DALE NI, REED-DAVIS R, LOFTHOUSE RN, ANDERSON C. Effectiveness of intermittent pneumatic leg compression for preventing deep vein thrombosis after total hip replacement. JAMA 263, 2313-231, 1990.

40. JOHNSON R, GREEN JR, CHARNLEY J. Pulmonary embolism and its prophylaxis following the Charnley total hip replacement. Clin Orthop 127, 123-132, 1977.

41. JORGENSEN PS, TORNHOLM C, KNUDSEN JB, BOENG L, JOSEFSON L, BJERREGAARD P, JORGENSEN PK, HAGEN K. Thromboprophylactic effect of a low molecular weight heparin (Fragmin) in acute hip fracture surgery. A placebo controlled study. Thromb Haemost 62, 525 (Abstr), 1989.

42. KAKKAR VV, FOK PJ, MURRAY WJ, PAES T, MERENSTEIN D, DODDS R, FARRELL R, CRELLIN RQ, THOMAS EM, MORLEY TR et al. Heparin and dihydroergotamine prophylaxis against thrombo-embolism after hip arthroplasty. J Bone Joint Surg (Br) 67, 538- 542, 1985.

43. KORNINGER C, SCHLAG G , POIGENFURST J, WILFING C, REDL H, PELINKA H, GAUDERNAK T, WELZEL D. Randomized trial of low molecular weight heparin versus low dose heparin / acenocoumarin in patients with hip fracture. Thromboprophylactic effect and bleeding complications. Thromb Haemost 62, 187 (Abstr), 1989.

44. KUJATH P, HORST B, SPANNAGEL U, HABSCHIED W. Thromboembolic risk in surgical outpatients with injuries of the lower limb. Thromb Haemost 65, 703 (Abstr), 1991.

45. LASSEN MR, BORRIS LC, CHRISTIANSEN HM, MOLLER-LARSEN F, KNUDSEN VE, BORIS P, NEHEN AM, DE CARVALHO A, JURIK AG, NIELSEN BW et al. Heparin / dihydroergotamine for venous thrombosis prophylaxis: Comparison of low dose heparin and low molecular weight heparin in hip surgery. Br J Surg 75, 686-689, 1988.

46. LASSEN MR, BORRIS LC, CHRISTIANSEN HM, MOLLER-LARSEN F, KNUDSEN VE, BORIS P, NEHEN AM, JURIK AG, DE CARVALHO A, NIELSEN BW et al. Prevention of thromboembolism in hip fracture patients. Comparison of low-dose heparin and low molecular weight heparin combined with dihydroergotamine. Arch Orthop 108, 10-13, 1989.

47. LASSEN MR, BORRIS LC, CHRISTIANSEN HM, BOLL KL, EISKJAER SP, NIELSEN BW, SCHOTT P, OLSEN AD, RODENBERG JC, LUCHT U. Prevention of thromboembolism in 190 hip arthroplasties. Comparaison of LMW heparin and placebo. Acta Orthop Scand 62, 33-38, 1991.

48. LEVINE MN, HIRSH J, GENT M, TURPIE AG, LECLERC J, POWERS PJ, JAY RM, NEEMEH J. Prevention of deep vein thrombosis after elective hip surgery. A randomized trial compairing low molecular weight heparin with standard unfractionated heparin. Ann Int Med 114, 545-551, 1991.

49. LEYVRAZ PF, RICHARD J, BACHMANN F, VAN MELLE G, TREYVAUD JM, LIVIO JJ, CANDARDJIS G. Adjusted versus fixed-dose subcutaneous heparin in th prevention of deep-vein thrombosis after total hip replacement. N Engl J Med 309, 954-958, 1983.

50. LEYVRAZ PF, BACHMANN F, VUILLEUMIER B, BERTHET S, BOHNET J, HALLER E. Adjusted subcutaneous heparin versus heparin plus dihydroergotamine in prevention of deep vein thrombosis after total hip arthroplasty. J of Arthroplasty 3, 81-86, 1988.

51. LEYVRAZ PF, BACHMANN F, HOEK J, BULLER HR, POSTEL M, SAMAMA M, VANDENBROEK MD. Prevention of deep-vein thrombosis after hip replacement: randomized comparison between unfractionated heparin and low molecular weight heparin. Brit Med J 303, 543-548, 1991.

52. LOTKE PA, ECKER ML, ALAVI A, BUKOWITZ H. Indication for the treatment o deep venous thrombosis following total knee replacement. J Bone Joint Surg (Am) 66, 202-208, 1984.

53. LOWE LW. Venous thrombosis and embolism. J Bone Joint Surg (Br) 63, 155-167, 1981.

54. LYNCH AF, BOURNE RB, RORABECK CH, RAUKIN RN, DONARD A. Deep vein thrombosis and continous passive motion after total knee arthroplasty. J Bone Joint Surg (Am) 70, 11-14 1988.

55. MANNUCCI PM, CITTERIO LE, PANAJOTOPOULOS N. Low-dose heparin and deep-vein thrombosis after total hip replacement. Thromb Hemost 36, 157-164, 1976

56. MATZSCH T, BERGQVIST D, FREDIN H, HEDNER U. Low molecular weight heparin compared with dextran as prophylaxis against thrombosis after total hip replacement. Acta Chir Scand 156, 445-450, 1990.

57. MATZSCH T, BERGQVIST D, FREDIN H et al. Comparison of the thromboprophylactic effect of a low molecular weight heparin versus dextran in total hip replacement. Thromb Hoemorrh Disorders 3/1, 25-29, 1991.

58. MONREAL M, LAFOZ E, NAVARRO A, GRANERO X, CAJA V, CACERES E, SALVADOR R, RUIZ J. A prospective double-blind trial of a low molecular weight heparin once daily compared with conventional low dose heparin three times daily to prevent pulmonary embolism and venous thrombosis in patients with hip fracture. J Trauma 29, 873-875, 1989.

59. MORRIS GK, HENRY APJ, PRESTON J. Prevention of deep-vein thrombosis by low dose heparin in patients undergoing total hip replacement. Lancet 2, 797-800, 1974.

60. MOSKOVITZ PA, ELLENBERG SS, FEFFER HL, KENMORE PI, NEVIASER RJ, RUBIN BE, VARMA VM. Low dose heparin for prevention of venous thromboembolism in total hip arthroplasty and surgical repair of hip fractures. J Bone Joint Surg (Am) 60, 1065-107, 1978.

61. OCKELFORD PA, CARTER CJ, CERSKUS A, SMITH CA, HIRSH J. Comparison of the in vivo hemorrhagic and antithrombotic effects of a low antithrombin III affinity heparin fraction. Thromb Res 27, 679-690, 1982.

62. OCKELFORD PA, CARTER CJ, MITCHELL L, HIRSH J. Discordance between the anti-Xa activity and the antithrombotic activity of an ultra-low molecular weight heparin fraction. Thromb Res 28, 401-409, 1982.

63. PAIEMENT G, WESSINGER SJ, WALTMAN AC, HARRIS WH. Low-dose warfarin versus external pneumatic compression for prophylaxis against venous thromboembolism following total hip replacement. J of Arthroplasty 2/1, 23-26, 1987.

64. PLANES A, VOCHELLE N, MAZAS F, MANSAT C, ZUCMAN J, LANDAIS A, PASCARIELLO JC, WEILL D, BUTEL J. Prevention of post-operative venous thrombosis: a randomized trial compaing unfractionated heparin with low molecular weight heparin in patients undergoing total hip replacement. Thromb Haemost 60, 407-410, 1988.

65. PLANES A, VOCHELLE N, SILSIGUEN M. Report for the European workshop on the prevention of thromboembolism. Windsor 1991 (In press).

66. ROBERTS TS, NELSON CL, BARNES CL, FERRIS EJ, HOLDER JC, BONE DW. The preoperative prevalence and post operative incidence of thromboembolism in patients with hip fractures treated with dextran prophylaxis. Clin Orthop 255, 198-203, 1990.

67. SANDLER DA, MARTIN JF, DUNCAN JS, BLAKE GM, WARD P, RAMSAY LE, LAMONT AC, ROSS B, SHERRIFF S, WALTON L. Diagnosis of deep-vein thrombosis: comparison of clinical evaluation, ultrasound, plethysmography and venoscan with X-Ray venogram. Lancet 2, 716-719, 1984.

68. SEVITT S, GALLAGHER NG. Prevention of venous thrombosis and pulmonary embolism in injured patients. Lancet 2, 981-989, 1959.

69. SHARROCK NE, HAAS SB, HARGETT MJ, URQUHART B, INSALL JN, SCUDERI G. Effects of epidural anesthesia on the incidence of deep-vein thrombosis after total knee arthroplasty. J Bone Joint Surg (Am) 73, 502-506, 1991.

70. STEVENS J, FARDIN R, FREEARK RJ. Lower extremity thrombophlebitis in patients with femoral neck fractures. J Trauma 8, 527, 1968.

71. STRINGER MD, STEADMAN CA, HEDGES AR, THOMAS EM, MORLEY TR, KAKKAR VV. Deep vein

thrombosis after elective knee surgery. An incidence study in 312 patients. J Bone Joint Surg (Br) 71, 492-497, 1989.

72. STULBERG BN, INSALL JN, WILLIAMS GW, GHELMAN B. Deep-vein thrombosis following total knee replacement. J Bone Joint Surg (Am) 66, 194-201, 1984.

73. TEN CATE JW. Low molecular weight heparins in the prophylaxis of venous thrombosis: a meta-analysis. International Symposium of low-molecular-weight heparins and related polysaccharides. Munich, june, 27-28, 1991.

74. THOMAS DP, MERTON RE, BARROWCLIFFE TW, THUNBERG L, LINDAHL U. Effects of heparin oligosaccharides with high affinity for antithrombine III in experimental venous thrombosis. Thromb Hoemost 47, 244-248, 1982.

75. TORHOLM C, BROENG L, SEEST JORGENSEN P et al. Thromboprophylaxis by low molecular weight heparin in elective hip surgery. J Bone Joint Surg (Br) 73, 434-438, 1991.

76. TURPIE AGG, LEVINE MN, HIRSH J, CARTER CJ, JAY RM, POWERS PJ, ANDREW M, HULL RD, GENT M. A randomized controlled trial of a low molecular weight heparin (Enoxaparin) to prevent deep-vein thrombosis in patients undergoing elective hip surgery. N Engl J Med 315, 925-929, 1986.

77. VAN DEN BERG E, RUMPF KD, FROHLICH H, WATERBUSCH G, MULLER-VAHL H, REILMANN H, GRAEN J. Vascular spasm during thromboembolism prophylaxis with heparin - dihydroergotamine. Lancet 2, 268-269, 1982.

78. Venous Thrombosis Clinical Study Group. Small doses of subcutaneous sodium heparin in the prevention of deep-vein thrombosis after elective hip operations. Br J Surg 62, 348-350, 1975.

79. WELIN-BERGER T, BYGDEMAN S, MEBIUS C. Deep vein thrombosis following hip surgery: relation to activated factor X inhibition activity effect of heparin and dextran. Acta Orthop Scand 53, 937-945, 1982.

80. WILLIAMS JW, EIKMAN EA, GREENBERG SH, HEWITT JC, LOPEZ-CUENCA E, JONES GP, MADDEN JA. Failure of low dose heparin to prevent pulmonary embolism after hip srugery or above the knee amputation. Ann Surg 188, 468-474, 1978.

81. WINTER CHRISTENSEN S, WILLE-JORGENSEN P, KJAER L, STADEAGER C, WIDDING A, VERSTERGAARD A, BJERG-NIELSEN A. Contract thermography, ^{99M} Tc-Plasmin Scintimetry and ^{99M} Tc-Plasmin Scintigraphy as screening methods for deep venous thrombosis following major hip surgery. Thromb Haemost 58, 831-833, 1987.

23

Hemostatic abnormalities, anticoagulation and anesthesia

G. Janvier, S. Winnock

The essential function of anesthesia is to allow pain-free surgery. There are two different techniques of anesthesia which may, under certain circumstances, be used together: general anesthesia where the patient loses consciousness, and regional anesthesia where the area to be operated undergoes analgesia.

The anesthetist frequently meets coagulation-linked problems in his daily work. Coagulation disorders may exist before surgery or be its result. They may stem from a pathological condition or be due to the prescription of anticoagulation therapy [5, 25, 29, 38, 43, 80]. Anticoagulation may be necessary during surgery to prevent surgical complications (clotting induced by vascular clamping and extracorporeal blood circulation, thromboembolism etc.) or to prevent thrombosis of prosthetic devices implanted in the patients (table I).

In these circumstances coagulation disorders may interfere with the choice of an anesthetic technique and induce abnormal perioperative bleeding.

Table I: Indications for anticoagulation

CONDITION	DURATION	
	PERMANENT	TEMPORARY
Thrombo-embolism	Deep venous thrombosis/ Pulmonary embolism	Deep venous thrombosis/ Pulmonary embolism
Foreign Body	Cardiac valve prosthesis	Cardiopulmonary bypass Haemodialysis Vascular suggery Arterials catheters
Prophylaxis	Atrial fibrillation Congestive heart failure recurrent pulmonary embolism recurrent venous thrombosis Malignancy	peroperative immobilization sepsis respiratory failure
Others	Cerebrovascular disease (Progressive strokes/transient ischaemic attacks) Mitral valve disease	Myocardial infarct Disseminated intravascular coagulation cardioversion

1. Preoperative anticoagulation and hemostatic disorders

The evaluation of coagulation disorders in a patient scheduled for surgery consists of several stages. The first is to screen for pathological or therapeutical coagulation abnormalities, allowing a precise diagnosis of the coagulation disorder presented by the patient. During the second phase an attitude toward this disorder must be adopted, depending on 3 factors: the nature of the disorder, the type of surgery to be undergone and the type of anesthesia which is required.

1.1 Detection of coagulation disorders [5, 53]

There is a large variety of circumstances under which a patient may present preoperative coagulation problems. Screening these problems requires anamnestic, clinical and laboratory data.

1.1.1 History

The aim of the history is to pinpoint any consequences of a coagulation disorder but also to look for pathologic conditions auspicious to the emergence of such a problem. Family and individual history of abnormal bleeding are looked for as well as any signs of disease which may lead to coagulation disorders. Prescription of drugs which may alter coagulation is also looked for, especially a self-prescription which may go unnoticed.

1.1.2 Physical examination

Its role is to screen for symptoms (eg. hepatomegaly or splenomegaly) of pathologies which could induce coagulation disorders.

1.1.3 Laboratory examinations

For economical reasons, laboratory examinations are prescribed whenever the history or physical examination is positive or when, for a variety of reasons, the interrogation is impossible to carry out or incomplete. Firstly, only screening tests are prescribed (bleeding time, prothrombin time, partial thromboplastin time and platelet count), they are sufficient to detect the majority of coagulation disorders. When positive, they must be complemented by more specific tests in order to make a precise diagnosis.

1.2 The nature of coagulation disorders

A great number of pathological conditions may lead to abnormal bleeding.

1.2.1 Platelet disorders

Platelet disorders can result from an alteration in number (thrombocytopenia) or function of the platelets. With platelet count under 40000 per mm3 bleeding may occur during or after surgery. Thrombocytopenia has multiple causes: production defect (medullary aplasia, neoplastic medullary infiltration), sequestration (splenomegaly), accelerated destruction (antibodies, infection, consumption, hemorrahge). Functional disorders of platelets result in a prolonged bleeding time. Such disorders include defective adhesion (Bernard-Soulier syndrome, complete afibrinogenemia), defective primary aggregation (thrombasthenia) or defective platelet release reaction (storage pool disease, aspirin etc...).

1.2.2 Plasma coagulation factors deficiency

- Fibrinogen deficiency

Deficiency of fibrinogen may be congenital or acquired: patients may be asymptomatic or display hemorrhagic syndromes. The defect is usually detected on a prolonged prothrombin time. Acquired deficiency of fibrinogen is seen in liver insufficiency or following administration of certain drugs. A reduction in fibrinogen is also present in disseminated intravascular coagulation and in fibrinolytic states.

- Hemophilia

Hemophilia is the most common congenital coagulation disorder. A low factor VIII procoagulant activity is responsible for a prolonged partial thromboplastin time. When activity is under 40 percent of the normal level, the patient is at risk for surgical bleeding. Factor IX insufficiency may also lead to severe hemorrhage, and the defect should be compensated when under 40 percent of the normal level.

- Von WILLEBRAND disease

Patients with von Willebrand disease may present hemorragic syndrome. In this disease laboratory findings include a prolonged bleeding time, a reduction in factor VIII antigenic and coagulant activities and abnormal platelet function.

- Liver insufficiency

In liver insufficiency a decreased liver protein synthesis and an increased plasma proteolytic activity tend to reduce the level of all plasmatic coagulation factors except factor VIII. In the absence of liver insufficiency a decrease in factors II, VII, IX and X is associated with vitamin K deficiency. Vitamin K deficiency may result from obstructive jaundice, biliary fistula, intestinal malabsorption syndromes or after prolonged oral administration of antibiotics. All these disorders are detected by a prolonged prothrombin time.

- Circulating anticoagulants

Patients with circulating anticoagulants to factors I, V, VIII, IX, X, XI and XIII have been reported. In these patients the defect is not corrected by replacement therapy. Some of these disorders are associated with bleeding risk, others with thrombotic risk.

1.2.3 Anticoagulant therapies [20, 29, 36, 48, 55, 77].

Heparin essentially induces an inactivation of thrombin which is appropriately monitored by the partial thromboplastin time. Coumarin therapy induces the same coagulation disorders as vitamin K deficiency. Other drugs referred as antiplatelet drugs interfere with platelet function. Ticlopidine a widely used antithrombotic therapy inhibits primary phase of ADP induced aggregation.

1.3 Assessment of the bleeding risk

Perioperative coagulation disorders may lead to an hemorrhagic state and eventually to an hematoma at the site of anesthetic puncture or of surgical entry. The consequences of the bleeding vary according to:

- the nature and the intensity of the coagulation disorder
- the type of surgery and of anesthesia.

1.3.1 Nature and intensity of the coagulation disorder

During therapeutical anticoagulation the bleeding risk is calculated and measured by regular monitoring [1, 2, 25]. Heparin anticoagulation (non-fractionated heparin) is easily handled, since this drug has a short half-life and is readily antagonized [20, 25]. On the other hand the effects of low molecular weight heparin coumarin K and of antiplatelet drugs are more difficult to control [36, 53, 55, 77, 80].

Pathological coagulation disorders are less predictable in terms of bleeding risk because of a discrepancy between the results of laboratory tests and clinical manifestations. Nonetheless a safety line has been drawn, for most coagulation factors, under which no potentially hemorrhagic surgery should be performed. In the same way a platelet count under 40.000 per mm^3 must be considered incompatible with surgery [80].

1.3.2 Type of surgery

The consequences of a coagulation disorder may be disastrous particularly during surgery of the ocular globes, the brain and during liver and traumatic surgery [80].

1.3.3 Type of anesthesia

General anesthesia is only rarely problematic in terms of compatibility with anticoagulation. Difficulties are most often encountered when there is need of invasive techniques such as placing a central catheter. Accidental puncture of a large vessel may result in hematoma whose localization and size eventually lead to severe complications. Epidural and spinal anesthesia are much more problematic in the presence of a coagulation disorder. These techniques may be complicated by peridural hematoma. Clinical manifestations include: back pain, sensitive or motor deficit of the lower limbs, urinary retention and abdominal distention. When the localization is subarachnoid the patient may present signs of meningeal hemorrhage [26, 57]. Diagnosis is made on myelography or computerized tomography of the lumbar spine. Recovery without any sequela is possible if the surgical treatment (laminectomy with hematoma evacuation) is carried out within a very short period following the emergence of the first neurological signs (less than 6 hours). These hematomas may appear even in the absence of anticoagulation or coagulation disorders. From 1952 to 1983, 18 publications reported 20 peridural hematoma occurring after peridural anesthesia, 7 of which occurred when the patient had not received anticoagulant or antiplatelet therapy beforehand. Indeed, 1/3 of peridural hematoma occurred in anticoagulated patients. In the other cases anticoagulants were not prescribed but there was coagulation disorder, vascular malformation or severe hemodynamic disorder. In fact, these hematomas occur frequently after spinal or epidural anesthesia, as shown by USUBIAGA [81] who reported 10% of peridural hematoma occurences in patients undergoing inter-vertebral disk surgery under peridural anesthesia. In many cases hematomas appear after traumatic or hemorrhagic puncture. However, the presence of hematoma in the peridural region does not necessarily lead to the appearance of neurological signs and the latter would only appear when a critical volume is reached.

The effect of anticoagulation is to increase the incidence and severity of post-lumbar puncture hematoma. Accordingly, WULF and STRIEPLIG [85] have shown in a post-mortem study carried out on 10 patients having undergone surgery under peridural anesthesia and, for 9 anticoagulated postoperatively anticoagulation using heparin, the presence of peridural hematoma in 4 cases. In 3 patients the catheter was still in place, in the fourth it had been removed 23 days earlier. DICKMAN et al. [21] report 2 peridural hematoma occurring after spinal anesthesia; one patient had received urokinase intra-arterially while the other had received systemic heparin. Development of a peridural hematoma following epidural anesthesia has been reported in patients receiving anticoagulant therapy before and after anesthesia [11, 17, 19, 32, 41, 42]. The overall incidence of hematomas is one in 10 000 spinal anesthesia and one in 15 000 epidural anesthesia [44]. Conversely, ODOOM [67] et RAO [70] have shown that anticoagulation therapy with heparin could be associated safely with spinal or peridural anesthesia.

1.4 Management of a patient with preoperative coagulation disorder [24, 30, 31, 33, 35, 50, 56, 59, 65, 67, 70, 75, 76, 79, 83, 86]

ln all cases the pathologic coagulation disorders should be corrected with appropriate therapy. Therapeutic anti- coagulation should be allowed only if it can be easily controlled. In most cases this entails discontinuing the prescription of antiplatelet drugs, low mocular weight heparins and coumarins, and replacing them with non-fractionated heparin. Surgery should not be performed before the effects of these drugs disappear. If emergency surgery is required appropriate antagonization of anticoagulation is necessary.

When spinal or epidural anesthesia is required, anticoagulation should be avoided in cases of traumatic lumbar puncture [68, 69, 81]. As difficult lumbar puncture may not be always anticipated, anticoagulation should not be started before anesthesia. RAO and EL-ETR [70] recommend a one hour delay between the lumbar puncture or the removal of a peridural catheter and the administration of heparin. Fibrinolytic drugs should not used when a spinal or peridural anesthesia has been performed [67]. In case of pathologic coagulation epidural anesthesia should not be administered. The minimal platelet count compatible with safe epidural anesthesia is thought to be 100 000 per mm^3 [10].

2. Hemostatic disorders and perioperative anticoagulation : effects on anesthesia

2.1 Perioperative anticoagulation

To avoid deep-vein thrombosis, some patients are maintained intraoperatively under prophylactic anticoagulation with nonfractionated heparin or low molecular weight heparin [7, 39, 52]. On the other hand full anticoagulation, which will totally suppress most hemostatic factors, is prescribed for certain types of surgery (vascular clamping) [82] or when dynamic or functional extracorporeal circulation (ECC) (vascular by-passes, hemodialysis, etc...) is required [6, 23].

When general anesthesia is administered on an anticoagulated patient, intramuscular and subcutaneous premedication must be avoided [80] Venous and arterial punctures must be meticulously carried out. Certain authors have even contraindicated direct catheterization of the central subclavicular vein. Orotracheal intubation is preferred to nasotracheal intubation so as to avoid severe epistaxis.

2.1.1 Vascular clamping [82]

Vascular clamping (aortic, carotid, etc...) carried out intraoperatively is essentially performed with non fractionated heparin whose effects are easily monitored and neutralized by protamine in case of necessity. Dosage varies from 50 $IU.kg^{-1}$ to 300 $IU.kg^{-1}$ according to the type surgery. When vascular declamping takes place, anticoagulation is optimal (see neutralization of heparin) [20]. This anticoagulation interferes only slightly with anesthetic techniques, apart from the consequences of possible surgical bleeding when anticoagulation is uncontrolled. The problems of associating a technique of spinal or epidural anesthesia with anticoagulation has been described above. Nerve blocks (of the upper or lower limbs), and intravenous regional anesthesia can be carried out under anticoagulation.

2.1.2 Extracorporeal circulation [6, 23, 80]

Non-fractionated heparin is administered during extracorporeal circulation to ensure total inhibition of the coagulation process. Prior to ECC the prescription of anesthetic drugs is adjusted to suit the surgical events (skin incisions, sternotomy, retractors, pericardiectomy, aortic canulation). Acute normovolemic hemodilution is usually foreseen in patients who have hematocrit higher than 40 % in order to save fresh autologous blood which will be used after ECC. Before connecting the ECC to the patient, anticoagulation must be carried out in a central venous catheter at a dosage of 3000-4000 $IU.kg^{-1}$ of non fractioneted heparin. This anticoagulation is started just prior to incision of the left internal mammary arteries or before the aortic or vena cava canulation. This prescripion is monitored by measuring the activated clotting time (ACT) or others appropriated lab tests three minutes after the infection of heparin [2, 23]. The values measured must be 4 or 5 times that of the control value.

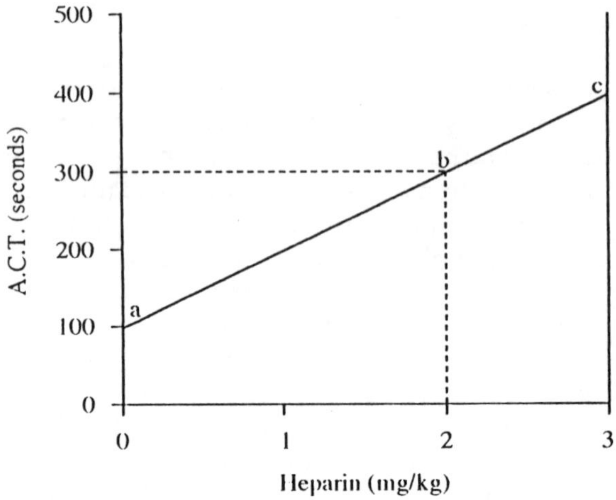

Figure 1: Heparin dose-response curve. Baseline ACT (a) and ACT after heparin 2 mg/kg body weight is given (b) are plotted.
The amount of heparin necessary to prolong the ACT to a given value (c) is extrapolated.

Patients with unstable angina who are under continuous heparin infusion are usually less responsive to heparin and need higher doses (higher than 4-5000 $IU.Kg^{-1}$ in order to obtain a prolonged ACT of over 400 seconds). A complementary dose of 100 $IU.Kg^{-1}$ is administered two hours after the initial dose and every following hour (figure 1). These doses are monitored by repeated PTT measures. There are 5 reasons why this standard method may not completely satisfactory:

- Available heparin preparations have variable activity.
- Hypothermia reduces heparin elimination
- The relationship between patient's weight and heparin distribution volume is not linear.
- The volume of blood circulating in the ECC varies with the ECC's device. It must be noted that "heparin-like" materials are available which totally modify the dosages of anticoagulation requirements. These materials need further clinical evaluation.
- There are individual and chronobiological variations of heparin activity.

For these reasons this therapy must be monitored repeatedly during ECC with ACT or by measuring the levels of circulating heparin, using titration with protamine (a difficult test to carry out) [19, 20, 38].

2.1.3 Neutralization of heparin [12, 23, 27, 63]

For neutralization of heparin protamine is administered after ECC is stopped and as soon as the patient's hemodynamic state is stable. 2500-5000 IU are injected over five minutes to detect any intolerance to the protamine injection (peripheral vasodilation and pulmonary hypertension), then the neutralizing dosage is 100-150 IU for 100 IU of circulating heparin. The half-life of heparin at 37°C is 90 minutes; the dose of circulating heparin is therefore the total dose administration administered less the metabolized amount (at 25°C, heparin is not metabolized). At the end of the admistration of protamine, ACT is checked so as to find a value which can be identical to control values.

Many recent works have shown that perfect monitoring of anticoagulant activity associated with large doses of aprotinin considerably reduces intra and postoperative blood losses. On the other hand it has also been proven that neutralizing protamine at the end of ECC could be responsible for the serious reactions provoked by the acute release of thromboxane, with severe pulmonary arterial hypertension and bronchoconstriction in some cases leading to a right ventricular failure. This complication is due to an activation of the complement by heparin-protamine complex, and is responsible for the aggregation and hyperactivity of leucocytes and platelets in the pulmonary circulation. Type I IgE are secreted during these accidents. Hypersensitivity can follow previous exposition to the drug or to a preparation containing protamine, such as late-acting insulin. It is well-known that diabetics receiving this type of insulin have high levels of IgE antiprotamine antibodies. Some patients allergic to fish and shellfish also present hypersensitive reactions to protamine [12].

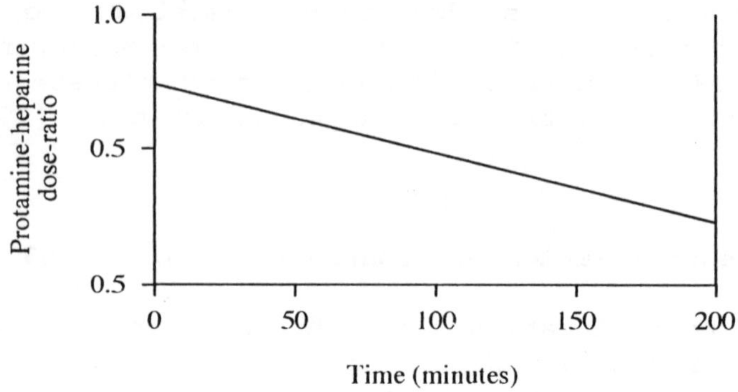

Figure 2: Protamine requirements decrease with time after the administration of heparin (modified from Dutton et al [27].

There is no means of predicting this complication. Recent work has been orientated towards safe preventive treatments such as short-lasting blockade of the thromboxane receptors. While waiting for these treatments to prove themselves, the present aim is to minimize the prescribed doses of protamine at the end of ECC (figures 2 and 3). Several methods are validated, among them DUTTON's which shows a linear relationship between heparinemia and the dose of neutralizing protamine as a function of the time passed after the administration of heparin. This relationship is not valid in children [27].

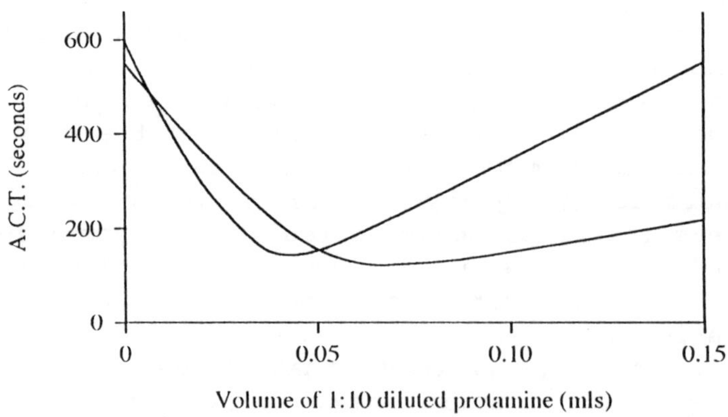

Figure 3: Protamine dilution curve: examples from two patients (modified from Dutton et al [27]).

Priming hemodilution of the ECC interferes with hemostatic and fibrinolytic factors. These symptoms differ according to the nature of the substitutes prescribed [28]. During ECC, anticoagulation and hemodilution may also induce intraoperative hemorrhage and hemodynamic disorders. Controlling them, means readjusting anesthetic techniques and intensive care therapies (changes in anesthetic agents, transfusion, inotropic drugs, vasoactive amines, etc...).

2.1.4 Functional extracorporeal circulation [80]

Functional extracorporeal circulation such as hemodialysis, when required is usually started before surgery. The aim is to take the patient into surgery without any hydroelectrolytic disorders (kaliemia less than 3-4 mmol/l). When surgery can lead to major hemodynamic disorder, e.g. liver transplant, heart and lung transplant, the best hemodialysing method is continuous veno-venous hemofiltration. This technique requires that anticoagulation doses be guided by methods adapted to the patient's hemorrahgic risks and to the prevention of clotting in the hemodialysis circuits; There are 2 modalities for prescription of anticoagulants (general heparinization of the patient or local anticoagulation of the device). A dose of non-fractionated heparin (15000 IU) or of low molecular weight heparin (3500 IU Anti-Xa) is administered to these ends. Continual perfusion of non-fractionated heparin doses of 50-120 $IU.h^{-1}$ is adjusted according to coagulation time (ACT carried out at the patient's bed). When direct anticoagulation of the circuits is administered locally, protamination after the device aims to neutralize half the injected dose of heparin.

This intra-operative technique palliates the absence of spontaneous diuresis. It helps to stabilize the hydroelectrolytic parameters and consequently prevents circulatory overloading. On the other hand it may lead to abnormal bleeding due to excessive anticoagulation. Hemofiltration modifies only slightly the pharmacokinetics of the anesthetic agents. Its main advantage from a hemodynamic stand-point is to minimize the cardiocirculatory variations of oliguric or anuric patients subject to aggressive surgery. Anticoagulation stability is always precarious during hemofiltration. Only repeated monitoring allows a precise adjustment of anticoagulant doses. When the patients is at high risk for hemorrhage, this technique may be carried without anticoagulation (with the risk of hemodialyzer circuit clotting).

2.2 Intraoperative hemostatic disorders responsible for a state of hypocoagulability

Two hyperfibronolytic states may be present in intraoperatively: fibrinolysis secondary to disseminated intravascular coagulopathy (DIC) and isolated primitive fibrinolysis [9, 80].

2.2.1 DIC

DIC is an intermediary pathological process due to the appearance of thrombin and fibrin in the blood stream. The process has two consequences; firstly it induces consumption of hemostatic factors; secondly hypocoagulability is responsible for bleeding along with the formation of thrombi in the microcirculation inducing secondary ischaemic necrotic injuries. DIC is a serious complication of numerous severe diseases.

Fifty to sixty percent of all DICs occur in various forms of aggressive surgery, with obstetrical etiology representing 80% of these (retroplacental hematoma, postpartum hemorrhaging and severe toxemia). The other surgical etiologies regroup traumatic shocks, fat embolisms, revascularization syndromes, severe acute pancreatitis, ruptured aneurysms of the aorta, hemorrhagic shocks.

The initial clinical signs of this disease is of an abnormal bleeding at the site of surgery or of venous punctures. The blood is incoagulable and the formation of clots is absent even after prolonged contact with an absorbent surface. This hemorrhage has no tendency to spontaneous recovery. Shock and hemolysis are associated in 70% and 20% of cases respectively. Other intraoperative clinical symptoms are inconstant; they appear in a second phase (visceral and skin symptoms:

kidney, liver, pulmonary, cardiac, neurological, etc...). Specific laboratory findings are indispensable to confirm the clinical suspicion and monitor the treatment. Hypofibrinogemia (less than 1 g), hypoprothrombinemia and thrombocytopenia (less than 100.000 per mm^3) are associated [3]. Reactional fibrinolysis is characterized by the soluble monomers of fibrin in the plasma, fibrin and fibrinogen degradation products, and a decrease of plasminogen level.

The treatment of this syndrome must lead, in the shortest time, to:

- Eliminating the cause of DIC (uterine evacuation, surgical hemostasis, antibiotics in septic states, etc...).
- Complementing the coagulation factor deficiency (fresh frozen plama, fibrinogen, platelets).
- Correcting the secondary fibrinolytic process by administration of antiplasmin of the aprotinin type [34, 40] under the protection of a therapy limiting the consumption of the hemostatic factors (antithrombin III and heparin) [49].

The efficacy of the therapy is judged on the evolution of the hemorrhagic syndrome and on the normalization of the coagulation tests.

This state of acquired hypocoagulability necessitates the use of a vigorous treatment whose chances of efficacy depend on its early clinical and biologic recognition.

2.2.2 Isolated primitive fibrinolysis [9, 22]

Isolated primitive fibrinolysis are rarer intraoperatively. They have been described during hepatic surgery, liver transplantation or post-transfusion hemolytic accidents. They differ from DIC in that although hemostatic clots are formed, they dissolve quickly. Biological diagnosis is based on a major fall in fibrinogen associated with an increase in FDP and plasmin and a secondary decrease in platelet count.

The treatment of these disorders consists of eliminating the triggering factors and the use of

Kunitz or Frey inhibiting antiproteases (aprotinin) [45].

These different types of hyperfibrinolysis with hypercoagulability necessitate a readjustment of anesthetic techniques according to their repercussions on the patient's general and specific visceral hemodynamics (lack of drug clearance, hypovolemia, etc...). The essential aim is to correct the hemorrhagic syndrome by substituting depleted factors while controlling blood volume and avoiding the perpetuation of consumption phenomena.

When the patient is under spinal or epidural anesthesia, the appearance of this type of complication must lead to the postoperative search for the existence of peridural hematoma, since these techniques may provoke local vascular wounds. It is also desirable to discontinue the injection of local anesthetic agents if bleeding by DIC or fibrinolysis occurs intraoperatively. The vasoplegia induced in the surgical site can only make the local hemorrhage more serious.

2.2.3 Massive transfusions [14, 16, 71]

During massive transfusions, diffuse bleeding may be observed. They are characterized by an "oozing" at the mucous membranes, surgical incision and puncture sites. These hemorrhagic diatheses step from a decrease of hemostatic factors due to consumption and dilution. A fall of fibrinogen below 0.5 $g.l^{-1}$, of factor V below 30%, platelets below 85000 / mm^3, with APTT 1.5 to 2 times the control justifies immediate supplies of fibrinogen, platelets, concentrated hemostatic factors, and according to certain authors, fresh blood [64].

During massive transfusion there is a close relationship between the fall in hemostatic factors and blood loss. The causes of these post-transfusion hemorrhagic diatheses are multiple (decrease in hemostatic factors, drop in ionized calcium, hypovolemia, etc.). MILLER showed in 1971 that thrombocytopenia associated with thrombasthenia are the principal factors [59].

3. Hemostatic disorders and postoperative anticoagulation

These intraoperative coagulation disorders may continue postoperatively or intensify. Their clinical expression is often more dramatic since the consequences of plurivisceral stress are added to the hemorrhagic syndrome. Their treatment respects the same rules as set out above intraoperatively.

Postoperative anticoagulation has a variety of indications (cardiovascular surgery, patient suffering from coronary insufficiency, prevention of thromboembolism and venous disease, etc.). Usually nonfractionated heparin or low molecular weight heparin is administered immediately after surgery, with the dosage adapted to suit the indications and the patient's thrombotic and hemorrhagic risk factors [6, 52].

Coumarins, more or less precociously, takes over from heparin treatment. These treatments may be responsible for hemorrhagic complications at the site of surgery, such as cellular spaces of the trunk (retroperitoneal hematoma), or as a gastric ulcer. These complications must be diagnosed early; if not, local mechanical disorders or serious hemodynamic instability may ensue. In some cases reoperation for hemostasis may be required. Hemorrhage linked to the prescription of anticoagulants must be controlled by antidotes or coagulation factors replacement, and the blood volume must be restored by red blood cell transfusion and fresh frozen plasma or plasma substitutes [72, 80].

3.1 Heparin-associated thrombocytopenia

If bleeding is the most common complication encountered when prescribing heparin, there is a side effect which is paradoxical but just as important. It is characterized by the appearance of thrombocytopenia, possibly accompanied by arterial or venous vascular thrombosis.

Two forms of heparin-associated thrombocytopenia have been described [4, 47, 51, 84]. The first, whose frequency varies from 0.6 à 30%, has an early appearance (1-3 days after installing the treatment). It is accompanied by a moderate drop in platelet count and is spontaneously reversible. The second, which is idiosyncratic has a lower incidence (0.18-1.6%) and a later onset (7-15 days) [7]. It is accompanied by a sharp drop in the number of platelets and is complicated by multiple thrombotic phenomena. This thrombocytopenia returns to normal 2-6 days after discontinuing the prescription of heparin. Low molecular weight heparins seem to interact less with platelets and are responsible for fewer accidents. Heparins of bovine origin would be more common sources of thombocytopenia than those of porcine origin [46].

The mechanism evoked is immunoallergic. IgG, whose anti-body Fab parts are linked to heparin, forms a complex where the Fc parts settle on the platelets PF4 receptors. In this way the platelets are consumed by aggregation and form white thrombi (white clot syndrome). These antiheparin antibodies may also interact with endogenous heparin. They also settle on the endothelial cells [47].

The diagnosis relies on clinical evolution and laboratory findings. The fall in the number of platelets is important enough to reach values lower than 50 $G.l^{-1}$. The specificity of antiplatelet antibodies is weak. The laboratory diagnosis is based on tests of in vitro platelet aggregation. If aggregation is 20% higher than control value, the test is considered to be positive. Their specificity is around 90% while their sensitivity is only 40%. A test based on the release of serotonin carbon 14 by the platelets is more sensitive but deserves to be validated [78].

The prevention of this complication is to avoid prolonged heparin treatment and to favor an early replacement of heparin by coumarins. The choice of a replacement anticoagulant is difficult. It is guided by the urgency of thrombotic consequences (dextran, coumarins, antiplatelet, thrombolytic drugs, specific immunoglobulins, etc.). Surgery may be necessary when severe vascular thrombosis occurs. In cardiac surgery and ECC, the appearance of this type of complication is formidable. In ECC it is advisable to use heparin of a different origin, associated with major antiplatelet drugs (prostacyclin) and coumarins.

4. Anesthesia and its effects on blood coagulation

In literature there is a consensus that spinal or epidural anesthesia reduces the incidence of postoperative deep venous thrombosis (DVT) with regard to general anesthesia. The incidence of postoperative DVT in orthopedics under general anesthesia is 54-75% (diagnosis carried out with phlebography), while is 20-40% with spinal or epidural anesthesia. The same pattern is true for pulmonary embolism [9, 60, 61].

In what ways do spinal or epidural anesthesia reduce the occurence of venous thromboembolism complications?

It acts directly on the sympathetic nerves system and speeds up the venous flow in the anesthetized region. It has been shown that spinal or epidural anesthesia reduces peripheral vascular resistance by 45-60% and consequently increases blood flow by 40-70% (1.44 to 2.36 ml/100 g of muscle per minute) during the duration of sympathetic blockade [7, 9, 22]. Conversely, peripheral blood flow falls by 10-20% in the first hour, and by 30% in the third hour during general anesthesia. Spinal or epidural anesthesia reduces intraoperative bleeding by 20-50% compared to general anesthesia. In this way transfusion requirement is reduced. BORG [8] AND HENNY [37] have shown on in vitro experimental models that certain local anesthetics at high concentration (25 $\mu g.ml^{-1}$ of lidocaine and bupivacaine hydrochloride) prevent platelet aggregation to collagen and PDA. In clinical practice the concentrations used are weaker (2 $\mu g.ml^{-1}$). However, ODOOM [67] and NIELSEN [66] have shown that spinal or epidural anesthesia inhibitits platelet aggregation to these concentrations. The mechanisms of local anesthesia on the platelets are not precise; that certain receptors are neutralized is probable (GII_b $GIII_a$). Local anesthetic drugs are known to slow down the secretion of catecholamines, whose influence on platelet aggregation has been demonstrated.

Concerning coagulation and fibrinolysis, reports comparing the influence of anesthetic techniques (general and spinal or epidural) are contradictory [61, 62]. General anesthesia reduced coagulation and activates fibrinolysis, whereas postoperatively fibrinolytic activity is reduced and coagulation is activated (acute phase response) [9, 13, 80]. Under local anesthesia the coagulant activity and the fibrinolysis remain unchanged, possibly reduced by the accompanying dilution at first, but then reactivated by a feed back phenomenon [18, 73]. The normalization is quicker postoperatively in concerning the levels of powerful coagulation inhibitors and in particular antithrombin III. Both anesthetic techniques are normally accompanied by hemodilution. In spinal or epidural anesthesia it is higher and systematic, and contributes in increasing the loading volume in order to control the anesthetized region's vasoplegia [28]. It must be noted that plasma substitutes, most often prescribed in hemodilution, play a non-negligible role on the hemostasis and fibrinolysis. Albumin is the most neutral product. On the other hand high molecular weight, hydroxyethyl starch (HES) and high molecular weight dextrans have a Von Willebrand-like activity when they are administered at volumes higher than 1.5 $g.Kg^{-1}$. Solutions of weak concentration or of the lowest molecular weights have fewer effects on the reduction of VIII Von Willebrand and VIII RCO factors. The fibrinolytic activity is most activated postoperatively when the patients are diluted [28]. tPA level increases more quickly than PAI, fibrinogen levels are lowered. The dextrans activate the passage of the fibrinogen in fibrin without modifying the intrinsic and extrinsic fibrinolysis.

Overall the intra and postoperative differences between the two techniques are negligible. They depend more on the conditions in which anesthesia is carried out, the nature of the plasma substitutes which are used and the volume of surgical blood losses. However, in clinical practice spinal or epidural anesthesia expresses a greater reduction in the occurrence of postoperative venous thrombosis in comparison with general anesthesia.

In conclusion, perioperative hemostasis disorders may be responsible for lifethreatening thrombotic or bleeding complications. The prevention of these complications requires early detection, a precise identification and an appropriate correction. The anesthetist is deeply involved in this process.

REFERENCES

1. AIACH M, FIESSINGER JN, CAPRON L, NUSSAS C, HOUSSET E, LECLERC M. Kinetic study of factor X during oral anticoagulation with acenocoumarol: potential value for the initiation of treatment. Thromb Haemost 47, 69-71, 1982.

2. ANSELL J, TIARKS C, HIRSH J, McGEHEE W, ADLER D, WEIBERT R. Measurement of the activated partial thromboplastin time from a capillary (fingerstick) sample of whole blood, a vew method for monitoring heparin therapy. Am J Clin Path 95, 222-227, 1991.

3. ARDLY NG, GLOW G, SCARTZ CJ. Influence of catecholamines on nucleotides induced platelet aggregation. Nature 212, 415, 1960.

4. BELL WR. Heparin-associated thrombocytopenia and thrombosis. J Lab Clin Med 111, 600-605, 1988.

5. BLERY C. Faut-il dresser un bilan de coagulation avant une anesthésie locorégionale chez un sujet ASA 1? Ann Fr Anesth Réanim 9, 371-374, 1990.

6. BOLDT J, ZICKMANN B, BALLESTEROS M, SCHOLZ D, DAPPER F, HEMPELMANN G. Does the preparation of heparin influence anticoagulation during cardiopulmnary bypass? Journal of Cardiothoracic and Vascular Anesthesia 5, 449-453, 1991.

7. BONEU B, CARANOBE C, CADROY Y, DOL F, GABAIG AM, DUPOUY D, SIE P. Pharmacokinetic studies of standard non-fractionated heparin, and low molecular weight heparins in the rabbit. Semin Thromb Hemostas 14, 18, 1988.

8. BORG T, MODIG J. Potential antithrombotic effects of local anesthetics due to their inhibition of platelet aggregation. Acta Anaesthesiol Scand 29, 739-742 ,1985.

9. BOUDAOUD S, EURIN B. L'anesthésie médullaire diminue-t-elle le risque thrombogène de la chirurgie de la hanche? STV 2, 631-633, 1990.

10. BROMAGE PR. Neurologic complication of regional anesthesia for obstetrics. Anesthesia for obstetrics. Second edition. Shnider SM, Levinson G (Eds). Baltimore, Williams and Wilkins. p 320, 1987.

11. BUTLER AB, GRENN CD. Hematoma following epidural anesthesia. Can. Anaesth. Soc J 17, 625-639, 1970.

12. CAMPBELL FW, GOLDSTEIN MF, ATKINS PC. Management of the patient with protamine hypersensitivity for cardiac surgery. Anesthesiology 61, 761-764, 1984.

13. CHIN SP, ABOU-MADI N, EURIN B, WITVOET J, MONTAGNE J. Blood loss in total hip replacement: extradural phenoperidine analgesia. Br J Anaesth 54, 491-494, 1982.

14. CIAVARELLA D, REED RL, COUNTS RB, BARON L, PAULIN E. Clotting factors levels and risk of diffuse microvascular bleeding in the massively transfused patient. Br J Haematol 67, 365-368, 1987.

15. CINES DB, TOMASKI A, TANNENBAUM S. Immune endothelial-cell injury in heparin-associated thrombocytopenia. N Engl J Med 316, 581-589, 1987.

16. COLLINS JA. Recent developments in the area of massive transfusion. World J Surg 11, 75-81, 1987.

17. DARNAT S, GUGGIARI M, GROB R, GUILLAUME A, VIARS P. Un cas d'hématome extradural rachidien au cours de la mise en place d'un cathéter épidural. Ann Fr Anesth Réeanim 5, 550-552, 1986.

18. DAVIS FM, McDERMOT E, HICKTON C, WELLS E, HEATON DC, LAURENSON VG, GILLEPSIE WJ, FOATE J. Influence of spinal and general anesthesia on hemostasis during total hip arthroplasty. Br J Anaest 59, 561-571, 1987.

19. DE ANGELIS J. Hazards of subdural and epidural anesthesia during anticoagulant therapy: A case report and review. Anesth Analg 51, 676-679, 1972.

20. DE SWART CAM, NIJMEYER B, ROELOFS JMM, SIXMA JJ. Kinetics of intravenously administered

heparin in normal humans. Blood 60, 1251, 1982.

21. DICKMAN CA, SHEDD SA, SPETZLER RF, SHETTER AG, SONTAG VKH. Spinal epidural hematoma associated with epidural anesthesia: complications of systemic heparinization in patients receiving peripheral vascular thrombolytic therapy. Anesthesioloiy 72, 947-950, 1990.

22. DONADONI R, BAELE G, DEVULDER J, ROLLY G. Coagulation and fibrinolytic parameters in patients undergoing total hip replacement: influence of the anesthesia technique. Acta Anaesthesiol Scand 33, 588-592, 1989.

23. DOUTREMEPUICH C, SIGONNEY R, BARON JP, REFAUVELET J, LESBURGERES C. Surveillance de l'hypocoagulabilité et de l'héparinémie en chirurgie cardiaque par le temps de coagulation activé. Les Cahiers de CECEC, 33, 23-30, 1990.

24. DRIPPS RD, VANDAM LM. Long-term follow-up of patients who received 10,098 spinal anesthetics: Failure to discover major neurological sequela. JAMA 156, 1486-1491, 1954.

25. DROUET L. Surveillance de l'héparinothérapie au doigt (mais pas à l'oeil). STV 3, 327-328, 1991.

26. DUPEYRAT A, DEQUIRE PM, MEROUAN A, MOULLIER P, EID G. Subrachnoid and spinal anesthesia. Ann Fr Anesth Réanim 9, 550-562, 1990.

27. DUTTON DA, HOTHERSALL AP, McLAREN AD, TAYLOR KM, TURNER MA. Protamine titration after cardiopulmonary bypass. Anaesthesia 38, 264-268, 1983.

28. DUVELLEROY M, DURUBLE M, VICAUT E. L'hémodilution normovolémique. STV 1, 281-286, 1989.

29. ELLISON N, OMINSKY AJ. Clinical considerations for the anesthesiologist whose patient is on anticoagulant therapy. Anesthesiology 39, 328-336, 1973.

30. FOOD, ROSSIER AB. Preoperative neurological status in predicting surgical outcome of spinal epidural hematomas. Surg Neurol 15, 389-401, 1981.

31. GINGRICH TF. Spinal epidural hematoma following continuous epidural anesthesia. Anesthesiology 29, 162-163, 1968.

32. GREENSITE FS, KATZ J. Spinal subdural hematoma associated with attempted epidural anesthesia and subsequent continuous spinal anesthesia. Anesth Analg 59, 72-73, 1980.

33. GROLLMUSS J, HOFF J. Spontaneous spinal epidural haemorrhage: Good results after early treatment. J Neurol Neurosurg Psychiatry 38, 89-90, 1975.

34. HARPER PL, LUDDINGTON RJ, JENNINGS I, REARDON D, SEAMAN MJ, CARELL RW, KLINK JR, SMITH M, ROLLES K, CALNE R. Coagulation changes following liver revascularization during liver transplantation. Transplantation 48, 603-607, 1989.

35. HELPERIN SW, COHEN DD. Hematoma following epidural anesthesia: Report of a case. Anesthesiology 35, 641-644, 1971.

36. HEMKER HC, FRANCK HLL. The mechanism of action to oral anticoagulants and its consequences for the pratice of oral anticoagulation. Haemostasis 15, 263-270, 1985.

37. HENNY CP, ODOOM JA, TEN CATE H, TEN CATE JW, OOSTERHOFF RJ, DABHOIWALA NF, SIH IL. Effects of extradural bupivacaine on the hemostatic system. Br J Anaesth 58, 301-305, 1986.

38. HIRSH J, GALLUS AS. Heparin. In: Hoffbrand AV, Brain MC, Hirsh J (Eds). Recent advances in hematology, Chap. 22. New York: Churchill, Liningstone, pp 453-466, 1967.

39. HOLM HA, ABILDGAARD U, KALVENES S, ANDERSSEN N, ANKER E, ARNESEN KE, BLIKOM D, DRIVENES A. The antithrombotic effect of heparin in deep venous thrombosis: relation to four heparin assays. Acta Med Scand 216, 287-293, 1984.

40. HUNT BJ, COTTAM S, SEGAL H, GINSBURG R, POTTER D. Inibition by aprotinin of tPA-mediated fibrinolysis during orthopedic liver transplantation. Lancet 336, 381, 1990.

41. JACK TM. Subdural hematoma as a complication of spinal anesthetic (letter). Brit Med J 285, 972, 1982.

42. JANIS KM. Epidural hematoma following postoperative epidural analgesia: A case report. Anesth Analg 51, 689-692, 1972.

43. JANVIER G, WINNOCK S, FREYBURGER G. Value of the activated partial thromboplastin time for preoperative detection of coagulation disorders not revealed by a specific questionnaire. Anesthesiology 75, 920-921, 1991.

44. KANE RE. Neurologic deficits following epidural or spinal anesthesia. Anesth Analg 60, 150-161, 1981.

45. KANG YG, MARTIN DJ, MARQUEZ JM, LEWIS JH, BONTEMPO FA, SHAW BW Jr, STARZL TE, WINTER PM. Intraoperative changes in blood coagulation and thromboelastographic

monitoring in liver transplantation. Anesth Analg 64, 888-896, 1985.

46. KAPPA JR, FISHER CA, TODD B, STENACH N, BELL P, CAMPBELL F, ELLISON N, ADDONIZIO VP. Intraoperative management of patients with heparin-induced thrombocytopenia. Ann Thorac Surg 49, 714-722, 1990.

47. KELTON JG, SHERIDAN D, SANTOS A, SMITH J, STEEVES K, SMITH C, BROWN C, MURPHY WG. Heparin-induced thrombocytopenia: Laboratory studies. Blood 72, 925-930, 1988.

48. LAFOREST MD, COLAS-LINHART N, GUIRAUD-VITAUX F, BOK B, BARA L, SAMAMA M, MARIN J, IMBAULT F, UZAN A. Pharmacokinetics and biodistribution of technetium 99m labeled standard heparin and a low molecular weight heparin (Enoxaparin) after intravenous injection in normal volunteers. Br J Haematol 77, 201-208, 1991.

49. LANGLEY PG, KEAYS R, HUGHES RD, FORBES A, DELVOS U, WILLIAMS R. Antithrombin III supplementation reduces heparin requirement and platelet loss during hemodialysis of patients with fulminant liver failure. Hepatology 14, 251-256, 1991.

50. LAURSEN J, FODE K, DAHLERUP B. Spinal epidural hematomas. Clin Neurol Neurosurg 89, 247-253, 1987.

51. LESECHE G, DENNINGER MH. Thrombopénies induites par l'héparine: difficultés diagnostiques, physiopathologiques et thérapeutiques. STV 3, 563-566, 1991.

52. LEYVRAZ PF, RICHARD J, BACHMANN F, VAN MELLE G, TREYVAUD JM, LIVIO JJ, CANDARDJIS G. Adjusted versus fixed dose subcutaneous heparin in the prevention of deep venous thrombosis after total hip replacement. N Engl J Med 309, 954-958, 1983.

53. LOELIGER EA, POLLER L, SAMAMA M, THOMSON JM, VAN DEN BESSELAAR AMHP, VERMYLEN J, VERSTRAETE M. Questions and answers on prothrombin time standardization in oral anticoagulant control. Thromb Haemost 54, 515-517, 1985.

54. LUCAS CH, LEDGERWOOD AM. Clinical significance of altered coagulation. Tests after massive transfusion for trauma. The American Surgeon 3, 125-130, 1981.

55. MAFFRAND JP. Nouvelles thérapeutiques antiagrégantes. STV 2, 175-177, 1990.

56. MAGUIRE T, MAYUMI T, DOLI S. Spinal subarachnoid haematoma after lumbar puncture in a patient receiving antiplatelet therapy. Anesth Analg 62, 777-779, 1983.

57. MAYUMI T, DOHI S. Spinal subarachnoid haematoma after lumbar puncture and heparinization. A case report, review of the literature, and discussion of anaesthetic implications. Anesth Analg 65, 1201-1207, 1986.

58. MESSER HD, FORSHAN VR, BRUST JCM, HUGHES JEO. Transient paraplegia from hematoma after lumbar puncture: A consequence of anticoagulant therapy. JAMA 235, 529-530, 1976.

59. MILLER RD, ROBBINS TO, TONG M, BARTON SR. Coagulation defects associated with massive blood transfusions. Ann Surg 174, 794-801, 1981.

60. MODIG J, MALMBERG P, KARLSTRÖM M. Effect of epidural versus general anesthesia on calf blood flow. Acta Anaesth Scand 24, 305-309, 1980.

61. MODIG J, HJELMSTEDT A, SAHLSTEDT B, MARIPUU E. Comparative influences of epidural and

general anesthesia on deep venous thrombosis and pulmonary embolism after total hip replacement. Acta Chir Scand 147, 125-130, 1981.

62. MODIG J, BORG T, BAGGE L, SALDEEN T. Role of epidural and of general anesthesia in fibrinolysis and coagulation after total hip replacement. Br J Anaesth. 55, 625-629, 1983.

63. MONTALESCOT G. Réactions gravissimes après neutralisation de l'héparine par la protamine. STV 1, 101-105, 1989.

64. MURRAY DJ, OLSON J, STRAUSS R, TINKER JH. Coagulation changes during packed red cell replacement of major blood loss. Anesthesiology 69, 839-845, 1988.

65. NEHLS DG, SHETTER AG, HODAK JA, WAGGENER JD. Chronic spinal epidural hematoma presenting as lumbar stenosis: Clinical, myelographic and computed tomographic features. Neurosurgery 14, 230-233, 1984.

66. NIELSEN TH, NIELSEN HK, HUSTED SE, HANSEN SL, OLSEN KH, FJELDBORG N. Stress response and platelet function in minor surgery during epidural bupivacaine and general anaesthesia: effect of epidural morphine addition. Eur J Anaesth 6, 409-417, 1989.

67. ODOOM JA, SIH IL. Epidural analgesia and anticoagulant therapy. Experience with one thousand cases of continuous epidurals. Anaesthesia 38, 254-259, 1983.

68. OWENS EL, KASTEN GW, HESSEL EA 2d. Spinal subarachnoid hematoma after lumbar puncture and heparinization. A case report, review of the literature, and discussion of anesthetic implications. Anesth Analg 65, 1201-1207, 1986.

69. PAN G, KULKARNI M, MACDOUGALL DJ, MINER ME. Traumatic epidural hematoma of the cervical spine: Diagnosis with magnetic resonance imaging. Case report. J Neurosurg 68, 798-801, 1988.

70. RAO TLK, EL-ETR AA. Anticoagulation following placement of epidural and subarachnoid catheters: An evaluation of neurologic sequela. Anesthesiology 55, 618-620, 1981.

71. REED RL, CIAVARELLA D, HEIMBACH DM, BARON L, PAULIN E, COUNTS RB, CARRICO CJ. Prophylactic platelet administration during massive transfusion. Ann Surg 203, 40-48, 1986.

72. REM J, FEDDERSEN C, BRANDT MR, KEHLET H. Post operative changes in coagulation and fibrinolysis independent of neurogenic stimuli and adrenal hormones. Br J Surg 68, 229-233, 1981.

73. RICHARD LC, BULLER HR, BOVILL J, TEN CATE JW. Influence of anesthesia on coagulation and fibrinolytic proteins. Br J Anaesth 55, 869-872, 1983.

74. ROLBIN SH, ABBOTT D, MUSCLOW E, PAPSIN J, LIE LM, FREEDMAN J. Epidural anesthesia in pregnant patients with low platelet counts. Obstet Gynecol 71, 918-920, 1988.

75. RUDEHILL A, GORDON E, RAHN T. Subdural hematoma. A rare but life-threatening complication after spinal anesthesia. Acta Anaesthesiol Scand 27, 376-377, 1983.

76. RUFF RL, DOUGHERTY JH. Complications of lumbar puncture followed by anticoagulation. Stroke 12, 879-881, 1981.

77. SAMAMA MM, BARA L, CHAPPEY O. Les héparines des bas poids moléculaire. STV 1, 107-117, 1989.

78. SHERRIDAN D, CARTER C, KELTON JG. A diagnostic tests for heparin-induced thrombocytopenia. Blood 67, 27-30, 1986.

79. STEPHANOV S, DE PREUX J. Lumbar epidural hematoma following epidural anesthesia. Surg Neurol 18, 351-353, 1982.

80. STOW PJ, BURROWS FA. Anticoagulants in anaesthesia. Can J Anaesth 34, 632-649, 1987.

81. USUBIAGA JE. Neurological complications of spinal and epidural analgesia. In: Saidman IJ, Moya F (Eds). Complications of anesthesia. Thomas, Springfield, pp 227-240, 1970.

82. VERHAEGHE R. Un traitement antithrombotique pour les prothèses vasculaires des membres? STV 2, 301-303, 1990.

83. WALDMAN SD, FELDSTEIN GS, WALDMAN HJ, WALDMAN KA, ALLEN ML. Caudal administration of morphine sulfate in anticoagulated and thrombocytopenic patients. Anesth Analg 66, 267-268, 1987.

84. WARKENTIN TE, KELTON JG. Heparin-induced thrombocytopenia. Prog Hemost Thromb 10, 1-35, 1991.

85. WULF H, STRIEPLIG E. Postmortem finding after epidural anaesthesia. Anaesthesia 45, 357-361, 1990.

86. ZILKHA A, IRWIN G, FAGELMAN D. Computed tomography of spinal epidural hematomas. AJNR 4, 1073-1076, 1983.

24

Anticoagulation and Audiology

C. Doutremepuich, M.C.Lalanne,

F. Azougagh Oualane

Hearing is the link between people and an important factor in social relationship. Hearing disorders are generally without jeopardy for the life of the patient, but are very uncomfortable and can have an extremely disruptive effect on the patient's day-to-day existence. The causes of hearing impairement are unknown in a large proportion of patients and current therapies are without effect in many cases. It is therefore necessary to search for new ways of comprehension of such phenomena, one approach being the determination of the role of hemostatic disorders.

1. Anatomy

The ear is an organ which includes 3 different parts: the external ear, the middle ear and the inner ear. The inner ear is very complex. It is formed by the bony and the membraneous labyrinths.
The bony labyrinth consists of a cavity (the vestibule), semicircular canals and the cochlea. The membraneous labyrinth which lies within in the bony labyrinth.

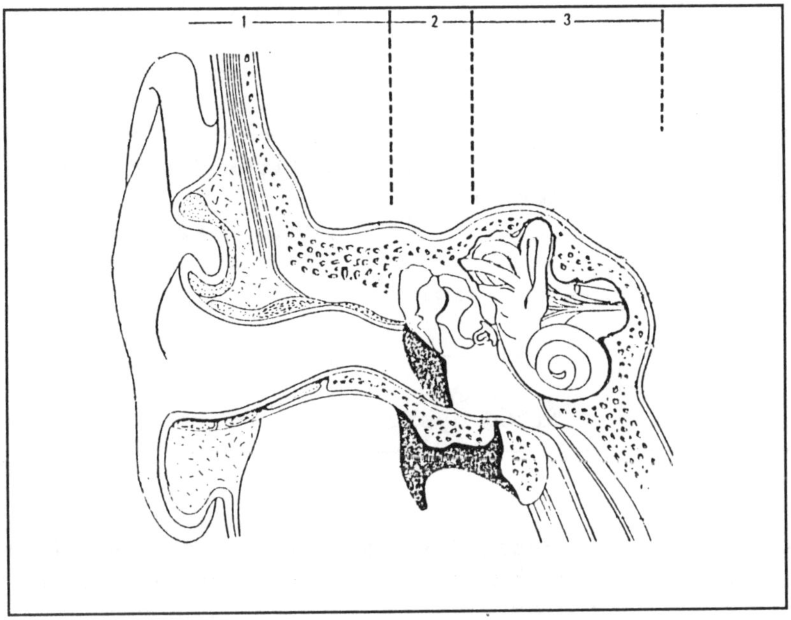

Figure 1: Anatomy of the ear

1: external ear; 2: middle ear; 3: inner ear.

is composed of sacculus and utriculus vestibuli, gives rise to the vestibular nerve (equilibrium), and of the Reissner membrane and the organ of Corti, origin of the cochlear nerve (audition).
Both nerves form the acoustic or vestibulo- cochlear which transmits stimuli to the brain.

2. Pathophysiology

The ear is involved in audition and equilibrium. Sound transmision is effected through the middle and the inner ear. Vibrations are passed on by the liquid of the labyrinth to the organ of Corti, which changes the vibrations into nervous impulses. Information is integrated in the nervous temporal centers.

Table I: Type and nature of audiologic illness

Type	Nature
Mechanical —> lesion —	—> otoliths (middle ear) —> cochleo-vestibular
Drugs ———> ototoxicity	
Vascular —	—> vessel —> ectopic localization —> blood dysfunction —> cell suffering

Equilibrium is determined by the perception of head movements. This perception begins in the vestibule and in the semicircular canals by displacement of the endolymphatic liquid and of little bony fragments, the otoliths, within it. Liquid displacemenIt and pressure variations are converted into nerve impulses.

Labyrinthine dysfunction provokes vertigo, sudden deafness and tinnitus. Mechanical causes of such disorders exist, like a faulty temporo-mandibular joint, an artery rubbing against the auditory nerve among others, but they can also be drug-related [10], noise-related, of central origin, or due to cochlear deterioration [1]. However, vascular modifications are also involved. For example, Ectopia of the jugular dome provokes venous forms of tinnitus, while internal carotid abnormalities (stenosis, tumor...) give rise to arterial forms of this symptom. When vascular abnormalities cause hearing losses and associated disorders, it could be presumed that qualitative modifications of blood components (erythrocytes, platelets or coagulation factors) (associated with trophic insufficiencies) will take an active part in such pathology. In fact, audiologic cells can suffer as a consequence of occlusion of the supplying irrigating vasculature, produced after modification of blood function (hyperviscosity and blood cell hyperactvity).

Hemostatic causes of audiological disturbances are commonly treated by antihistamines or vasodilators, which dilate both arteries and veins. However, if capillary blood function is disturbed such therapy would be insufficient and could be usefully replaced by anticoagulant drugs.

3. Anticoagulant drugs

3.1 Coagulation and thrombosis

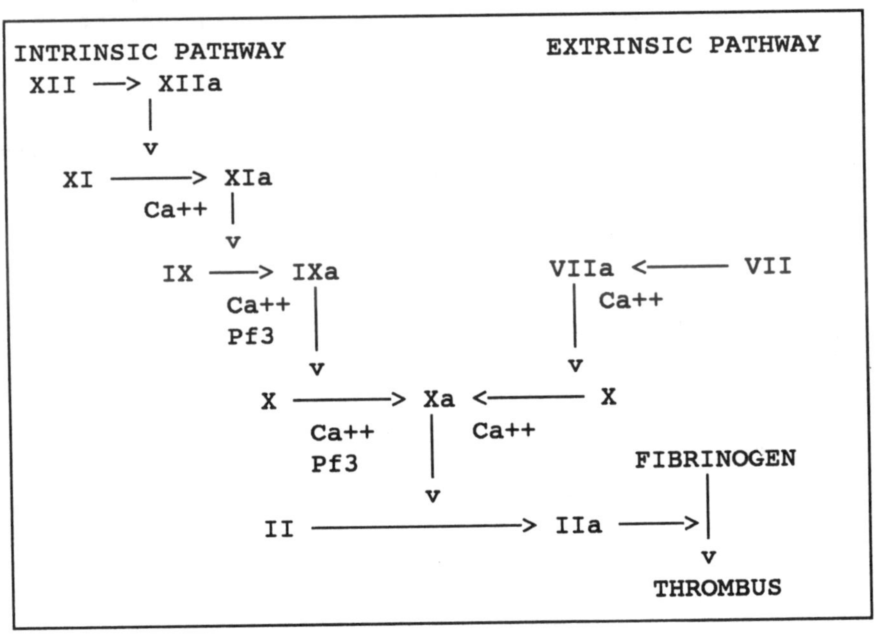

Figure 2: Coagulation cascade

Ca++: Calcium; Pf3: Platelet factor 3

Blood coagulation is a cascade of enzyme reactions initiated through two pathways (extrinsic and intrinsic) after vessel injury. This phenomenon is generally limited by a system of physiological regulation including various factors (mainly activated protein C and antithrombin III (ATIII)).
Deficiencies in this system provoke the appearance of abnormal thrombus formation.

3.2 Vitamin-k antagonists

Vitamin-k catalyzes the carboxylation of τ-carboxyglutamic acid constituents which are very important for phospholipids and calcium binding of coagulation factors. This vitamin k-dependent carboxylase requires the reduced or hydroquinone form of vitamin k, which is converted to its 2,3 epoxide in the course of promoting prothrombin synthesis. Vitamin-k antagonists appear to function by blocking the subsequent reduction of vitamin k epoxide to its hydroquinone form by inhibiting another enzyme, vitamin K epoxide reductase, thus reducing the activity of vitamin k-dependent carboxylase.

3.3 Heparins

Heparin is the most commonly employed drug in antithrombotic therapy. It displays effects on primary hemostasis, reinforces the inhibition of coagulation (ATIII, HCII) and favours fibrinolysis by the release of tPA from endothelial cells. In recent years, new heparin compounds (low molecular weight heparins or LMWH) have been used in humans for their antithrombotic effect, which seems more effective than that obtained with unfractionated heparin at the same dosage [7].

4. What relationship between audiologic disturbances and coagulation ?

A study was performed on seventy-nine patients (45 men, 34 women) suffering from audiologic disorders. Mean age was 61.04 ± 14.06 years. They were investigated by audiograms, electrocochleography and doppler. Four kinds of pathologies were determined using these observations and selected for the study. They were: sudden deafness, presbyacusia, tinnitus and vertigo.

4.1 Hemostatic evaluations

4.1.1 Blood collection and treatment

Blood was collected by venepuncture. The first milliliters were discarded to avoid coagulation. Blood was then drawn into plastic tubes containing either trisodium citrate 3.8% (1:9 V/V) for coagulation and aggregation tests or EDTA, for blood filtration. Part of the citrated blood was then centrifuged for 20 minutes at 1000 rpm to obtain platelet-rich-plasma (PRP) and then, 10 minutes again at 5000 rpm to obtain platelet-poor-plasma (PPP). Blood in EDTA was conserved in a mild warm bath (37°C). Several parameters of the hemostatic system were explored using 3 check-ups: coagulation, primary hemostasis (platelet aggregation) and red cells deformability.

4.1.2 Coagulation check-up

Common tests of coagulation can be used. They are: Prothrombin time (Neoplastine[R], Stago), APTT (CK Prest[R], Stago Laboratories, France), thrombin clotting time (Houdé Laboratories, France), fibrinogen level (Fibritest[R], Stago Laboratories, France) and by the thromboelastogram potential index (or TPI) determined on whole blood (normal value: 6-10) [6].

4.1.3 Platelet aggregation

Two kinds of protocol exist to assess platelet aggregation on plasma using the Born method and on whole blood using Cardinal's device. Aggregation is always measured on an aggregometer (VS 500, Chronolog[R] Coultronics SA - France).

- Aggregation on whole blood

The model chosen was an electrical model [4]. An electrode was mounted in a cap that fits over the top of the cuvette. The conductance between the two electrodes was constant. The temperature of the aggregation module was set at 37°C and a stirring bar was introduced into the test tube. Stirring speed was 1100 r/min. The aggregating reagents were collagen (20 μg/ml final concentration) and ADP (10 μM final concentration, Stago Laboratories, France). Changes (impairment) of conduction between the two electrodes were recorded and analyzed using MERAP[R] software (Coultronic SA, France).

- Aggregation on plasma

The model chosen was the optical method described by Born [2]. The temperature of the aggregation module was set at 37°C and a stirring bar was introduced into the test tube. Stirring speed was 1100 r/min. Upon addition of the aggregating reagent collagen (40 μg/ml final concentration) and ADP (1 and 2 μM final concentration - Stago Laboratories, France), the platelets aggregated and light transmission increased. The changes in light transmission were recorded and the data were automatically analyzed using MERAP[R] software (Coultronic SA, France).

4.1.4 Red cell deformability

Red cell deformability way estimated using the Reid-Dormandy apparatus. One milliliter of whole blood was filtered through a Millipore[R] membrane, under 20 cm water pressure and the filtration time was determined.

4.2 Statistics

Statistical analysis included measurement of means and standard deviation of the mean in each type of pathology (PCSM Deltasoft software, France). Determination of correlation was performed using linear regression. A $p<0.05$ was considered significant.

4.3 Results

Patients were divided into two groups according to the biological observations made.

In group 1, patients presented no hemostatic disorder, while, in group 2, they have one or more defects (table II).

Frequency of abnormal biological haemostatic function increased according to the number of clinical defects. They was a very good correlation ($p<0.01$) between the number of audiologic defects and the number of biological disturbances.

Table II: Frequencies (in %) of biological observations according to the number of audiologic abnormalities

Biological groups	Normal Gr. 1	Abnormal Gr. 2			
		Agg.	Visc.	Coag.	all
		alone or in association			
Clinical defects	(%)	(%)	(%)	(%)	(%)
1 defect observed	47	18	21	14	53
2 defects assoc.	20	26	23	31	80
3 defects assoc.	11	26	10	53	89
4 defects assoc.	0	0	100	0	100

Agg.: aggregation; Visc.: viscosity; Coag.: coagulation; assoc.: associated

No statistical variation was observed in platelet count, hematocrit, fibrinogen level or any other coagulation test except TPI. Examination of biological evaluation in these patients showed that biological defects were observed in 70% of the patients studied.

5. Place of anticoagulant therapy in audiologic disturbances

A most commonly-held concept in medicine is that illness has "large" pathophysiological origins like trauma, lesions or thrombosis in main vessels, etc. However, it appears that from this study tiny modifications in microcirculation, like capillaries occlusion, is also capable of producing serious pathology. In a previous study [9], we already demonstrated that occlusion of microvessels, perhaps by catecholamine- dependent anoxia, provokes a decrease of the trophic blood flow in the ear. In this study on 20 patients suffering from Menière's disease, coagulation was disturbed in 90% of cases. Normalization of TPI by calcium heparin treatment led to the disappearence of vertigo. Recent work has demonstrated the involvement of hyperlipidemia and hyperviscosity in audiological disturbances. As shown in the current study, hypercoagulability was the most frequently present defect [5] and reinforces the value of anticoagulant treatment in this type of illness. Heparin is indicated in that it presents both anticoagulant and antilipidemic effects [3, 11]. However, it has the disavantage of a greater risk from hemorrhage and is more uncomfortable in daily use than low molecular weight heparins. Association of heparin fractions and anti-aggregating drugs (like aspirin) at a low dose to reduce bleeding risk could be a good alternative when coagulation and platelet activation have been observed.

A new area of research is then open and could bring new solutions to an old problem: what do in audiologic disorders when classical treatments have no effect?

REFERENCES

1. ALLEVA M, LOCH W, PAPARELLA M. Tinnitus. Prim.Care, 17 (2), 289-297, 1990.

2. BORN G, CROSS M. The aggregation of blood platelets. J Physiol (London) 168, 176-195, 1963.

3. BROWNING G, GATEHOUSE S, LOWE G. Blood viscosity as a factor in sensorineural hearing impairment. Lancet 1, 121-123, 1986.

4. CARDINAL D, FLOWER R. The electronic aggregometer: a novel device for assessing platelet behaviour in blood. J Pharmacological methods, 135-158, 1980.

5. COURTENEY-HARRIS R, FORD G, INNES A, COLIN J. Pulsatile tinnitus: three cases of arteriovenous fistula treated by ligation of the occipital artery. J Laryngol Otol 104(5), 421-422, 1990.

6. DOUTREMEPUICH C. A propos de l'étude biologique de la maladie de Ménière et du syndrome mébiériforme: note préliminaire. Rev Laryng 95 (1-2), 45-48, 1975.

7. DOUTREMEPUICH C, LALANNE MC, DOUTREMEPUICH F, PUYAL C. Low molecular weight heparins today: pharmacological considerations. In: "Low molecular weight heparins in clinical practice". Marcel Dekker, New York, pp 85-96, 1992.

8. HAZELL J, JASTREBOFF P. Tinnitus I: Auditory mechanisms: a model for tinnitus and hearing impairment. J Otolaryngol 19(1), 1-5, 1990.

9. PORTMANN M, DOUTREMEPUICH C, BEBEAR JP, VAZEL P. Données complémentaires sur l'étude de la maladie de Ménière et des syndromes méniériformes. Rev Laryng 96 (5-6), 45-48, 1975.

10. STYPULKOWSI P. Mechanisms of salicylate ototoxicity. Hear Res 46 (1-2), 113-145, 1990.

11. ZHANG O. Mechanism of inner ear damage to hyperlipidemia. Chung Hua Erh Pi Yen Hou Ko Tsa Chih 24 (2), 75-78, 1989.

25

Use of anticoagulants and antithrombotics in dermatology

O. Gauthier

The cutaneous vascular network is the area into which the arterial circulatory flow spreads and is the origin of the return venous circulatory flow. In addition, the skin possesses its own vascular network which makes it the predominant domain for microcirculation. Thus, in patients with skin diseases one meets the consequences of disorders of the systemic circulation and also specific disorders of the cutaneous circulation itself.

A patient suffering from a dermatological complaint is also often found to be suffering from another disorder requiring treatment which we shall call non-specific and which one can find in any other branch. The dermatologist is thus confronted with non-dermatological indications for use of anticoagulants and true dermatological indications.

1. Non-specific indications

Concern the classic use of anticoagulants such as in the prevention of thromboembolic events or in the treatment of a general cardiovascular disorder and is usually only a continuation of a course of treatment prescribed by another specialist.

2. As to actual cutaneous disorders we shall look at various uses of anticoagulant treatments

2.1 The Kasabach-Merrit syndrome or thrombopenia-hemangioma syndrome is one case where conventional hematological treatment is required

Here we have a complication occuring in infants or small children where large angioma suddenly present signs of inflammation and take on an ecchymotic and distended aspect evoking thrombosis. The platelet count shows a thrombopenia of around 30 000 platelets. There is a phenomenon of sequestration, activation and platelet consumption occuring inside the vascular malformation. In capillaro-venous malformations, phenomena of disseminated intravascular coagulation syndrome can occur locally with evocative biological signs and require urgent heparinotherapy whereas this is not usually the case with hemangiomes. This infrequent disorder aside, indications requiring the use of anticoagulants or antithrombotics essentially consist of disorders of microcirculation.

2.2 Cutaneous microcirculation disorders

Non-fractioned heparin has been used for a long time, especially for its anti-inflammatory and healing properties, but since treatment was constrictive it was, and remains, little used.

There are almost no indications for Antivitamin K.

Low Molecular Weight Heparins constitute an interesting but recent acquisition and we will developed this aspect farther on in the article.

There will most certainly be indications for the use of fibrinolytics, especially the new preparations which are easier to handle and carry fewer risks, but their use has still to be codified [3].

Disorders in microcirculation of the dermis are indications where Low Molecular Weight Heparins can be used. Apart from their antithrombotic and anticoagulant properties, Low Molecular Weight Heparins activate tissue, as does non-fractioned heparin but it would seem in a more marked way, in particular tissular mechanisms [4] in endothelial cells and this can be exploited in the treatment of microangiopathies, in particular their antithrombogenic activity. This activity is the result of the three-way interaction of Low Molecular Weight Heparins with endothelial cells: they increase the synthesis or liberation of t-PA whence a local profibrinolytic effect; they increase the synthesis or liberation of prostacyclin metabolites; they interact with the thrombine fixed on the endothelial cells.

Heparin is in part fixed by the endothelial cells and takes part in their intense physiological activity in several ways. Endothelial cells, platelets and fibrinoleucocytary film and glycocalix combined make up a functional ensemble whose roles and complexity we are starting to understand. The endothelial cell and its environment [1] thus participate in several physiological processes: hemostasis, coagulation, fibrinolysis; exchanges with plasma and the sub-endothelial extracellular matrix, in particular by its action on fibrinogen IV and fibronectin; action on angiogenesis and thus on the processes of tissular healing. In this respect, the importance of the angiogenic cofactors of heparin - thrombine, platelet growth factor, fibroblast growth factor, macrophage growth factor, protein C and its cofactor of endothelial origin, Factor S and thrombomodulin - must be noted.

The action concerning inflammation and immunity brings into play interleukines, prostaglandins, adhesion molecules or integrins, immunoglobulines and endothelial leucocyte adhesion molecules, cells of circulating blood, in particular monocytes and polynuclears. In addition, Low Molecular Weight Heparins react with numerous plasmatic proteins and play a role in the phosphorylation of cell receptors. It is possible to imagine that Low Molecular Weight Heparins, used therapeutically, might have an action linked to its effect on hemostasis and fibrinolysis and also to its effect on microcirculation, and the hinge it constitutes in the tissular processes of nutrition, gas exchange, neoangiogenesis and healing, and in the processes of inflammation and immunity.

Indications for this type of treatment in microangiopathies are essentially:

- necrotic angiodermititis,
- microangiopathies of diabetes with ulceration,
- ulcers occuring during hypertension and inflammatory vascularitis, such as in rheumatoid arthritis,
- ulcers on "atrophie blanche" [2]

2.2.1 Necrotic angiodermititis with cutaneous ulcers or gangrene in superficial patches is a consequence of cutaneous microinfractions by thrombosis in arterial or venous vessels in the middle dermis or at the junction of dermis and hypodermis. The usual etiology is senile microangiopathy (atherosclerosis) occuring in elderly patients outside of any major arterial disease. The physiological hypercoagulability of the elderly could be one of the favoring factors. The ulcerated zone often appears following a traumatism which would appear to trigger an extensive process of cutaneous necrosis. This necrosis concerns superficial cutaneous and subcutaneous layers and can extend as far as the apeunoris and superficial tendon and is accompanied by considerable pain, recurring nocturnally. The necrosis evolves with no sign of regression for several weeks, abraded away at one edge of the lesion while on other patches it stops without any particular reason and spontaneous healing occurs. This type of necrotic angiodermititis occurs on the legs and the lesions can often spread round the whole member before their progress stops spontaneously. Numerous types of treatment have been proposed, including heparin, antisludge platelets and nonsteroidal anti-inflammatory, but without any conclusive results.

2.2.2 The same type of leg ulcers caused by necrotic angiodermititis can be found as a complication in diabetes, arterial hypertension and in number of inflammatory processes such as rheumatoid arthritis and other disorders [6].

Protocol for use of Low Molecular Weight Heparins:

Various Low Molecular Weight Heparins can be used. Among those which are at present available in France we used the following:

- Fraxiparine: 0.6 ml per day, or 15000 U anti-Xa IC,
- Enoxaparine: (Lovenox): 0.8 ml/day, or 8000 U anti-Xa IC,
- Fragmine: 0.4 ml/day, or 5000 U anti-Xa IC.

The product was injected subcutaneously in a single daily injection. The duration of treatment was from 20 to 30 days, depending on the particular case.

The results were essentially judged on clinical criteria: effect on pain, on the extension of necrosis, on signs of healing. In this latter case the effects were particularly favorable and very rapid. As early as the third or fourth day of treatment, pain which is usually intolerable began to subside and necrosis began to stop its progression. Around the tenth day progression had entirely ceased and signs of healing had begun to appear and were confirmed in the following days. Progressive healing required a variable amount of time depending on the extent of the lesions and the general condition of the patient but seemed to be largely favorably influenced by this treatment in comparison with what experience has shown of spontaneous evolution. The result appears to be dose-dependent. Trial treatment using lower doses (0.3 ml/SC per day of Fraxiparine, 0.2 ml/SC per day of Enoxaparine) showed favorable results but less clearly marked. The use of higher doses than those prescribed for preventive treatment does not seem to have any drawback, except perhaps for some temporary bleeding in layers around the lesions in a few, rare patients (especially noted with the use of Enoxaparine).

The biological tests carried out did not show any anomalies at the tolerance level and did not seem to contraindicate treatment of elderly patients.

Insofar as ulcers caused by diabetic microangiopathy, hypertensive ulcers and those caused by inflammatory microangiopathy in patients with rheumatoid arthritis are concerned, the results were also favorable, with cessation of the extension of necrosis and evolution towards healing in a much shorter time that is usually observed.

2.2.3 Ulcers on "atrophie blanche"

"Atrophie blanche" is a dermatosis which occurs on the legs and is often complicated by very painful ulcerations which tend to drag on.

It is characterized by the appearance on the skin of small white lesions which are slightly sunken and ivory white, surrounded by a pigmented ring with dilated capilliaries grouped in patches. These lesions correspond to the obstruction of the superficial vessels of the dermis by deposits of fibrin. These deposits are clearly visible under the electronic microscope. A rare, primitive form has been described as occuring in young women and it is characterised by the onset of recurring ulcerations of the legs with no apparent cause. Of the secondary forms, which are more frequent and which have various etiologies, the most common forms are venous circulatory problems and stasis. The primum movents appears to be an early form of fibrinolysis caused by the non liberation of the activator of plasminogen which causes cutaneous ischemia and its attendant atrophy.

The protocol used:

The same Low Molecular Weight Heparins, at the same doses and for the same duration. The favorable clinical effects were evident in the ulcerated areas. Alleviation of pain appeared in a few days and healing of lesions rapidly thereafter. The area healed using this treatment showed a good quality skin appearance and not the white, atrophied and fragile area left after spontaneous evolution. The patches of "atrophie blanche" neighbouring the ulcerated zone did not seem to evolve much during the time we had the patients under observation.

3. Cutaneous complications in circulatory problems of the veins

Apart from "atrophie blanche", circulatory problems in the veins of the lower limbs (varicosis, and epecially post-phlebitic disorders) are usually complicated by inflammatory cutaneous and subcutaneous disorders. These are cases of inflammatory hypodermatitis evolving to envelop cutaneous sclerosis and sometimes towards interstitial calcinosis. It is in these zones that the ulcerations appear subsequently.

In a good number of the patients treated, the Low Molecular Weight Heparins used following the same protocol brought improvement, especially on the level of acute pain and inflammation, without however resolving all the problems.

4. Varicose phlebitis

The frequent complications of varicosis are characterized by the sudden onset of inflammatory phenomena on a superficial varicose segment which is thrombosed. The varicose vein looks like a bright red cord and is extremely painful.

The protocol consisted of daily subcutaneous injections of Low Molecular Weight Heparins in the doses already mentioned, over a period of ten days and outside of all concomitant treatment. The patient could go about his normal activities.

Results :

Favorable results can be noted within a few days: pain is alleviated, inflammation diminishes progressively. The biopsy of the thrombosed fragment taken on the tenth day of treatment showed evident signs of repermeabilization of the vein. Normally, it is not necessary to carry out a phlebotomy to remove the clots and sometimes the varicosis repermeabilizes and reconstitutes itself spontaneously. A short course of treatment seems to be enough. The various properties of Low Molecular Weight Heparins seem to be put to good use in this indication.

5. Exceptional problems

Some disorders pose problems which still have to be solved but the use of anticoagulants or the new types of fibrinolytics would appear to be possible here.

Behçets syndrome would appear to be in part due to problems of local liberation of t-PA, especially insofar as cases of superficial phlebitis are concerned.

Our experience is limited to a single case of superficial phlebitis of the veins of the forearm after venous puncture. The use of Low Molecular Weight Heparins at previously mentioned doses over a period of 10 days enabled almost complete recovery in two weeks.

Antiphospholipid Syndrome is of interest to the dermatologist especially in cases of Sneddon's disease, the anomalies of factors of hemostasis being outside of our domain.

Sneddon's disease is characterized by the appearance of livedo reticularis and the onset of multiple vascular events. Its prognosis is not good.

Histology shows thrombosis in both veins and arteries of the dermis with no major signs of inflammation but with characteristic anomalies of the endothelial cells [7]. These cells are rich in Weibel-Palade corpuscles and have a "hobnail" aspect.

The appearance of antiphospholipid antibodies directed against the endothelial cells and platelets would appear to be responsible for the livedo. This should enable early diagnosis and thus a course of treatment which will have to be defined and codified.

Treatment of other rarer disorders which are also characterized by thrombosis of microcirculation could be envisaged but this is the realm of the future.

6. Conclusion

Current use of anticoagulants and antithrombotics in dermatology is more especially centered around disorders of microcirculation and Low Molecular Weight Heparins.

Their efficiency has been proved in the case of necrotic angiodermititis and microangiopathic ulcerations. Superficial varicose phlebitis are also an excellent indication.

Repeat treatments can be envisaged since the short duration of prescription offers little chance of complications appearing, if one excepts risk of thrombopenia.

The fibrinolytic properties of these Low Molecular Weight Heparins enable vascular repermeabilization of the venous network which is of great interest. The disabling sequellae of phlebitis could perhaps be diminished if Low Molecular Weight Heparins were used in their treatment.

REFERENCES

1. CLAUDY AL. La vascularisation cutanée. Angiogénèse. Structure et fonction des cellules endothéliales. Ann Dermatol Vénéréol 118, 61-68, 1991.

2. GAUTHIER O, LEROUX E. Utilisation d'une héparine de bas poids moléculaire dans le traitement des ulcères de jambe par microangiopathie. Nouv Dermatol 7, 637-640, 1988.

3. LABLANCHE JM. Les thrombolytiques. La Revue du Praticien 39(3), 259-262, 1989.

4. MOLHO P, TOBELEM G. L'héparine hier et aujourd'hui. Médecine/Science 85(1), 74-79.??

5. PRIOLLET P. Atrophie blanche. Ann Dermatol Vénéréol 114, 1005-1008, 1987.

6. RISPAL-CASTANO J. Utilisation d'une héparine de bas poids moléculaire: la Fraxiprine dans le traitement des ulcères de jambe par microangiopathie et des thrombophlébites veineuses superficielles. Thesis. Bordeaux, n° 34, 1989.

7. SMITH KJ, SKELTON HG 3d, JAMES WD, ANGRITT P, SCHERBENSKE J, VAUGHAN K, LUPTON GP. Cutaneous Histopopathologic Findings in "Antiphospholipid Syndrome". Correlation with disease, including human immunodeficiency virus disease. Arch Dermatol 126, 1176-1183, 1990.

26

Anticoagulation and hepatocellular disfunction

L. Schouler, G. Janvier, P. Couzigou

1. Liver function in hemostasis

1.1 Hepatic synthesis

The liver plays a major role in the synthesis of coagulation and fibrinolytic factors [30]. Majority of clotting factors (I, II, V, VII, IX, X, XI, XIII prekallickrein, light molecular weight kininogen), inhibitors of both coagulation and fibrinolysis (protein C, protein S, antithrombin III, heparin cofactor II and antiplasmin) and fibrinolytic proteins (plasminogen) are principally synthetized by liver cells.

Factor VIII and factor Willebrand are produced by vascular endothelial cells [7, 63]. However, the low molecular weight procoagulant part of factor VIII (VIII: C) seems to be synthetized by liver [50].

Extrinsic pathway inhibitor (factor VIII a tissue factor complex and factor Xa) could be produced by endothelial cells [2].

Synthesis of vitamin K dependent factors (II, VII, IX, and X) is dependent on both liver production and vitamin K. This vitamin is necessary for the insertion of a second carboxyl group into the gamma-carbon of glutamic acid residues, which confers coagulant activity on the precursor proteins [13].

Des-gamma-carboxy prothrombine (DCP) is a protein induced by vitamin K absence or antagonist (PIVKA), and can be detedted in plasma [5, 38, 44]. DCP is found in blood of vitamin K's deficient patients or receiving vitamin K antagonist or suffer from hepatocellular carcinoma [38, 44]. DCP can be equaly found, at lower level, in serum of cirrhotic patients [28, 52].

1.2 Hepatic clearance of clotting factors

Liver cells are also responsible of coagulation factors clearance, with elimination of activated clotting factors and fibrinogen degradation product [19, 32].

2. Hemostasis abnormalities during hepatic diseases "spontaneous anticoagulation"

2.1 Disease synthesis of coagulation and inhibitor factors

All clotting factors production could be defective in hepatopathy, especially in fulminant hepatic insufficiency or in cirrhosis, because of deficient hepatic synthesis.

Biological traduction of this abnormality, because of extrinsic factors deficiency, is a prolonged prothrombin time in 70 percent of cirrhotic patients [18]. Owren's thrombotest which explores factors II, VII, IX and X, normotest which is not affected by

PIVKA presence in the plasma and cephalin or partial thromboplastin time are also frequently abnormal in severe liver disease. Prothrombin time is commonly considered as the more useful clinical screening test to appreciate liver hemostatic factors production and hepatopathy liver function. Vitamine K dependant factors could be more decreased than factor V in cirrhosis probably in part because of associated cholestasis. However, factor V is more specific, as independant vitamine K factor to appreciate the liver function [13].

Fibrinogen level, without disseminated intravascular coagulation (DIC) or fibrinolysis is low only in 15 percent cirrhosis [15]. So decrease rate of this clotte factors is not a specific or early sign of hepatocellular defect [46]. Prolonged thrombin time is frequent in severe liver disease despite normal fibrinogen level [24]. Impaired function of fibrinogen, linked with structural modification is described, even with normal quantity of fibrinogen. One hypothesis, is an impairement of fibrin polymerization may be due to excess of sialic acid in ß and α fibrinogen chains [42].

Factors of contact phase of intrinsic coagulation (factors XI, XII, prekallikrein and kininogen) are also deficient in liver disease. The more severely affected and earliest decreased is prekallikrein which has been proposed as a useful test in hepatic failure [20, 64].

On the contrary, factor VIII (coagulant activity and related antigen) and factor Willebrand levels are raised in alcoholic and non alcoholic cirrhosis [23, 47]. To explain this increase, a diminution of hepatic clearance seems more probable than an increment of production [30, 36].

Plasma proteins inhibitors (antithrombin III, protein C) are also decreased during cirrhosis [1, 61, 66]. The most important of them (antithrombin III) could be at a very low level and severely umbalanced activators and inhibitors factors of coagulation with major risk of hemorrhage or thrombotic diathesis [14].

2.2 Decrease hepatic clearance

Hepatic clearance of clotting factors is also impaired during liver disease, with an important result on haemostasis. So, when coagulation factors are activated, survival in plasma of these factors is abnormaly lengthened and expose to DIC [14]. The best demonstration of the decrease of hepatic catabolism is the evidence of thrombosis and DIC in case of cirrhosis patients who received concentrates which contain activated clotting factors [6, 49].

3. Fibrinolysis and disseminated intra-vascular coagulation

Accelerated lysis of clotted blood from cirrhotic patients, in vitro, is well known [22, 32, 58]. The explanation is probably a reduction of clearance plasminogen activators [21] and an impairement of synthesis fibrinolytic inhibitors [32, 58].

In vivo, authors found and elevated level of plasminogen activator antigen (T-PA) in blood of cirrhotic individuals with accelerated fibrinolysis [8, 26]. They supposed that some patients with liver disease have an insufficient inhibition of T-PA activity, responsible of exagerated fibrinolysis.

Accelerate fibrinolysis, raised of fibrinogen degradation product (FDP), low clotting factor levels, and thrombocytopenia are frequent biological facts in cirrhosis.

That is the reason why many authors suggested a permanent low-grad of disseminated intravascular coagulation during cirrhosis [10].

This concept is supported by the reversal of such abnormalities with heparin therapy [29, 59]. In fact, other studies demonstrate only a pronlongation of fibrinogen's survival, but not of platelets with heparin treatment [53].

The mecanism of DIC in hepatocellular deficiency is controversial, but it seems that low rate of antithrombin III could play an essential part in this phenomenon [13, 15, 36, 41, 62].

This concept is contested in a recent revue [10]. DIC is considered as an unusual component in coagulation cirrhosis. An argument in favor of limited cases of DIC in severe liver disease, is a serie of 184 autopsies of cirrhotic patients that show up only 4 thrombosis disease [45]. The main critic of this study is the possibility of post-mortem fibrinolysis.

In the same way, level reduction of extrinsic pathway inhibitor has been described in patients with DIC, but not in patients with severe liver disease [2]. This discovery suggests that DIC is not a component of cirrhosis's coagulopathy. However, abnormal coagulation of this patients is an increased risk for DIC [10]. The evidence for increased risk is the frequency of DIC during infection [12], hemorrhage [10] or after peritoneo-jugular shunt [9].

Another study of 35 cirrhotic patients, demonstrated no proof of plasmin degradation fragments in plasma or serum, for 80 percent of them. The remaining 20 percent patients had circulating plasmin degradation fragments and an additional illness (sepsis, shock or pancreatic carcinoma) to liver disease [60].

The detection of DIC of patients with hepatocellular dysfunction is not easy. Diagnosis can be established by the decrease of fibrinogen level and correlative rise of FDP and D-dimer levels [10, 11].

Primary haemostasis abnormalities :

Thrombocytopenia is common during cirrhosis [15], With intravascular platelet half-life decrease [53, 57]. Increased spleen sequestration, in link with portal hypertension, is the major factor of low platelets count. Other possible causes of thrombopenia in liver disease are defective folic acid and vitamin B_{12} [53], megakaryocyte depression in alcoholic patients and immunological factors [4, 34].

At low rate, trombocytopenia in cirrhosis contribute in hemorrhage predisposition. In contrast, role of defective platelet function is not clear and very controversial.

Studies report defective platelet aggregation and prolonged bleeding time with bleeding manifestation in cirrhosis individuals [55, 56]. An explanation is the inhibiting role of FDP accumulation in cirrhotic plasma [55]. Another cause, would be a membrane phosphatid lipid abnormality with deficiency prostaglandin synthesis [33].

However, other study including 60 cirrhotic patients failed to demonstrate significant platelet defect function [3].

4. Therapy by coagulation inhibitors and hepatopathy

4.1 Invasive procedure or major surgery and hepatopathy

In case of compensated hepatopathy with normal haemostasis, heparin and/or antivitamin K may be used, sometimes for a prolonged prescription of antivitamin K for example, in case of major cardiac surgery for valvulopathy.

In case of abnormal haemostasis, antithrombin III supplementation reduces heparin requirement and also platelet loss during hemodialysis of patients with hepatic failure [36]. Antithrombin III therapy is also benefit in invasive techniques requiring anticoagulation in patients whth hepatopathy and decreased coagulation protein. Before prothrombin complexes infusion, antithrombin III will be administered. The eventual therapeutic role of protein S and C in similar situations is not well known. Heparin administration in disseminated intravascular coagulation is not recommended. Although heparin therapy combined with plasma infusions may correct the coagulation disturbance, heparin itself may cause massive bleeding [27]. However if in general disseminated intravascular coagulation may not be clinically significant in liver disease, it is of importance in patient with peritoneojugular shunt [25], Aprotinin, naturally occurring inhibitor of human plasmin and kallikrein, has a great potential in hepatic surgery, especially in orthotopic liver transplantation [40]. In case of abnormal primary hemostasis, desamino D arginyl vasopressin (DDAVP) is useful. Platelet concentrates should be given to correct severe thrombocytopenia (less than 70000/mm^3) and problems of platelet dysfunction. Epsilon aminocaproïc acid also may be given to patients who show active fibrinolysis.

4.2 Therapy for haemorrhage in liver disease

Fresh frozen plasma supplies all the missing clotting factors but has the potential risk of viral transmission. Prothrombin complexes have a more important risk of thromboembolic episodes due to the presence of actived coagulation factors. Association with antithrombin III is useful: antithrombin III concentrates have been effective in disseninated intravascular coagulation, fulminant hepatitis and also to prevent thrombosis after liver transplantation in children. So antithrombin III administration must precede infusion of prothrombin complexes or has to be realize if fresh frozen plasma administration excede 2 liters/24h. Fibrinolysis inhibitor may be useful, as tranexamic acid which has proven efficacy in severe gastrointestinal bleeding treatment with vitamin K should be give if there is evidence of vitamine K deficiency but should be discontinued if there is no further reponse after two days treatment. Platelet concentrates should be given to correct severe thrombocytopenia (less than $70000/mm^3$) and problems of platelet dysfunction.

Desamino D arginyl vasopressin (DDAVP) cause a rise of factor VIII C and von Willebrand factor levels. DDAVP has been shown to return the prothrombin time to normal in cirrhotics and to shorter or normalize the bleeding time.

5. liver toxicity of anticoagulant drugs

5.1 Parenteral anticoagulation

HEPARIN: Two studies reported moderate transaminase elevation with heparin used [43, 51]. This abnormality occured in more of 70 percent of cases, with normalization despite continuation of therapy.

None severe or clinical manifestation of hepatitis was attributed to heparin.

5.2 Enteral anticoagulation

PHENINDIONE: is the major, prothrombin synthesis inhibitor which can induce hepatic injury [37, 39]. Generalized hypersensitivity manifestation with nephropathy occured in 1 to 3 percent with hepatic injury in about 10 percent of these cases [48]. Liver injury is both cytotoxic and cholestative but never sufficiently severe to cause liver failure [65]. This anticoagulant has been generaly abadonned in favor of the coumarin derivatives [54].

WAFARIN: is responsive of experimental steatosis in animals and perhaps implicated in severe liver injury cases, but only when it was taken in overdose [65].

COUMARIN: was occasionaly incrimined in liver injury, but not conclusively. In a recent study [16], 2 cases of transaminase elevation during coumarin therapy were observed in 2173 treated patients (0.37 %). Jaundice after phenprocoumon therapy with recurrence after re-exposure has been reported [17].

REFERENCE

1. AUROUSSEAU MH, D'ANGELIS JI, JOSSO F. Antithrombine III versus prothrombin in liver cirrhosis. Haemostasis 10 , 104-107, 1981.

2. BAJAJ MS, RANA SU, WYSOLMERSKI RB, BAJAJ SP. Inhibition of the factor VII a tissues factor complex is reduced in patients with dissiminated intravascular coagulation but not in patient with severe hepatocellular disease. J Clin Invest 79, 1874-1878, 1987.

3. BALLARD HS, MARCUS AJ. Platelet aggregation in portal cirrhosis. Ann Intern Med 136, 316-319, 1976.

4. BARRISON IG, KNIGHT ID, VIOLA L, BOOTS MA, MURRAY-LYON IM, MITCHELL TK. Platelet associated immunoglobulins in chronic liver disease. Br J Haematol 48, 347-350, 1981.

5. BLANCHARD RA, FURIE BC, JORGENSEN M., KRUGER SF, FURIE B. Aquired vitamin K - dependent carboxylation deficiency in liver disease. N Engl J Med 305, 242-248, 1981.

6. BLATT PM, LUNDBLAD RL, KINGDON HS, MC LEAN G, ROBERTS HR. Thrombogenic materials in prothrombin complex concentrates. Ann Int Med 81, 766-770, 1974.

7. BLOOM AL, PEAKE IR, GIDDINGS JC, SHEARN SAM, TUDDENHAM EGD. Endothelial cells and factor VIII related protein. Lancet 1, 46, 1976.

8. BOKS A, BROMMER EJP, SCHALIN SW, VAN VLIET HH. Hemostasis and fibrinolysis in severe liver failure and their relation to hemorrhage Hepatology 6, 79-86, 1986.

9. BÜLLER HR, TEN CATE JW. Antithrombin III infusion in patients undergoing pertitonio-venous shunt operation: failure in the prevention of disseminated intravascular coagulation. Thromb Haemost 49, 128-131, 1983.

10. CARR JM. Disseminated intravascular coagulation in cirrhosis. Hepatology 10, 103-110, 1989.

11. CARR JM, McKINNEY M, McDONAGH J. Diagnosis of DIC: role of D-dimer. Am J Clin Pathol 91, 280-287, 1989.

12. CASH JD. Disseminated intravascular coagulation. In: Poller L (Ed). Recent advances in blood coagulation. Edimburgh, London and New-York, Churchill Liningstone, pp 293-311, 1977.

13. CHILSHOW M. Hematological disorders in liver disease. In: Wright R, Millward-Sadler GH, Alberti KGMM, Karraud S (Eds). Liver and biliary disease: pathophysiology, diagnosis,

management. Philadephie, Saunders WB, pp 189-214, 1985.

14. COLMAN RW, RUBIN RN. Blood coagulation. In: Arias IM, Jakoby WB, Popper H, Schachter D, Shofritz DA (Eds). The liver: Biology and pathobiology. New-York, Raven Press, pp 1033-1042, 1988.

15. CONARD J, CERTIN M, SAMAMA M, OPOLON P. Les troubles de la coagulation au cours des cirrhoses et leur traitement. In: Loygue J (Ed). Traitement des cirrhoses du foie. Paris, Masson, pp 188-200, 1975.

16. COX D, O'KENNEDY R, THORNES RD. The rarety of liver toxicity in patients treated with coumarin (1,2 - Benzopyrone). Hum Toxicol 8, 501-506, 1989.

17. DE-MAN RA, WILSON JH, SCHALM SW, TEN-KATE FJ, VAN-LEER E. Phenprocoumon induced hepatitis mimicking non A, non B hepatitis. J Hepathol 11, 318-321, 1990.

18. DEUTSCH E. Blood coagulation changes in liver diseases. Prog Liver Dis 2, 69-83, 1966.

19. DEYKIN D, CHUN R, LOPEZ A, SILVERSMITH P. The role of the liver in serum induced hypercoagulability. J Clin Invest 45, 256-263, 1966.

20. FISHER A, SCHMAIER AH, ADDONIZO V, COLMAN RW. Assay of plasma prekallikrein: comparison of amidolytic, esterolytic coagulation and immunological assay. Blood 59, 963-970, 1982.

21. FLETCHER AP, BIERDERMAN O, MOORE D et al. Abnormal plasminogen-plasmin system activity (fibrinolysis) in patients with hepatic cirrhosis: its cause and consequences. J Clin Invest 43, 681-695, 1964.

22. GOODPASTURE EW. Fibrinolysis in chronic hepatic insufficiency. Johns Hopkins Hosp Bull 25, 330-336, 1914.

23. GREEN AJ, RATNOFF OD. Elevated anti haemophiliac factor (AHF factor VIII) procoagulant activity and AHF - like antigen in alcoholic cirrhosis of the liver. J Lab Clin Med 83, 189-197, 1974.

24. GROLWICK HR, GIVERBER H, ABRAMS E. Dysfibrinogenemiea associated with hepatoma. Increased carbohydrate content of the fibrinogen molecule. N Engl J Med 299, 221-226, 1978.

25. HARMAN et al. Ann Int Med 90, 774, 1979.

26. HERSCH SL, KUNELIS T, FRANCIS RB Jr. The pathogenesis of accelerated fibrinolysis in liver cirrhosis: a critical role for tissue plasminogen activator inhibitor. Blood 69, 1315-1319, 1987.

27. HILLENBRAND P, PARBLHOO SB, TEDRYCHOWSKI A, SHERLOCK S. Significance of intravascular coagulation and fibrinolysis in acute hepatic failure. Gut 15, 83-88, 1974.

28. HO CH, LEE SD, CHANG HT, WU JC, TSAI VT, LO KJ. Application of des-gamma-carboxy prothrombin as a complementary tumor marker with α-fetoprotein in the diagnostic of hepatocellularcarcinoma. Scand J Gastroenterol 29, 235-240, 1989.

29. HORDER MH. Consumption coagulopathy in liver cirrhosis: Thrombosis and diathesis. Haemorrhagica 36 (Suppl), 397-401, 1969.

30. KELLY DA, SUMMERFIELD JA. Hemostasis in liver disease. Sem Liver Dis 7, 182-191, 1987.

31. KRONINGER C, STARSEN JM, COLLEN D. Turnover of human extrinsic (tissue type) plasminogen

activator in rabbits. Thromb Haemost 46, 658-661, 1981.

32. KWAAN HC, McFADZEAN AJS, COOK J. Plasma fibrinolytic creativity in cirrhosis of the liver. Lancet 1, 132-136, 1956.

33. LAFFI G, COMINELLI F, RUGGIERO M, FEDI S, CHIARUGI V, GENTILINO P. Molecular mechanism underlying impaired platelet responsiveness in liver cirrhosis. FEBS lett 220, 217-219, 1987.

34. LANDOLFI R, LEONE G, FEDELI G. Platelet associated igG in acute and chronic hepatic disease. Scand J Haematol 25, 417-422, 1980.

35. LANGLEY PG, HUGHES RD, WILLIAMS R. Increased factor VIII complex in fulminant hepatic failure. Thromb Haemost 54, 693-696, 1985.

36. LANGLEY PG, KEAYS R, HUGHES RD, FORBES A, DELVOS U, WILLIAMS R. Antithrombin loss hemodialysis of patients with fulminant hepatic failure. Hepatology 14, 251-256, 1991.

37. LEVINE WG. Anticoagulant, antithrombotic and thrombolytic drugs. In: Goldman LS, Gilman A, Koell AG(Eds). The pharmacological basis of therapeutics, 5th Ed. Macmillan, New-York, p 1350, 1968.

38. LIEBMAN HA, FURIE BC, TONG MJ, BLANCHARD RA, LO KJ, LEE SD, COLEMAN MS, FURIE B. Des - gamma - carboxy (abnormal) prothrombin as a serum marker of primary hepatocellular carcinoma. N Engl J Med 310, 1427-1431, 1984.

39. MAKAUS N, VAANDER VEER JB. Severe drug sensitivity to phenindione (phenyl-indanedione) JAMA 155, 739-741, 1954.

40. MALLET SV, COX D, BURROUGHS AK, ROLLES IC. Aprotinin and reduction of blood loss and

transfusion requirements in orthotopic liver transplantation. Lancet 336, 886-887, 1990.

41. MANNUCCI E, DIAGUARDI N, EL NINNO E, MANNUCI PM. Value of thrombotest and antithrombine III in the assessment of liver function. Scand J Gastroenterol 19 (suppl), 103-107, 1973.

42. MARTINEZ T, KEANE PM, GILMAN PB. The abnormal carbohydrate composition of the dysfibrinogenimia associated with liver disease. A NY Acad Sci 408, 388-396, 1983.

43. MINAR, EHRINGER H, HIRSCHL M, INGERLE H, KONECHY U, MAROSI L, ENDLER T, GABL F, DEUTSCH E. Transaminasenaustieg: eine weitgehend unbekannte nebenwirkung der heparinotherapie. Dtsch Med Wochenschr 105: 1713-1717, 1980.

44. NAKAO A, SUZUKI Y, ISSHIKI K, KIMURA Y, TAKEDA S, KIHIMOTO W, NONAMI T, HARADA A, TAKAGI H. Clinical evaluation for plasma abnormal prothrombin (des - gamma - carboxy prothrombin) in hepatobiliary malignancies and other diseases. Am J Gastroenterol 86, 62-66, 1991.

45. OKA K, TANAKA K. Intravascular coagulation in autopsy cases with liver diseases. Thromb Haemost 42, 564-570, 1979.

46. OLIVER JM, GRUEL Y, BACQ Y. Anomalies de l'hémostase au cours des hépatopathies. Gastroenterol Clin Biol 15, 679-688, 1991.

47. OUTRYVE M, VAN BAELE G, WEERDI GA, BARBIER F. Antihaemophilic factor A (F VIII) and serum fibrin - fibrinogen degradation products in hepatic cirrhosis. Scand J Haematol 11, 148-152, 1973.

48. PERKINS J. Phenindione sensitivity. Brit Med J 1, 127-130, 1962.

49. RUBIN RN. Disseminated intravascular coagulatin. Transfusion 17, 198-201, 1977.

50. SHAW E, GIDDING JC, PEAK IR, BLOOM AL. Synthesis of procoagulant factor VIII, factor VIII related antigen and other coagulation factors by the prolated perfused rat liver. Br J Haematol 41, 585-596, 1979.

51. SONNENBLICK M, OREN A, JACOBSONN W. Hypertransaminasemia with heparin therapy. Brit Med J 3, 77, 1975.

52. SOULIER JP, GOZIN D, LEFRERE JJ. A new method to assay des - gamma - carboxy prothrombin as a serum marker of primary hepatocellular carcinoma. Gastroenterology 91, 1258-1262, 1986.

53. STEIN SF, HORKER LA, Kinetic and functional studies of platelets, fibrinogen, and plasminogen in patients with hepatic cirrhosis. J Lab Clin Med 99, 217-230, 1982.

54. STRICKER BHC, SPOELSTRA P. Drug induced disorders. Vol 1 Drug Induced hepatic injury. Elsevier Amsterdam - New York - Oxford , pp 112-116, 1985.

55. THOMAS DP. Abnormalities of platelet aggregation in patients with alcoholic cirrhosis. Am NY Acad Sci 201, 243-250, 1972.

56. THOMAS DP, REAM VJ, STUART RK. Platelet aggregation in patient with Laennec's cirrhosis of the liver. N Engl J Med 264, 1344-1348, 1967.

57. TOGHILL AJ, GRENN S. Platelet dynamics in chronic liver disease using the 111 Indium oxine label. Gut 24, 49, 52, 1983.

58. TYTGAT G, COLLEN D, DE VREKER R et al. Investigation on the fibrinolytic system in

liver cirrhosis. Acta Haematol 40, 265-274, 1968.

59. TYTGAT GM, COLLEN D, VERSTRAETE M, Metabolism of fibrinogen in cirrhosis of the liver. J Clin Invest 50, 1690-1701, 1971.

60. VAN DE WATER L, CARR JM, McDONAGH J. Analysis of elevated fibrinogen degradation product levels in patients with liver disease. Blood 67, 1468-1473, 1986.

61. VIGANO S, MANNUCI PM, D'ANGELO A, RUMI MG, VIGANO P, DEL NINNO E, CARGNEL A, COLOMBO M, PODDA M. The significance of protein C antigen in acute and chronic liver biliary disease. Am J Clin. Pathol 84, 454-458, 1985.

62. VON KAULLA E, VON KAULLA KN. Antithrombine III and diseases. Am J Clin Pathol 48, 69-80, 1967.

63. WION KL, KELLY D, SUMMERFIELD JA, TUDDENHAM ED, LAWN RM. Distribution of factor VIII in RNA and antigen in human liver and other tissues. Nature 317, 726-729, 1985.

64. WONG PY, COLMAN RW, TALAMO RL, BABIOR BM. Kallikrien bradykinin system in chronic liver disease. Am Intern Med 77, 205-207, 1981.

65. ZIMMERMAN HJ. Hepatotoxicity, Appleton - Century - Crofts, New-York, p 510, 1978.

66. ZURBORN KH, KIRCH W, BROHN HD. Immunological and functional determination of the protease inhibitors, protein C and antithrombine III, in liver cirrhosis and in neoplasia. Thromb Res 52, 325-336, 1988.

27

Anticoagulation and the kidney

C. Combe, M. Aparicio

Activation of local and systemic coagulation processes are induced by several renal diseases and may require specific anticoagulation therapy. The first parts of this chapter are devoted to these topics, including the influence of hemostasis and anticoagulation on the course of renal failure.

The last sections of the chapter deal with the implication of hemostasis and anticoagulation in therapies used in patients with renal failure, namely hemodialysis, peritoneal dialysis, and kidney transplantation.

1. Local and systemic hemostasis in kidney diseases

Activation of blood coagulation and fibrin deposition are common events in some forms of human and experimental glomerulopathies (GN) and are thought to play an important pathogenetic role in the development and the progression of the disease [31, 38, 40, 41]. On the other hand, chronic renal failure is associated with several disorders of platelet function and the coagulation pathway which induce a bleeding tendency in uremic patients [3, 18, 36, 55]. In this section, we will discuss first the pathophysiological aspects of local and systemic hemostasis disorders associated with different types of clinical of experimental nephropathies; the second part of this section will be devoted to the analysis of the disorders of hemostasis and coagulation associated with uremia.

1.1 Local hemostasis and fibrinolysis in glomerular diseases

The hemostatic system within the renal glomerulus

Procoagulant and anticoagulant compounds are both synthesized in the normal unstimulated glomerulus [38]. Thromboplastin, which is necessary for the activation of the extrinsic coagulation pathway, has been found in glomeruli isolated from normal rat [17], rabbit [33], and human [74] kidneys. Both epithelial and mesangial glomerular cells are able to produce thromboplastin [21, 81]. This synthesis can be stimulated by TNFα in cultured mesangial cells [81]. Other factors which have a putative hemostatic effect are found in the normal glomerulus, such as extra-cellular matrix or glomerular basement membrane components like collagen, heparan sulfate and fibronectin [38], or other factors involved in the hemostatic process like von Willebrand factor [75] or thrombospondin (60).

Lipid mediators are produced within renal glomeruli [14, 54]. The synthesis of prostacyclin, which can inhibit platelet aggregation, is stimulated by vasoconstricting agents [5]. On the other hand, an increase in the production of thromboxane within the glomerulus has been advocated in the pathogenesis of glomerular thrombosis such as in the hemolytic uremic syndrome [61]. The aggregation of platelets is also stimulated by platelet activating factor (PAF), the synthesis of which by isolated glomeruli can be enhanced by several agonists [14].

The presence of several components of the fibrinolysis system within the kidney, particularly in the glomerulus is well documented [4, 38, 67]. The effect of factors of fibrinolysis like urokinase and tissue- type plasminogen activators [4, 67] is balanced by the antifibrinolytic activity of other compounds such as plasminogen activator inhibitors [44].

In conclusion, several components which can modulate platelet function, coagulation and fibrinolysis are found in the normal glomerulus. Their synthesis can be influenced by several agonists, particularly mediators of inflammation. These mediators can be generated as a consequence of the infiltration of glomeruli by blood-borne leukocytes in several human or experimental GN, leading to the activation of local coagulation and the formation of glomerular fibrin deposits [38].

The role of intraglomerular coagulation in the progression of chronic renal failure

Chronic renal insufficiency, once established, tends to progress to end-stage renal failure [42]. Although several factors contribute to this progression, such as abnormal intrarenal physical forces, systemic hypertension, hyperlipidemia, calcium and phosphate deposits, factors released by infiltrating inflammatory cells and by intrinsic glomerular cells [42], intra- glomerular coagulation may also contribute to the progression of glomerular sclerosis. In an experimental model consisting in rats subjected to subtotal nephrectomy, the administration of heparin reduces glomerular sclerosis [58]. Because heparin affects clotting, it has been suggested that local activation of the coagulation process may play a part in glomerular sclerosis. Nevertheless, this protective effect of heparin may also be explained by its antiproliferative properties, particularly on glomerular mesangial cells [15].

Experimental and human renal diseases with fibrin deposits in the glomeruli or in the renal vessels

Glomerular fibrin deposits are found in several types of acute nephropathy. In acute renal failure due to bilateral cortical necrosis, a rare affection in man, microthromboses in the glomeruli and renal vessels are constant and extensive [38, 41]. On the contrary, when acute tubular necrosis underlies the mechanism of acute renal failure, glomerular fibrin is seldom found [38]. Acute renal failure may arise during the course of several disorders associated with disseminated intra-vascular coagulation, which can worsen the course of renal failure. This is the case of obstetric complications such as pre-eclamptic toxemia [41], and of acute renal failure due to pancreatitis of septicemias.

Intra-glomerular fibrin deposists are found in various types of experimental GN such as Masugi's nephritis [79] chronic serum sickness nephritis [8], or auto-immune nephritis in NZB mice [45]. Human GN are accompanied by less fibrin deposits than experimental animal GN; the mechanisms leading to the deposits of fibrin seem to be related to alterations in renal fibrinloysis. Extracapillary fibrin deposits in human GN contain significant amounts of the plasminogen activator inhibitor type I [66]; in another study, both plasminogen activator and urokinase activity were reduced in the urine of patients with renal function impaired by various types of GN [16].

1.2 Systemic hemostasis in patients with the nephrotic syndrome

The most striking abnormalities of hemostasis have been described in patients presenting the nephrotic syndrome but without renal failure [37, 56]. This condition is accompanied by an increased tendency to thrombosis first reported by Addis in 1948 [1]. Since then, thrombotic complications have frequently been observed in nephrotic patients in both venous and arterial systems [1], with a high frequency of renal vein thrombosis, now to be considered as a complication of the nephrotic syndrome, while in the past it was considered as a cause [1]. Renal vein thrombosis is a superimposed feature of a number of GN, chiefly membranous GN, mesangiocapillary GN, and of lupus nephritis and amyloidosis accompanied by the nephrotic syndrome [28]. The tendency of nephrotic patients to thrombotic episodes has been attributed to a state of hypercoagulability [28]. There may be an increase in fibrinogen levels and an elevation of the levels of factors V, VII, VIII-Von Willebrand, and X, with a mild increase in the platelet count and a significant increase in platelet adhesiveness and aggregation [56]. Antithromin III (heparin cofactor) levels may be normal or greatly reduced [19, 56], especially in patients with severe hypoalbuminemia, probably because of urinary losses. Protein C and protein S levels are usually normal or increased in the nephrotic syndrome, but the functional activity of these proteins may be reduced, contributing to the hypercoagulable state [28]. Urokinase inhibitors and antiplasmins were found increased not only after, but also before a venous occlusion test [56]. Fibrinogen degradation products have been found in the urine of nephrotic patients, but not in their sera [56]. Unfortunately, there is currently no evidence that one or several particular abnormalities are responsible for thrombogenesis or that factors permitting to predict the risk of thrombosis in the individual nephrotic patient exist [38].

1.3 Hemostasis in chronic renal failure

Bleeding is a common complication of uremia [3, 18, 22]. The modern management of renal failure has greatly reduced the incidence of severe hemorrhages, but bleeding still presents a problem for uremic patients, particularly during surgery or invasive procedures. Most of the problems are due to platelet dysfunction and abnormalities in the interaction of platelets and the vessel wall. There is a direct correlation between prolongation of the bleeding time and reduced platelet adhesion with clinical bleeding in uremic patients. Neither platelet count nor platelet half-life are significantly altered in uremia [3]. In contrast, defects in platelet function have consistently been reported [3, 18, 19]; both platelet adhesive- ness and aggregation in response to various agonists (thrombin, adenosine diphosphate, and epinephrine) are impaired. The availability of platelet factor 3 (PF3) is diminished [22]. Several studies have demonstrated abnormal prostaglandin metabolism in the platelets of uremic patients, with a deficient synthesis of thromboxane B2 and a functional cyclo- oxygenase defect [3, 19, 62]. These modifications of platelet cyclooxygenase metabolism are potentiated by modifications of vascular production of cyclooxygenase products [63]. In uremia, although concentrations of von Willebrand factor (vWF) and factor VIII are normal, modified platelet membrane receptors for vWF binding may explain the impaired platelet-vessel wall interaction and the bleeding tendency [22]. More recently, Remuzzi has suggested that endothelium-derived relaxing factor (nitric oxyde) can also be a mediator of the bleeding tendency of uremia [64].

Uremic factors are also probably involved in the genesis of the platelet defect of uremic patients [3]. Platelet function is improved, although not normalized, by intensive dialysis [46]. Guanidinosuccinic acid, phenols and phenolic acid inhibit platelet aggregation at concentrations approximating those found in uremic patients [34, 59]. Increased levels of parathyroid hormone, associated with the secondary hyperpathyroidism of chronic renal insufficiency, has been implicated as a contributing cause of uremic platelet dysfunction [36].

Several methods have been used to correct the bleeding tendency of uremic patients. The most important is hemodialysis: as stated above, uremic factors are implicated in the pathogenesis of platelet dysfunction. Although there is no close relationship between blood urea nitrogen (BUN) levels and bleeding complications, the risk of bleeding increases when BUN concentrations exceed 100 mg/dl [3]. Thus, dialysis may be helpful by lowering BUN levels and removing other putative factors affecting bleeding tendency [3, 19]. A synthetic analogue of antidiuretic hormone, 1-deamino-8-D-arginine vasopressin (DDAVP), shortens the bleeding time of uremic patients [3, 18, 48] presumably by relasing factor VIII vWF from the vascular endothelium. In patients with severe uremic bleeding, a correction of the bleeding tendency has been achieved with the infusion of cryoprecipitate [18, 35]. Ten bags of cryoprecipitate are generally sufficient to make the bleeding time return to its original value within 24 hours [35]. The hematocrit also affects platelets function. Transfusion of red cells to raise the hematocrit above 30% shortens the bleeding time, as does the correction of renal anemia by treatment with recombinant human erythropoietin [2, 22, 50].

2. Anticoagulation in patients with renal diseases

2.1 Influence of anticoagulation on the course of glomerulonephritis

Although in several types of experimental animal nephropathies, the administration of antiplatelet or anticoagulant drugs has been shown beneficial [38, 42, 58], no clearly convincing data have been demonstrated in human GN despite logical arguments to treat these diseases with anticoagulants [28, 38]. For example, since fibrin-related antigens are frequently demonstrated in the lesions of idiopathic crescentic GN type I, the use of anticoagulants in conjunction with steroids and cytotoxic agents has theoretical merit [28]. Nevertheless, patients with anti glomerular basement antibody disease may be at special risk because of the possible presence of pulmonary hemorrhage and the coagulation disorders present in uremia; the need to perform a renal biopsy may pose an additional problem [28]. In acute extracapillary GN with fibrin deposits heparin appears at best as an adjuvant to the immunosuppressive therapy [38]. Uncontrolled therapeutic trials with the defibrinating agent ancrod have given encouraging results in severe lupus nephritis [39] and in other types of GN [38], but have to be confirmed. In chronic GN, few therapeutic trials of antiplatelet or anticoagulant agents have been performed. In a trial in patients with primary IgA GN (Berger's disease), a combination of aspirin and dipyridamole was not any more effective than placebo in preserving renal function [28]. Two studies have been carried out in patients with membrano-proliferative GN [20, 84]. In the first one [84], patients were treated with a combination of dipyridamole and warfarin for one year, and with placebo for another year. Renal function determined from the slope of the reciprocal of serum creatinine values versus time remained stable in the treatment period, but worsened during the control period. In a prospective, randomized, double- blind, placebo-controlled trial, treatment with a combination of dipyridamole and aspirin induced less progression to end-stage renal disease and a higher glomerular filtration rate than in the placebo group [20]. In a short term study including patients with membranous GN, mesangial IgA GN and segmental and focal hyalinosis, dipyridamole induced a significant decrease of proteinuria, compared to placebo, but no significant effect on renal function was demonstrated [12].

In conclusion, despite a certain involvement of platelet activation and intraglomerular coagulation in various GN, the results of the clinical studies conducted so far are controversial and do not allow conclusions about the efficacy of anticoagulant and antiplatelet agents in the progressive renal disease.

2.2 Anticoagulation in patients with nephrotic syndrome

As stated above, there is an increased frequency of deep venous thrombosis in patients with nephrotic syndrome. Nevertheless, the prevention of venous thrombosis in these patients is debated, notably because one cannot reliably predict the patients who are at the highest risk for thrombotic events [38]. Some authors recommend to begin anticoagulant therapy when serum albumin concentration is lower than 15 g/l [38, 13].

The prognosis of any GN may be worsened by a superimposed acute renal vein thrombosis, but it is not yet certain whether the slow development of chronic renal vein thrombosis accelerates the rate of progression of chronic renal insufficiency [28].

In acute renal vein thrombosis, there is no discussion about the necessity of anticoagulant therapy, since these patients are exposed to an increased risk of pulmonary emboli. However, the choice of the drug may be difficult [38]. In case of very low plasma antithrombin III concentration and high α-2-macroglobulin concentration, heparin may be inefficient and may even diminish the antithrombin activity of the latter [24]. On the other hand, the use of antivitamin K drugs may be difficult in case of variations of albumin concentration, to which they are bound [13].

In cases of chronic renal vein thrombosis, anticoagulation has little effect on renal function, and thrombosis may reoccur in the recanalized vessels when anticoagulants are discontinued [28]. Anticoagulants are mainly prescribed to prevent pulmonary thrombotic emboli.

2.3 Anticoagulation in patients with chronic renal failure

Renal insufficiency per se is not an indication for anticoagulation. Nevertheless, patients with renal failure, whether acute or chronic, may need anticoagulation therapy. Impaired renal elimination of drugs can modify their therapeutic efficacy. This can be the case with anticoagulants.

Influence of renal failure on the metabolism of standard heparin

The metabolism of standard unfractionated heparin relies on two mechanisms. The first one is a saturable mechanism depending on the reticuloendothelial system and endothelial cells. Heparin is metabolized by this cellular system and its metabolites are excreted in urine; at high heparin doses, the cellular system is saturated and heparin is excreted directly in urine by a second mechanism [29]. However, the doses of heparin used in clinical practice are below the saturation limit of the cellular system of elimination and therefore heparin metabolism does not necessitate renal intervention [29]. In summary, the utilization of standard heparin in patients with renal failure requires no other adaptations then those necessitated by the increased risk of bleeding of these patients. The efficacy of the anticoagulation will be monitored exactly as it is in other patients.

Low molecular weight heparins (LMWH) and renal failure

The metabolism of LMWH is different from that of standard heparin. The cellular system of elimination of LMWH is saturated at low concentrations. Therefore, renal elimination plays a major role in the clearance of LMWH [7, 29]. Studies of LMWH in patients with chronic renal failure have demonstrated variable alterations of the pharmacokinetic parameters with the impairment of renal function. The elimination of CY 216 has been found not to depend on renal function [29] while the elimination of enoxaparine has been found delayed in patients with chronic renal insufficiency [11]. Nevertheless, the half-life of disappearance of the antifactor Xa activity was significantly prolonged with both types of LMWH. Therefore, the utilization of LMWH in patients with chronic renal failure requires a close monitoring of antifactor Xa activity to avoid a possible accumulation phenomenon [29].

Coumarin-type drugs and renal failure

After absorption in the stomach and jejumum, coumarin drugs are bound to albumin and distributed in the intravascular and interstitial spaces. Free drug is then taken up by hepatocytes where it blocks vitamin K metabolism. The coumarins are inactivated by hepatic microsomal enzymes and the resulting coumarin metabolites are either excreted into the bowel by the enterohepatic circulation or filtered and excreted by the kidneys [32]. Renal function does not influence the activity of coumarin drugs, since an impairment in renal function affects only the excretion of inactive metabolites. Never- theless, renal diseases accompanied by hypoalbuminemia, like the nephrotic syndrome, can increase the proportion of the free drug in the blood, and therefore increase its effectiveness [32]. The dose of coumarin derivatives in patients with hypoalbuminemia must be decreased; the daily dose should be adjusted according to the usual laboratory tests (such as the prothrombin time).

3. Hemostasis and anticoagulation in dialysis patients

Anticoagulation in patients on dialysis is a complex multifaceted problem. First, patients who need to be hemodialyzed present the specific defects of platelet function and coagulation linked to uremia. We have previously underlined the partial correction of the bleeding tendency in uremia achieved by hemodialysis. Second, dialysis alters coagulation through the exposition of blood to an extracorporeal circuit and the artificial membranes of the dialyzer. This interaction is thrombogenic, therefore the hemodialysis procedure requires an efficient anticoagulation procedure. Third, hemo- dialysis may modify the pharmacokinetics of anticoagulants, and thereby their therapeutic efficacy. Lastly, patients who need to be hemodialyzed have an increased risk of bleeding, particularly in cases of acute renal failure. These different aspects of anticoagulation in dialysis will be discussed in the following sections.

3.1 Effect of dialysis on coagulation

During hemodialysis, the blood is exposed to several artificial components, including the dialyzer membrane and extracorporeal circulation tubing. Plasma proteins adsorb to the hemodialysis membrane, and this in turn can lead to the activation of the intrinsic blood coagulation system [49]. When the fibrinogen layer exceeds 200 nm in thickness, the modified surface promotes platelet adhesion, leading to the formation of platelet aggregates and release of coagulation factors, including the potent phospholipid factor [43]. Thrombin is also adsorbed on hemodialysis membranes in a biologically active form, and can further enhance the activation of platelet adhesion and aggregation. During the platelet release reaction which follows platelet-foreign surface contact, platelet factor 3 is released and amplifies the classical coagulation pathway [47]. The subsequent adhesion of leukocytes and erythrocytes can lead to the formation of a mural thrombus in the artificial circuit [47, 49]. The type of dialyzer membrane determines the range of activation of coagulation during hemodialysis. Less biocompatible membranes (of a cellulosic type) induce a greater activation of coagulation than do biocompatible membranes made of such synthetic polymers as polyacrylonitrile, polysulfone [71, 80]. The activation of coagulation which occurs during a dialysis session is correlated with other so-called biocompatible events such as thrombocytopenia and leukopenia [49, 80]. In summary, the contact of blood with artificial materials, particularly dialyzer membranes, leads to the activation of coagulation, of various intensity according to the biocompatibility of the membrane.

3.2 Effect of dialysis on the elimination of anticoagulants

The dialysis procedure has little effect on the metabolism of the most commonly used anticoagulants. The elimination of heparin is not modified by hemodialysis, since its clearance does not rely on renal function [6]. LMWH are not eliminated by dialysis either, because they are linked to Antithrombin III, the molecular weight of which is 65,000 daltons, above that of ultrafiltered molecules. Since they are normally excreted in part by the kidney, their elimination is delayed in patients on dialysis [11, 72]. Antivitamin K drugs are not eliminated by dialysis, because of the high proportion of drug bound to albumin [47].

3.3 Anticoagulation in dialysis

Systemic heparin anticoagulation for chronic hemodialysis

Heparin is the most commonly used anticoagulant during hemodialysis. Never- theless, it is not an ideal anticoagulant. Heparin has no inhibitory effect on the platelet-foreign surface interaction [43, 47]. It has been demonstrated that heparin administered alone can even augment platelet adhesion [77]. Thrombus formation can take place upon the membranes of the artificial kidney in spite of adequate systemic heparinization. The nature of the dialysis membrane and the geometry to which that membrane conforms are important [47, 71].

Anticoagulation of patients during a dialysis session is usually achieved by a loading dose of heparin, followed by a constant infusion through the venous line of the extracorporeal circuit. The dosage varies within the dialysis population. It can not be estimated solely upon the basis of the patient's body weight [47]. To determine the minimal effective heparin dose, repeated measurements of the whole blood activated clotting time (WBACT) are performed during dialysis. Mathematical models of the utilization of heparin during dialysis have been developed, but they are not routinely used in clinical practice [23, 69]. When the patient is established on a regular hemodialysis schedule, the WBACT is monitored monthly to adapt heparin dosage. As a matter of fact, heparin requirements of a given patient can vary with time, for example because of the correction of the bleeding tendency of uremia by dialysis [3, 19]. If any untoward clotting or hemorrhagic tendency appears, urgent reassessment of the heparinization schedule should be made [47]. If clotting episodes occur despite adequate WBACT, the platelet function of the patient should be determined, particularly the release of platelet factor 4 and its heparin neutralizing activity. If the activity of the platelets is enhanced, the patient should be treated with an antiplatelet agent, such as aspirin at a low dose [47]. Heparin-induced immunologically mediated thrombocytopenia is a rare event in patients on regular hemodialysis. This is the indication of anticoagulation by alternative approaches.

Low molecular weight heparins for chronic hemodialysis

LMWH have a weaker anticoagulant activity and a longer half-life than standard heparin [51, 72]. These properties permit the use of a single dose injected at the beginning of the dialysis session. The clinical effectiveness is determined by assessing the quality of the restitution of the blood contained in the extracorporeal circuit at the end of the dialysis session. As a matter of fact, the determination of the anti-X-activated activity cannot be performed as easily as WBACT can be in the monitoring of heparin anticoagulation.

The efficacy of LMWH and heparin in preventing clotting in the extracorporeal circuit is equivalent [70]. Fibrinopeptide A levels in the plasma, which reflects the transformation of fibrinogen into fibrin [82], have been found equivalent with LMWH and heparin [51].

The main advantage of LMWH versus heparin resides in the use of a single injection for dialysis anticoagulation. Nevertheless, the higher cost of these heparins reduces their utilization.

Anticoagulation for dialysis in patients at high hemorrhagic risk

Strategies have been developed to perform dialysis in patients with a high hemorrhagic risk, for instance uremic patients with digestive bleeding, surgical patients, patients with intracranial hematoma...

Minimal heparinization is based on the utilization of half of the usual heparin dose required by a given patient, with a termination of the infusion 30 min before the end of the dialysis session [47]. Close monitoring of the WBACT and of the extracorporeal circuit avoids massive clotting of the circuit.

Regional heparinization requires the continuous infusion of protamine before the blood returns to the patient. This technique also requires a close monitoring of WBACT to avoid a clotting of the circuit, and the utilization of a low dose of protamine to avoid an "heparin rebound" phenomenon at the end of dialysis [47]. Protamine can also be used at the end of dialysis in hemorrhagic situations.

Dialysis can be performed without any anticoagulation. The extracorporeal circuit and the dialyzer need to be flushed with 0.9% saline every 15 min to detect partial clotting and to prevent hemoconcentration [47, 68]. If partial clotting can not be avoided, minimal heparinization must be performed.

Prostacyclin, a naturally occuring metabolite of arachidonic acid produced by vascular endothelia, raises the level of platelet cyclic adenosine monophosphate and thereby inhibits platelet aggregation and the release of platelet coagulation factors [43]. It has been successfully used to prevent clotting during dialysis, alone [73, 85] or in combination with heparin [43]. Its clinical use is limited because of its high cost and induction of hypotension due to its vasodilating properties. Regional citrate anticoagulation has been used for patients considered at risk for bleeding and in those with sensitivity to heparin resulting in thrombocytopenia [25, 57]. Citrate acts by binding the ionised calcium, thus making it unavailable to participate in the clotting cascade. The potential secondary effects of citrate anticoagulation are metabolic alkalosis and hypocalcemia.

4. Anticoagulation in patients treated by peritoneal dialysis

Peritoneal dialysis is increasingly used in the treatment of end-stage renal failure. Intraperitoneal fibrin formation induces peritoneal adhesions and catheter obstructions that jeopardize the long-term use of peritoneal dialysis [27, 76]. Heparin is added to the inflow dialysate to prevent fibrin formation and catheter obstruction [76]. Intraperitoneal fibrin formation can be inhibited even during peritonitis by the intraperitoneal infusion of heparin [30].

5. Hemostasis and anticoagulation in kidney transplant patients

Severe kidney allograft rejection is associated with local vascular thrombosis, interstitial fibrin deposits, and eventually with evidence of systemic intravascular coagulation [38]. In 17 irreversibly rejected human renal allograft, Rondeau et al. found that the glomerular fibrinolytic activity was decreased in the 5 cases in which tissue damage was maximal [66].

Renal endothelium is the first target of anti-HLA antibodies or of alloactivated cells during kidney rejection, with subsequent release of thromboplastin, platelet adhesion and activation [38]. T cells may release cytokines which activate the release of various cytokines and modify the local equilibrium between thromboxane and prostacyclin. Isolated glomeruli from chronically rejected kidneys synthetise larger amounts of procoagulant thromboxane B_2 than glomeruli from normal kidneys [26]. Among several cytokines implied in allograft rejection, TNFα stimulates the procoagulant activity of the endothelium [53].

In summary, coagulation is activated during kidney allograft rejection because of specific immune mechanisms (anti-HLA antibodies and alloactivated T cells), and of non specific mechanisms of renal inflammation (secretion of cytokines and imbalance in the production of prostaglandins).

Cyclosporine A (CsA), the major immuno- suppressive drug used in organ transplantation since the early eighties, has several adverse effects; among them, an increased tendency to deep vein thrombosis and pulmonary embolism in patients receiving the drug has been reported [78]. This may be linked to the elevation of von Willebrand factor and thrombomodulin induced by CsA [10, 83], or to the inhibition of the synthesis of PGI_2 by endothelial cells [52]. CsA also induces a disequilibrium within kidney allograft between prostacyclin and thromboxane production in favor of the latter, which can activate local coagulation [9].

There is no specific indication of anticoagulation therapy during kidney allograft transplantation, besides the treatment of thromboembolic complications.

REFERENCES

1. ADDIS T : Glomerular nephritis. Mac MILLAN, New-York 1948.

2. AKIZAWA T, KINUGASA E, KITAOKA T, KOSHIKAWA S. Effects of recombinant human erythropoietin and correction of anemia on platelet function in hemodialysis patients. Nephron 58, 400-406, 1991.

3. ANDRASSY K, RITZ E. Uremia as a cause of bleeding. Am J Nephrol 5, 313-319, 1985.

4. ANGLES CANO E, RONDEAU E, DELARUE F, HAGEGE J, SULTAN Y, SRAER JD. Identification and cellular localization of plasminogen activators from human glomeruli. Thromb Haemost 54, 688-692, 1985.

5. ARDAILLOU N, HAGEGE J, NIVEZ MP, ARDAILLOU R, SCHLONDORFF D. Vasoconstrictor evoked prostaglandin synthesis in cultured human mesangial cells. Am J Physiol 248, F240-F246, 1985.

6. BONEU B, BUCHANAN MR, CARANOBE C, GABAIG AM, DUPOUY D, SIE P, HIRSH J. The disappearance of a low molecular weight heparin fraction (CY 216) differs from standard heparin in rabbits. Thromb Res 46, 845-853, 1987.

7. BONEU B, CARANOBE C, SIE P. Pharmacokinetics of heparin and low molecular weight heparin. In: Hirsch J (Ed). "Antithrombotic therapy". Baillière-Tindall, London, vol 3, pp 531-534, 1990.

8. BORDER WA, WILLSON CB, DIXON FJ. Failure of heparin to affect two types of experimental glomerulonephritis in rabbits. Kidney Int 8, 140-148, 1975.

9. BROWN Z, NEILD GH. Cyclosporine inhibits prostacyclin production by cultured human endothelial cells. Transplant Proc 19, 1178-1180, 1987.

10. BROWN Z, NEILD GH, WILLOUGHBY J et al. Factor VIII related antigen (FVIIIRAg) levels in renal allograft recipients taking cyclosporine (CS). Thromb Haemost 54, 292, 1985.

11. CADROY Y, POURRAT J, BALADRE MF, SAIVIN S, HOUIN G, MONTASTRUC JL, VERNIER I, BONEU B. Delayed elimination of enoxaparin in patients with chronic renal insufficiency. Thromb Res 63, 385-390, 1991.

12. CAMARA I, DE LA CRUZ JP, FRUTOS MA et al. Effects of dipyridamole on the short-term evolution of glomerulonephritis. Nephron 58, 13-16, 1991.

13. CAMERON JS. Coagulation and thromboembolic complications in the nephrotic syndrome. Adv Nephrol 13, 75-114, 1984.

14. CAMUSSI G. Potential role of platelet-activating factor in renal pathophysiology. Kidney Int 29, 469-477, 1986.

15. CASTELLOT JJ Jr, HOOVER RL, HARPER PA, KARNOVSKY MJ. Heparin and glomerular epithelial cell-secreted heparin like species inhibit mesangial cell proliferation. Am J Pathol 120, 427-435, 1985.

16. COLUCCI M, SEMERARO N, MONTEMURRO P, CHIUMARULO P, TRIGGIANI R, MORRONE LF, SCHENA FP. Urinary procoagulant and fibrinolytic activity in human glomerulonephritis. Relationship with renal function. Kidney Int 39, 1213-1217, 1991.

17. DEPROST D, KANFER A. Quantitative assessment of procoagulant activity in isolated rat glomeruli. Kidney Int 28, 566-568, 1985.

18. DEYKIN D. Uremic bleeding. Kidney Int 24, 698-705, 1983.

19. DI MINNO G, MARTINEZ J, McKEAN ML, DE LA ROSA J, BURKE JF, MURPHY S. Platelet dysfunction in uremia multifaceted defect partially corrected by dialysis. Am J Med 79, 552-559, 1985.

20. DONADIO JV Jr, ANDERSON CF, MITCHELL JC 3d, HOLLEY KE, ILSTRUP DM, FUSTER V, CHESELBRO JH. Membranoproliferative glomerulonephritis. A prospective clinical trial of platelet-inhibitor therapy. N Engl J Med 310, 1421-1426, 1984.

21. DRAKE TA, MORRISSEY JH, EDGINGTON TS. Selective cellular expression of tissue factor in human tissues. Implications for disorders of hemostasis and thrombosis. Am J Pathol 134, 1087-1097, 1989.

22. ESCHBACH JW, ADAMSON JW. Hematologic consequences of renal failure. In: Brenner BM, Rector FC (Eds). "The kidney". Saunders, Boston, pp 2019-2035, 1991.

23. FARRELL PC, WARD RA, SCHINDHELM K, GOTCH FA. Precise anticoagulation for routine hemodialysis. J Lab Clin Med 92, 164-176, 1978.

24. FISHER AM, TAPON-BRETAUDIERE J, BROS A, JOSSO F. Respective roles of antithrombin III and α-2-macroglobulin in thrombin inactivation. Thromb Haemost 45, 51-54, 1981.

25. FLANIGAN MJ, VON BRECHT J, FREEMAN RM et al. Reducing the hemorrhagic complications of dialysis: a controlled comparison of low dose

heparin and citrate anticoagulation. Am J Kidney Dis 9, 147-153, 1983.

26. FRIEDLANDER G, MOULONGUET-DOLERIS L, KOURILSKY O, NUSSAUME O, ARDAILLOU R, SRAER VD. Prostaglandin synthesis by isolated glomeruli from normal and chronically rejected human kidneys. Contr Nephrol 41, 20-22, 1984.

27. FURMAN KI, GOMPERTS ED, HOCKLEY J. Activity of intraperitoneal heparin during peritoneal dialysis. Clin Nephrol 9, 15-18, 1978.

28. GLASSOCK RJ, ADLER SG, WARD HJ, COHEN AH: Primary glomerular diseases. In: Brenner BM, Rector FC (Eds). "The Kidney". Saunders, Boston, pp 1182-1279, 1991.

29. GOUDABLE C, SAIVIN S, HOUIN G, SIE P, BONEU B, TONTHAT H, SUC JM. Pharmacokinetics of a low molecular weight heparin (Fraxiparine) in various stages of chronic renal failure. Nephron 59, 543-545, 1991.

30. GRIES E, PAAR D, GRABEN N, BOCK KD. How much heparin intraperitoneally is necessary in CAPD? Nephron 49, 256, 1988.

31. HANCOCK W, ATKINS RC. Activation of coagulation pathways and fibrin deposition in human glomeulonephritis. Semin Nephrol, 5, 69-77, 1985.

32. HANDIN RI, LOSCALZO J. Hemostasis, thrombosis, fibrinolysis, and cardiovascular disease. In: Braunwald E (Ed). "Heart disease". Saunders, Philadelphia, vol 3, pp 1758-1781, 1988.

33. HOLDSWORTH SR, TIPPING PG. Macrophage-induced glomerular fibrin deposition in experimental glomerulonephritis in the rabbit. J Clin Invest 76, 1367-1374, 1985.

34. HOROWITZ HI, STEIN IM, COHEN BD, WHITE JG. Further studies on the platelet-inhibitory effect of guanidinosuccinic acid and its role in uremic bleeding. Am J Med 49, 336-345, 1970.

35. JANSON PA, JUBELIRER SJ, WEINSTEIN MJ, DEYKIN D. Treatment of the bleeding tendency in uremia with cryoprecipitate. N Engl J Med 303, 1318-1322, 1980.

36. JUBELIRER SJ. Hemostatic abnormalities in renal disease. Am J Kidney Dis 5, 219-225, 1985.

37. KANFER A. Coagulation factors in nephrotic syndrome. Am J Nephrol 10, 63-68, 1990.

38. KANFER A, RONDEAU E, PERALDI MN, SRAER JD. Coagulation in renal diseases: the role of the glomerular hemostasis system and implications for therapy. In: Andreucci VE, Fine LG (Eds). "International Yearbook of Nephrology 1992". Springer-Verlag, London, pp 3-54, 1992.

39. KANT KS, POLLAK VE, DOSEKUN A, GLAS-GREENWALT P, WEISS MA, GLUECK H. Lupus nephritis with thrombosis and abnormal fibrinolysis: effect of ancrod. J Lab Clin Med 33, 55-60, 1985.

40. KINCAID-SMITH P. Coagulation and renal disease. Kidney Int 2, 183-190, 1973.

41. KINCAID-SMITH P. Participation of intra-vascular coagulation in the pathogenesis of glomerular and vascular lesions. Kidney Int 7, 242-253, 1975.

42. KLAHR S, SCHREINER G, ICHIKAWA I. The progression of renal disease. N Engl J Med 318, 1657-1666, 1988.

43. KUZNIEWSKI M, SULOWICZ W, HANICKI Z, KUS J, NOWOGRODZKA-ZAGORSKA M, KOSTKA-TRABKA E,

BIERON K, DEBINSKA-KIEC A. Effect of heparin and prostacyclin/heparin infusion on platelet aggregation in hemodialyzed patients. Nephron 56, 174-178, 1990.

44. LACAVE R, RONDEAU E, OCHI S, DELARUE F, SCHLEUNING WD, SRAER JD. Characterization of a plasminogen activator and its inhibitor in human mesangial cells. Kidney Int 35, 806-811, 1989.

45. LAMBERT PH, DIXON FJ. Pathogenesis of the glomerulonephritis of NZB/W mice. J Exp Med 127, 507-518, 1978.

46. LINDSAY R, FRIESEN M, ARONSTAM A, ANDRUS F. Improvement of platelet function by increased frequency of hemodialysis. Clin Nephrol 10, 67-70, 1978.

47. LINDSAY RM, SMITH AM. Pratical use of anticoagulants. In: Maher JF (Ed). "Replacement of renal function by dialysis". Kluwer, Dordrecht, pp 246-275, 1989.

48. MANUCCI P, REMUZZI G, PUSINERI F, LOMBARDI R. Deamino-8-d-arginine vasopressin shortens the bleeding time in uremia. N Engl J Med 308, 8-12, 1983.

49. MOHAMMAD SF. Extracorporeal thrombogenesis: mechanisms and prevention. In: Maher JF (Ed). "Replacement of renal function by dialysis". Kluwer, Dordrecht, pp 229-245, 1989.

50. MOIA M, VIZZOTTO L, CATTANCO M, MANUCCI PM, CASATI S, PONTICELLI C. Improvement in the haemostatic defect of uremia after treatment with recombinant erythropoietin Lancet i, 392-394, 1987.

51. MORINIERE P, DIEVAL J, BAYROU B, et al. Low-molecular-weight heparin Fraxiparin[R] in chronic hemodialysis. A dose-finding study. Blood Purif 7, 301-308, 1989.

52. MYERS BD. Cycloporine nephrotoxicity. Kidney Int 30, 964-974, 1986.

53. NAWROTH PP, STERN DM. Modulation of endothelial cell hemostatic properties by tumor necrosis factor. J Exp Med 163, 740-745, 1986.

54. NORRIS SH. Renal eicosanoids. Sem Nephrol 10, 64-68, 1990.

55. PANICUCCI F, SAGRIPANTI A, PINORI E, VISPI M, LICHINI L, BARSOTTI G, GIOVANETTE S. Comprehensive study of haemostasis in chronic uremia. Nephron 33, 5-8, 1983.

56. PANICUCCI F, SAGRIPANTI A, VISPI M, PINORI E, LECCHINI L, BARSOTTI G, GIOVANETTI S. Comprehensive study of haemostasis in nephrotic syndrome. Nephron 33, 9-13, 1983.

57. PINNICK RV, WEIGMANN TB, DIEDERICH DA. Regional citrate anticoagulation for hemodialysis in the patient at high risk for bleeding. N Engl J Med 308, 258-261, 1983.

58. PURKERSON ML, TOLLEFSEN DM, KLAHR S. N-desulfated/acetylated heparin ameliorates the progression of renal disease in rats with subtotal renal ablation. J Clin Invest 81, 69-74, 1988.

59. RABINER SF, MOLINAS F. The role of phenol and phenolic acids on the thrombocytopathy and defective platelet aggregation of patients with renal failure. Am J Med 49, 346-351, 1970.

60. RAUGI GJ, LOVETT DH. Thrombospondin secretion by cultured human glomerular mesangial cells. Am J Pathol 129, 364-372, 1987.

61. REMUZZI G, HUS and TTP. Variable expression of a single entity. Kidney Int 32, 292-302, 1987.

62. REMUZZI G, BENIGNI A, DODESINI P, SCHIEPATTI A, LIVIO M, DE GAETANO G, DAY JS, SMITH WL, PINCA E, PATRIGNANI P, PATRONO C. Reduced platelet thromboxane formation in uremia. J Clin Invest 71, 762-768, 1983.

63. REMUZZI G, MARCHESI D, CAVENAGHI AE, LIVIO M, DONATI MB, DE GAETANO G, MECCA G. Bleeding in renal failure: a possible role for vascular prostacyclin (PGI_2). Clin Nephrol 12, 127-131, 1979.

64. REMUZZI G, PERICO N, ZOJA C, CORNA D, MACCONI D, VIGANO G. Role of endothelium-derived nitric oxide in the bleeding tendency of uremia J Clin Invest 86, 1768-1771, 1990.

65. RONDEAU E, DELARUE F, KANFER A, NUSSAUME O, SRAER JD. Profibrinolytic and procoagulant activities of human glomeruli from normal kidneys and rejected allograft. Fibrinolysis 2, 251-257, 1988.

66. RONDEAU E, MOUGENOT B, LACAVE R, PERALDI MN, KRUITHOF EKO, SRAER JD. Plasminogen activator inhibitor in renal fibrin deposits of human nephropathies. Clin Nephrol 33, 55-60, 1990.

67. RONDEAU E, OCHI S, LACAVE R, HE CJ, MEDCALF RL, DELARUE F, SRAER JD. Urokinase synthesis and binding by glomerular epithelial cells in culture. Kidney Int 36, 593-600, 1989.

68. SANDERS PW, TAYLOR H, CURTIS J. Hemodialysis without anticoagulation. Am J Kidney Dis 5, 32-35, 1985.

69. SARGENT JA, GOTCH FA. Principles and biophysics of dialysis. In: Maher JF (Ed). "Replacement of renal function by dialysis". Kluwer, Dordrecht, pp 87-143, 1989.

70. SCHRADER J, STIBBE W, ARMSTRONG VW, KANDT M, MUCHE R, KOSTERING H, SEIDEL D, SCHELER F. Comparison of low molecular weight heparin to

standard heparin in hemodialysis/hemofiltration. Kidney Int 33, 890-896, 1988.

71. SCHMITT GW, MOAKE JL, RUDY CK, VICKS SL, HAMBURGER RJ. Alterations in hemostatic parameters during hemodialysis with dialyzers of different membrane composition and flow design. Am J Med 83, 411-418, 1987.

72. SIE P, BONEU B. Low molecular weight heparin half-life is prolonged in haemodialysis patients. Thromb Res 43, 1-5, 1986.

73. SMITH MC, DANVIRIYASUP K, CROW JW, CATO AE, PARK GD, HASSID A, DUNN MJ. Prostacyclin substitution for heparin in long-term hemodialysis. Am J Med. 73, 669-678, 1982.

74. SRAER J, WOLF C, OUDINET JP, BENS M, ARDAILLOU R, SRAER JD. Human glomeruli release fatty acids which stimulate thromboxane synthesis in platelets. Kidney Int 32, 62-68, 1987.

75. STRIKER GE, SODERLAND C, BOWEN-POPE DF, GOWN AM, SCHMER G, JOHNSON A, LUCHTEL D, ROSS R, STRIKER LJ. Isolation, characterization and propagation in vitro of human glomerular endothelial cells. J Exp Med 160, 323-328, 1984.

76. TABATA T, SHIMADA H, EMOTO M, MORITA A, FURUMITSU Y, FUJITA J, INOUE T, MIKI T, NISHIZAWA Y, MORII H. Inhibitory effect of heparin and/or antithrombin III on intraperitoneal fibrin formation in continuous anbulatory peritoneal dialysis. Nephron 56, 391-395, 1990.

77. THOMSON C, FORBES CD, PRENTICE CR. The potentiation of platelet aggregation and adhesion by heparin in vitro and in vivo. Clin Sci Mol Med 45, 485-494, 1973.

78. VANRENTERGHEM Y, ROELS L, LERUT T, GRUWEZ J, MICHIELSEN P, GRESLE P, DECKMYN H, COLUCCI M, ARNOUT J, VERMYLEN J. Thromboembolic complications and haemostatic changes in cyclosporin-treated cadaveric allograft recipients. Lancet i, 999-1002, 1985.

79. VASSALLI P, McCLUSKEY RT. The pathogenic role of the coagulation process in rabbit Masugi nephritis. Am J Pathol 45, 653-673, 1964.

80. VERBEELEN D, JOCHMANS K, HERMAN AG, VAN DER NIEPEN P, SENNESAEL J, DE WAELE M. Evaluation of platelets and hemostasis during hemodialysis with six different membranes. Nephron 59, 567-572, 1991.

81. WIGGINS RC, NJOKU N, SEDOR JR. Tissue factor production by cultured rat mesangial cells. Stimulation by TNFα and lipopoly saccharide. Kidney Int 37, 1281-1285, 1990.

82. WILHELMSSON S, ASABA H, GUNNARSSON B, KUDRY KB, ROBINSON D, BERGSTROM J. Measurement of fibrinopeptide A in the evaluation of heparin activity and fibrin formation during hemodialysis. Clin Nephrol 15, 252-258, 1981.

83. YOSHIDA M, KOZAKI M, IOYA N, KAJI N, TAMAKI T, HIRAISHI S, ISHII H, KAZAMA M, FUKUTOMI K, NAGASAWA T. Plasma thrombomodulin levels as an indicator of vascular injury caused by cyclosporine nephrotoxicity. Transplantation 50, 1066-1069, 1990.

84. ZIMMMERMAN SW, MOORTHY AV, DREHER WH, FRIEDMAN A, VARANASI U. Prospective trial of warfarin and dipyridamole in patients with membranoproliferative glomerulonephritis. Am J Med 75, 920-927, 1983.

85. ZUSMAN RM, RUBIN RH, CATO AE, COCCHETTO DM, CROW JW, TOLKOFF-RUBIN N. Hemodialysis using prostacyclin instead of heparin as the sole

antithrombotic agent. N Engl J Med 304, 934-939, 1981.

28

Haemorrhages and anticoagulants the responsibility of the patient

F. Toulemonde

Even using sophisticated methods like monograms for heparin and (INR-ISI) system for OA, the risk of bleeding persists during antithrombotic treatments. In most of the cases, it is reported to an overdosage, and that is true in some cases.

But in some others, the patient is correctly anticoagulated i.e. in the therapeutic range, and yet bleeding is observed.

Then some change or trouble in the patient condition may be suspected.

The aim of this study is to collect - from the main published clinical trials - some usefull observations of bleeding mainly due to the patient conviction.

I - Perioperative prophylaxis with heparins

The most commonly used drugs in this indication are heparins. An interesting point is that the different treatments have been compared to placebo in several studies.

1. Low dose heparin prophylaxis (with unfractionnated heparin UFH)

a) In a general overview of 14 double blind placebo controlled trials, including around 3000 patients on prophylaxis in general surgery, Levine [32] stated "there was no statistical difference detected between treatment groups in any of the studies". For instance, there were two fatal haemorrhages in the heparin groups versus three in the placebo group.

b) In orthopedic surgery
In the same paper, their conclusions are: "there is no evidence that heparin prophylaxis leads to excessive fatal or major bleeding in hip surgery (fractures and elective) although there is a strong suggestion that minor bleeding and total blood loss is increased by heparin prophylaxis in elective hip surgery.

2. Low molecular weight heparin fractions (LMWH)

a) In a recent meta-analysis, Lassen [29] in general surgery showed that when compared to placebo, no difference in safety variables was recorded ; when compared to low dose heparin (tid) no bleeding complications were observed in these studies (n=8).

b) In hip surgery, studies comparing LMWH versus placebo (n=4), showed that in two of theses studies, the mean blood loss was increased by only 150 ml on average, which is of little importance. Major haemorrhages occurred less frequently in the LMWH group (3.3 %) as compared to UFH (5.7 %) in a recent survey [32].

3. Heparins, in general, present a very good safety in the two last largest studies in surgery

- STEP study [44] in 4498 patients compared LMWH to placebo: from 26 deaths, none was to be attributed to bleeding. Prophylaxis was discontinued for bleeding in 0.22 % in the LMWH group and 0.04 % in the placebo group (NS).

- Wolf [54] in 11561 patients compared LMWH versus UFH: from 51 deaths recorded, none was due to haemorrhage. Prophylaxis was discontinued, due to adverse events, in 0.4 % in the LMWH group and 0.84 % in the UFH group (p = 0.003).

4. To date

- The standard fixed best dosage (SFBD) [49] being established accurately for each LMWH, monitoring does not appear to be of some help and, quite recently, in the ISTH heparin subcommittee (Amsterdam, June 1991), it was agreed that there is little or no correlation between the results of in vitro assay (A-Xa value) and the clinical outcome (bleeding and thrombosis) in prophylaxis, as well as in treatment.

- Comparison of LMWH in a double blind manner is the ideal way to determine the role of the drug compared to placebo in bleeding determination. Three studies in general surgery [40, 41, 44], four in orthopedic surgery [20, 48, 50] and one in medical patient [5] were published; as pointed out by Hirsh [19] in a recent review, in no case there is a difference in major bleeding between LMWH treated and placebo treated groups.

These results obviously exclude the role of LMWH as a cause of the small percentage of bleeding observed, suggesting other reasons.

5. The patient's role itself is suspected in some cases

- J. Harenberg gives an excellent example [16]: In patients treated with LMWH he found only one single severe haemorrage, which was in relation with an undetected colon carcinoma.

- Individual sensitivity to heparin has been described.

In 1985, Mottironi showed that subcutaneous injection of 10 000 IU UFH increases the APTT (normal 25 sec) over 78 sec in 3 % of 258 patients tested before operation [37]. Heiden showed in 1981 that IV bolus dose of 100 IU/kg of heparin increases the bleeding time (BT) (normal = 5.3 min) over 20 minutes in 15 % of 46 healthy volonteers. In some of the volnteers, in whom heparin did not increase the BT, combination with aspirin produced a striking bleeding time prolongation, greatly exceeding that produced by aspirin alone [17]. Later, the role of aspirin already mentioned by Glazier [14] in 1976 has been clearly identified as a factor in post-prostatectomy haemorrage [52]. These unexpected individual sensitivities could lead to haemorrages.

Thus, even with soft anticoagulation, some underlying conditions may play a role in haemorrages. These conditions will act more actively in the two next chapters.

II - Treatment of thromboembolic diseases with heparins.

1. The present situation for heparin is not yet fully satisfactory

- From previous studies on heparin, it appears that intermittent IV administration should be dropped, inducing a too high risk of bleeding (14-30 %) [8].

- The two available routes (IV perfusion and SC) induce a rather mean low risk of major haemorrages (5.6 % versus 4.3 %) with comparable efficacy [32].

- The necessary monitoring is not yet precisely standardised and still not completly effective. This means that even in the "therapeutic range", a major bleeding may occur [4, 11] and quite recently. Poller (Amsterdam ISTH Heparin Sub-Commitee 1991) claimed evidence of the present unsatisfactory nature of the currently advised therapeutic range of 1.5 to 2.5 APTT ratio.

Moreover, there is sometimes a long way betwween intention to monitor and effective monitoring.

2. Here is the reason for the increasing interest for LMWH

- The heparin experience has given the way for their subcutaneous administration.

- Animal studies have shown a much weaker hemorragic potential versus heparin even given in high dosages [9].

- A more stable state in anticoagulation is observed, thus less controls appear necessary [1, 10, 16].

- Tolerance has been found to be equal or better as compared to heparin.

3. However, for heparin as for LMWH, some particular events could lead to individual bleeding.

a) A patient given, for study purpose or by mistake, a too high dosage is more at risk of bleeding.
That is true for LMWH [16] as well as for heparin [36].

b) An individual patient may present particular conditions favouring bleeding.

- In case of thromboembolism, when a patient presents an additional inflammatory syndrome (Fibrinogen level > 4 g), he needs almost twice more doses adjustment due to large variations in blood levels [6].
- In 1972 Salzman experienced 33 % major bleeding in DVT patients treated with intermittent IV heparin; of these 17 patients: 6 presented an identifiable wound or injury, 2 had been given antiplatelet agents, 7 had both risks and only 2 presented no predisposing cause [8]; obviously no correlation between bleeding with control of heparin therapy was observed.
- In 1977, Mant, in a similar study, concluded "Bleeding complications are more closely related to duration of therapy, age, sex and surgical trauma than to method of administration" [35]. Neither heparin level nor APTT results could be related to these complications.
- In 1979, Wilson, in a similar study detected, before treatment, 15 patients at risk of bleeding into areas of tissue trauma of vascular damage. Eight of these developed bleeding complications (53 %) in contrast to 18 % in 65 patients were not at similar risk ($p < 0.02$) [53].

This factor looks more important than the mode of heparin administration, the mean dosage of heparin being the same in bleeders and non bleeder groups. These particular conditions have also been later evoked by many others [14, 32, 51, 53].

d) The most precise informations can be found in a very recent work from a Dutch group [1, 38] comparing

LFH and LMWH. It presents an utmost interest because of its perfect quality with a large number of patients (196) and particular criteria in inclusion. Patients have been classified from the start into two groups according to the conventional criteria of bleeding risk. The high risk group was defined as: women over 60, men over 70, surgery within 10 days, renal insufficiency (creatinine level>400 µmol/l), recent intracranial bleeding or stroke, active peptic ulcer, arterial hypertension, recent cardiac ressucitation (<10 days) history of bleeding (intracranial or diathesis) and general heavy disability (WHO score 4). The low risk groups included all other patients. Thus, there was no exclusion for any bleeding risk and it is the reason why much more major bleeding occurred than usually ; for an equal mean A-Xa level (0.48 - 0.55 UI/ml): 6 major in the low risk and 17 in the high risk group. The univariate analysis ranked the parameters in the following order: WHO performance status (patients with WHO grade 4 had eight-fold increase in risk of bleeding compared with WHO grade 1), history of bleeding tendancy, cardiac ressucitation, recent trauma or surgery. In multivariate regression anlysis, it appears that the WHO performance status was the most important factor.

In addition it has been observed that the described risks factors are the same during UFH and LMH therapy. There is no difference indeed between mean values of A-Xa in bleeders and non bleeders but, after the inital bolus, the bleeding risk is 10 % if < 0.8 U/ml and 60 % if > 1 U/ml for both groups. Moreover, during the course of the treatment, for a mean A-Xa > 0.8 IU/ml, the bleeding risk increases from 11 to 40 % , if the mean A-Xa is < 0.8 IU/ml, no correlation has been found. Finally, the importance of some classical risk factors of bleeding have not been confirmed: age, sex, cancer, alcohol, antiinflammatory drugs, anemia.

Thus it is clear there exist several individual factors leading to bleeding in spite of a correct anticoagulation, yet their respective importance is not yet clearly defined (alcohol, antiinflammatory drugs).

III - Anticoagulation with oral anticoagulants (OA)

1. The main progresses are:

- The use of international normalised ratio (INR) to express thromboplastin time (TP) value as a function of reagent sensibility, as proposed in 1979 [23].
- The trend, from clinical experience, to use less intense therapy leading to equivalent efficacy but less bleeding.
- The possibility in reversing a strong anticoagulation state with a low dose of vitamin K IV (0.5 mg/Kg) without disturbing deeply the coagulation equilibrium [47].

2. But the field of indications is rather decreasing

a) Immediate prophylaxis with OA decreases [2] mostly due to LMWH increasing usage.

In general surgery, there are unsufficient data to support the use of OA for thromboembolism prophylaxis and adjusted doses are not recommended due to cost.

In orthopedic surgery, fixed minidoses are ineffective and are not recommended; adjusting the dosages to a desired range INR improves efficacy, but is difficult to manage.

b) Secondary prophylaxis

The use of INR facilitates a more precise adjustment of the dosages according to the disease. But, as it has been pointed out recently, a result comparison between studies (using and not using INR) are not easy, conversions of the reported tests results into the INR lead to approximate results [31].

Levine reported recently several studies [31, 33, 34] leading to the following observations:

- The disease to be treated with OA plays a major role in bleeding (up to tenfold).
- There are also obvious differences between studies in the same area.
- Bleeding frequently occrred when the PT was within the therapeutic range.

Thus, other additional reasons may interfere to increase the risk; they are mostly individual, for example:

1. The patient may have an individual sensitivity to OA. Rarely genetic, more often somatic, modifying the metabolism (reduced intake of vitamin K in fasting, cellular hepatic insufficiency) or particular disease leading to hypercatabolism of coagulation factors (fever, cancer, hyperthyroïdism) [12].

2. The patient may have an individual characteristic (known or unknown) which is a contraindication to OA. There is a much extensive classical list of contraindication to OA than to heparin [7]; whether any possible reduction due to less intense therapy is unknown.

3. The patient may be given, or has forgotten to warn the physician he takes drugs which interfer with OA. In contrast to heparin, the effect of OA is influenced by a large number of drugs which may dramatically alter the response of the patient [22].

4. The longer the treatment, the higher the risk for the patient to bleed: the risk increases almost linearly: 10 % for 12 weeks, 18 % for 1 year, 26 % for 2 years and 41 % at five years, as observed with rather intense therapy after venous thromboembolism [42].

5. The patient may present an instable anticoagulant state. In venous thromboembolism experience, it must be emphasized that the range can be attained in only 50-70 % of the time because of

variations in diet, vitamin K absorption and patient compliance with medication [22].

6. Patient may present a neglected or unknown underlying disease.

In the study comparing different intensities of OA, Hull [21] (prior to INR) found the same percentage of major haemorrages (4 %) in the two compared groups (intense versus less intense anti- coagulation). These four patients had an underlying disease (2 unsuspected ulcers - 2 surgery). In addition to 9 minor bleeding (without underlying disease), all the 13 patients were overdosed, another evidence of the spontaneous variations of the PT.

7. Two main recent studies investigated the risk factors for bleeding in very large trials and may be considered as a general overview.

7.1 1010 patients/years of AO were reviewed with regard to major bleeding complications by Launbjerg [30] in 1991 in patients with INR 2-4.

From 19560 PT assays, 11.5 % were above and 9.5 below the therapeutic range.

Multivariate analysis showed the major role of age > 75 years, overdosage (INR > 7),arterial hypertension, thiazide administration (independently) and cimetidine (ulcero-dependent) in bleeding occurence.

7.2 The most important contribution comes from the Boston group. They studied the bleedings both in hospital and in outpatients using sophisticated method.

Firstly, a retrospective analysis of a large cohort of patients for major bleeding risk factors determination, then calculation of a bleeding risk index. Finally, an evaluation of this index prospectively. All possible factors, indeed, have not been evaluated, but only the main one.

First step: In hospital studies (staring treatments) [25, 27].

Different factors have been identified and classified as: known at the start of treatment:

specific comorbid conditions (other than the indication for OA), cardiac, liver, kidney diseases, cancer, anemia, and heparin usage prior to OA in elderly patients.

Factors developping during therapy, in the other hand were overdosage and worsening liver function.

Two main observations can be done:

- Firstly, the role of comorbid processes is obvious. Patients with none of the four identified risks had only 1 % probability of MB; those with two or more of these processes had nearly 20 times that risk, as evidenced in controlled discriminant analysis.

- Secondly, the bleeding risk index integrated with physician's predictions led to more accurate prediction of MB than achieved by physicians alone. Moreover, a better management in hospital could reduce the % of MH in at least 80 % of the bleeding patients (equivocal indications, excessive anticoagulation, platelets interfering drugs, surgical procedures) suggesting bleeding could be prevented in many cases.

Second step: Outpatients studies [26, 28].

At the end of hospital stay and at the time of beginning long term OA, several independant risk factors have been, in the same manner as previously, identified and quoted (multivariate regression analysis). They were:

- Age >65 years,
- History of stroke,
- History of gastro-intestinal bleeding,
- Serious co-morbid conditions,
- arterial fibrillation.

These 5 items are independtly associated risk factors, which are the basis for a predictive score. Other factors have been identified such as systolic blood pressure > 160 (RR 2.8) and PT ratio at discharge: 1.2-1.5 (RR: 1.5); 1.5-2 (RR: 2.1); > 2 (RR: 3.1) but they have not been included into the scoring index.

Relationship between score group and MB are presented in Figure 3 which present cumulative

incidences in 3 groups defined on the basis of the five independent predictors.
0 point=low risk; 1 or 2 points=middle risk; 3 or more points=high risk.

The following main observations (on 565 patients) can be made.

First, major bleeding occurred in 12 % of the patients, with a cumulative risk of 22 % at 48 months. In one third of the cases,bleeding was fatal or life threatening. Second, the monthly risk decreased sharply from the first month of therapy, 3 % then 0.3 % per month after the first year of treatment, in contrast to other authors [12]. Third, five factors known at the start of outpatient therapy were independently associated with subsequent MB. Fourth, comorbid associations play an important role. Their role has already been evoked by several investigators [19, 43, 45].

It is of great interest to note the relationship between PT ratio and origin of bleeding (known or unknown). In most cases, PT ratio raised sharply during the week prior to bleeding in patients without known lesion (overdosage?) but not in patients with already known lesion. In other words, if a patient with rather low anti-coagulation (ratio < 1.5) bled, he has 73 % chances to bleed from a yet unknown lesion. If ratio is over 1.5, such probability is 16 %.

The frequency of these unknown bleeding lesions is high. In the total group, 130 haemorrages occured (65 majors and 65 minors). From these, in 49 cases there was an important lesion; 27 of them were already known and 22 were discovered after bleeding.

8. Regarding the particular case of intracerebral hematomas (ICH) during OA treatment, classical monitoring suffers many failures.

From a group of 71 patients, sampling at admission showed 15 overdosed, 11 underdosed and 45 in the therapeutic range. The authors [13] conclude there was no significant relation between the degree of anticoagulation and ICH occurrence. Moreover, no significant difference between the degree of anticoagulation in patients with ICH compared to OA patients without ICH.

IV. Conclusion

Many actors play a role in bleeding occurence: it is well known that the surgeon itself, well experienced or less, may be at the origin of variable bleeding frequency; in the same way the patient itself plays a role in the bleeding occurence whatever the anticoagulant drug used.

Known diseases for which patients are anticoagulated induce various degree in the risk. Unknown diseases at the origin of other bleeding, even in patients properly anticoagulated, like individual characteristics, (sentitivity).

A carefull history and examination of the patient would reduce the frequenc of these accidents [24, 46] together with laboratory control [3]. It is amazing to note that acute gastroduodenal lesions are found as high as in 16 % of DVT patients and even 38 % of PE patients [39].

It is probably one of the reasons why meta-analysis result in so disturbe ry results, one showing an increased risk of bleeding due to LMW compared to heparin, the other showing no significant difference between the two treatments.

The unavoidable risk of bleeding is real but low, it is the counterpart of so many avantages. In some cases paradoxically, haemorrhage is of benefit as it allows the diagnostic of unknown lesions like cancer.

REFERENCES

1. ALBADA J, NIEUWENHUIS HK, SIXMA JS. Treatment of acute venous thrombo-embolism with low molecular weight heparin (fragmin) - Results of a double-blind randomized study. Circulation 4, 935-940, 1980.

2. ARCELUS JI, CAPRINI JA, TRAVERSO CI. International perspective on venous thromboembolism prophylaxis in surgery. Semin Thromb Haemostas 4, 17, 322-325, 1991.

3. BIEMER JJ. Control of oral anticoagulant therapy. Ann Clin Lab Sci 18, 6, 421-428, 1988.

4. CONTI S. Letter to editor. The West J Med 137(1), 81, 1982.

5. DAHAN R, HOULBERT D, CAULIN C, CUZIN E, VILTART C, WOLER M, SEGRESTAA JM. Prevention of deep venous thrombosis in elderly medical patients by a low molecular weight heparin: a randomized double blind trial. Haemostasis 16, 159-164, 1986.

6. DEMICHELIS C, COHEN S, BRAGUER D, JUHAN-VAGUE I, AILLAUD MF. Utilité de la surveillance biologique de l'héparinothérapie à visée curative. J Pharm Clin 3, 3-4, 367-373, 1984.

7. DERLON A, FRESSINGER JN. Coordinators. Utilisation des antivitamines K en pratique médicale courante. Recommandations du GEHT. STV (Suppl 3), 5, 11-15, 1991.

8. DEYKIN D, SALZMAN EW, MAYER R. Prospective study of complications of heparin therapy ISTH Congrès - Washington D.C. 1972.

9. DOUTEMEPUICH C, TOULEMONDE F, BOUSQUET F, BONINI F. Comparison of the haemorragic effects of unfractionated heparin and a low molecular weight heparin fraction, CY 216, in rabbits. Thromb Res 43, 691-695, 1986.

10. ETUDE MULTICENTRIQUE FRANCAISES. Traitement des thromboses veineuses profondes constituées - Etude comparative d'un fragment d'héparine de bas poids moléculaire (fragmine) par voie SC et de l'héparine standard administrée par voie veineuse continue. Rev Med Interne 10, 375-381, 1989.

11. FAIVRE R, NEUHART Y, KIEFFER Y, APFEL F, MAGNIN D, DIDIER D, TOULEMONDE F, BASSAND JP, MAURAT JP. Un nouveau traitement des thromboses veineuses profondes, les fractions d'héparine de bas poids moléculaire - Etude randomisée. Presse Med 17, 197-200, 1988.

12. FORFAR JC. A 7 year analysis of haemorrhage in patients on long term anticoagulant treatment Biol Mol J 42, 128-132, 1979.

13. FRANKE CL, de JONGE J, VAN SWIETEN JC, OP de COUL AAW, VAN GIJN J. Intracerebral hematomas during anticoagulant treatment. Stroke 21(5), 726-730, 1990.

14. GLAZIER RL, CROWELL EB. Randomized prospective trial of continuous versus intermittent heparin therapy. JAMA 236(12), 1365-1367, 1976.

15. HARENBERG J, HUCK K, BRATSCH H, STEHLE G, DEMPFE CE, MALL K, BLAUTH M, VSADEL KH, HEENE DL. Therapeutic application of subcutaneous LMWH heparin in acute venous thrombosis. Haemostasis 20 (Suppl 1), 205-219, 1990.

16. HARENBERG J, LEBER G, DEMPFLE CE, HEENE DL, ZIMMERMANN R, KUBLER W. Long term anticoagulation with low molecular weight heparin in out patients with side effects on oral anticoagulants. Nouv Rev Fr Hematol 31, 363-369, 1989.

17. HEIDEN D, RODVIER R, HAROLD MIELKE C. Heparin bleeding, platelet dysfunction and aspirin. JAMA 216(4), 330-333, 1981.

18. HIRSH J, LEVINE MN. Low molecular weight heparin. Blood 79(1), 1-18, 1992.

19. HIRSH J. Oral anticoagulant drugs. N Engl J Med 324, 1865-1875, 1991.

20. HOEK J, NURMOHAMED MT, TEN CATE H, TEN CATE JW, BULLER HR. Prevention of deep vein thrombosis following total hip replacement by a low-molecular-weight heparinoid (Org 10172). Thromb Haemost 62, 520 (Abstr.), 1989.

21. HULL R, HIRSH J, JAY R, CARTER C, ENGLAND C, GENT M, TURPIE AG, McLOUGHLIN D, DODD P, THOMAS M, RASKOB G, OCKELFORD P. Different intensities of oral anticoagulant therapy in the treatment of proximal vein thrombosis. N Engl J Med 307, 1676-1681, 1982.

22. HYERS TM, HULL RD, WEG JG. Antithrombotic therapy for venous thromboembolic disease. Chest 92(2), 375-515, 1989.

23. ICTH-ISTH. Report of the expert panel on oral anticoagulant control. Thromb Haemost 42, 1073-1114, 1979.

24. KHER A, TOULEMONDE F. Examen simplifié de l'hémostase in pré-operatoire. Gaz Med de France 81, 1877-1883, 1974.

25. LANDEFELD C,S COOK EF, FLATLEY M, WEISBERG M, GOLDMAN L. Identification and preliminary

validation of predictors of major bleeding in hospitalized patients starting anticoagulant therapy. Am J Med 82, 703-713, 1987.

26. LANDEFELD CS, GOLDMAN L. Major bleeding in out patients treated with Warparin: incidence and prediction by factors known at the start of out patient therapy. Am J Med 87, 144-152, 1989.

27. LANDEFELD CS, McGUIRE E, ROSENBLATT MW. A bleeding risk index for estimating the probability of major bleeding in hospitalized patients starting anticoagulant therapy. Am J Med 89, 569-578, 1990.

28. LANDEFELD CS, ROSENBLATT MW. Bleeding in out patients heated with Warparin: relation to the prothrombin time and important remediable lesions. Am J Med 87, 153-159, 1989.

29. LASSEN MR, BORRIS LC, CHRISTIANSEN HM, SCHOTT P, OLSEN AD, SORENSEN JV, RAHR H, JENSEN HP. Clinical trials with low molecular weight heparins in the prevention of postoperative thrombo-embolic complications - A meta-analysis. Semin. Thromb Haemost 17(Suppl 3), 284-290, 1991.

30. LAUNBJERG J, EGEBLAD H, HEAF J, NIELSEN NH. Bleeding complications to oral anticoagulant therapy: mulivariate analysis of 1010 treatment years in 551 out patients. J Int Med 229, 351-3555, 1991.

31. LEVINE MN, HIRSH J. Hemorrhagic complications of anticoagulant therapy. Semin Thromb Haemostas 12(1), 39-57, 1986.

32. LEVINE MN, HIRSH J, KELTON JG. Heparin induced bleeding. In: Lane D, LindhahlU (Eds). Heparin: - Chemical and Biol. properties, - Clinical applications. E. Arnold, London, pp 517-531. 1989.

33. LEVINE MN, RASKOB G, HIRSH J. Hemorrhagic complications of long term anticoagulant therapy. Chest 89(2), 163-255, 1986.

34. LEVINE MN, RASKOB G, HIRSH J. Hemorrhagic complications of long term anticoagulant therapy. Chest 95(2), 265-365, 1989.

35. MANT MJ, O BRIEN BD, THONG KL, HAMMOND GW et al. Haemorrhagic complications of heparin therapy. Lancet 8022, 1133-1136, 1977.

36. MORABIA A. Heparin doses and major bleedings. Lancet 1, 8492, 1278-1279, 1986.

37. MOTTIRONI SC, SELZ Y. Hypersensibilité à l'héparine ou le chirurgien et les hématomes. Med et Hyg 43, 2659-2660, 1985.

38. NIEUWENHUIS HK, ALBADA J, BANGA JD, SIXMA JJ. Identification for risk factors for bleeding during treatment of acute venous thromboembolism with heparin or LMWH. Blood 78(9), 2337-2343, 1991.

39. NITTER-HANGE S, DALE J. High complication and failure rates of anticoagulant therapy are unavoidable. Z Kardiologie 75(Suppl 2), 293-297, 1986.

40. OCKELFORD PA, KESTEREN PJ, PATTERSON J, BRAND N, JOHNS A. A double blind placebo controlled trial to study the efficacy and safety of a low molecular weight heparin fragment (Fragmin) in patients having major elective hip surgery. Thromb Res (Suppl. VII-B) 23, 19, 1987.

41. OCKELFORD PA, PATTERSON J, JOHN AS. A double blind randomized placebo controlled trial of thrombo-prophylaxis in major elective general surgery using once daily injections of LMW heparin fragment (Fragmin). Thromb Haemostas 62(4), 1046-1049, 1989.

42. PETITTI DB, STORM BL, MELMON KL. Duration of Warparin anticoagulant therapy and the probabilities of recurrent thrombo-embolism and hemorrhage. Am J Med 81, 225-259, 1986.

43. PEYMAN M. The significance of hemorrhage during the treatment with Coumarin anticoagulants. Acta Med Scand 162, 339, 1-62, 1958.

44. PEZZUOLI G, NERI SERNERI GG, SETTEMBRINI PG, STEP Study Group. Effectiveness and safety of the LMWH CY 216 in the prevention of fatal pulmonary embolism and thrombo-embolic death in general surgery. Haemostasis 20(Suppl 1), 193-204, 1990.

45. POLLARD JW, HAMILTON MJ, CHRISTENSEN NA, ACHOR RWP. Problems associated with long-term anticoagulant therapy. Circulation 25, 311-317, 1962.

46. SAMAMA CM. Bilan d'hémostase pré-opératoire: Quoi de neuf? JEPU - Arnette Paris 105-112, 1990.

47. SHETTY HGM, BACKHOUSE G, BENTLEY DP, ROUTLEDGE PA. Effective reversal of Warparin-induced excessive anticoagulation with low dose vitamin K1. Thromb Haemost 67(1), 13-15, 1992.

48. TORHOLM C, BROENG L, SEEST JORGENSEN P et al. Thromboprophylaxis by low-molecular-weight heparin in elective hip surgery. J Bone Joint Surg (Br) 73, 434-438, 1991.

49. TOULEMONDE F. Can the bleeding potential of low molecular weight heparins be assessed and minimized in post surgery prophylaxis ? Semin Thromb Haemostas 17(Suppl 4), 351-356, 1991.

50. TURPIE A, LEVINE MN, HIRSH J, CARTER CJ, JAY RM, POWERS PJ, ANDREW M, HULL RD, GENT M. Arandomized controlled trial of a low

molecular weight heparin (Enoxaparine) to prevent deep-vein thrombosis in patients undergoing elective hip surgery. N Engl J Med 315, 925-929, 1986.

51. WALKER AM, JICK H. Predictors of bleeding during heparin therapy. JAMA 244(11), 1209-1212, 1980.

52. WATSON CJE, DEANE AM, DOYLE PT, BULLOCK KN. Identifiable factors in post-prostatectomy haemorrhage: the role of aspirin Brit J Urol 66, 85-87, 1990.

53. WILSON JR, LAMPMAN J. Heparin therapy: a randomized prospective study. Am Heart J 77(2), 155-158, 1979.

54. WOLF H, ENCKE A, HAAS S, WELZEL D. Comparison of the efficacy and safety of Sandoz LMW heparin and unfractionated heparin: interim analysis of a multicenter trial. Semin Thromb Haemostas 17(Suppl 4), 343-346, 1991.